Understanding Body Movement

Hedda Lausberg (ed.)

Understanding Body Movement

A Guide to Empirical Research on Nonverbal Behaviour

With an Introduction to the NEUROGES Coding System

PL ACADEMIC RESEARCH

Bibliographic Information published by the Deutsche Nationalbibliothek
The Deutsche Nationalbibliothek lists this publication
in the Deutsche Nationalbibliografie; detailed bibliographic
data is available in the internet at http://dnb.d-nb.de.

Library of Congress Cataloging-in-Publication Data

Understanding body movement : a guide to empirical research on nonverbal behaviour : with an introduction to the NEUROGES coding system / Hedda Lausberg (ed.).
pages cm
ISBN 978-3-631-58249-7
1. Movement, Psychology of. 2. Body language. 3. Nonverbal communication.
I. Lausberg, Hedda, 1964-
BF295.U53 20123
153.6'9—dc23
2013033385

ISBN 978-3-631-58249-7 (Print)

Internationaler Verlag der Wissenschaften
Frankfurt am Main 2013

PKL Academic Research is an Imprint of Peter Lang GmbH.

Peter Lang – Frankfurt am Main · Bern · Bruxelles · New York · Oxford · Warszawa · Wien

www.peterlang.com

This book is dedicated to our colleague

Uta Sassenberg

Dr. rer. nat. BSc. MSc.

(April 21, 1975 - November 20, 2011)

Editor and list of contributors

Editor

Lausberg, Hedda, Prof. Dr. med., Neurologist, Specialist in Psychosomatic Medicine and Psychotherapy, Psychiatrist, Dance Movement Therapist, Head of the Department of Neurology, Psychosomatic Medicine, and Psychiatry, Institute of Health Promotion and Clinical Movement Science, German Sport University Cologne
Am Sportpark Müngersdorf 6, 50933 Köln
h.lausberg@dshs-koeln.de

Contributors

Bryjovà, Jana, Dipl.-Psych., Psychologist, University Fribourg, Department of Psychology, 2, Rue de Faucigny, CH-1700 Fribourg/Switzerland
jana.bryjova@unifr.ch

Dvoretska, Daniela, Dipl.-Psych., Psychologist, Department of Neurology, Psychosomatic Medicine, and Psychiatry, Institute of Health Promotion and Clinical Movement Science, German Sport University Cologne
Am Sportpark Müngersdorf 6, 50933 Köln
d.dvoretska@dshs-koeln.de

Helmich, Ingo, Dipl.-Sportwiss.,Graduate in Sports Science, Department of Neurology, Psychosomatic Medicine, and Psychiatry, Institute of Health Promotion and Clinical Movement Science, German Sport University Cologne
Am Sportpark Müngersdorf 6, 50933 Köln
i.helmich@dshs-koeln.de

Hogrefe, Katharina, PhD, Clinical Linguist, Neuropsychological Research Group (EKN), Clinic for Neuropsychology, Hospital
Schwabing, Kölner Platz 1, 80804 München
Katharina.Hogrefe@extern.lrz-muenchen.de

Holle, Henning, Dr., Lecturer, Department of Psychology, University of Hull, HU6 7RX, Hull, U.K.
h.holle@hull.ac.uk

Kryger, Monika, Dipl.-Sportwiss. Graduate in Sports Science at the German Sport University Cologne. Student of English Studies at the RWTH Aachen
monikakryger86@googlemail.com

Lausberg, Hedda, Prof. Dr. med., Neurologist, Specialist in Psychosomatic Medicine and Psychotherapy, Psychiatrist, Dance Movement Therapist,
Head of the Department of Neurology, Psychosomatic Medicine, and Psychiatry, Institute of Health Promotion and Clinical Movement Science, German Sport University Cologne
Am Sportpark Müngersdorf 6, 50933 Köln
h.lausberg@dshs-koeln.de

Petermann, Kerstin, Dipl.-Dolmetscherin, PhD candidate, University of Leipzig, Institute of Applied Linguistics and Translatology,
Beethovenstr. 15, 04107 Leipzig
kerstinpetermann@hotmail.de

Rein, Robert, PhD, Graduate in Sports Science, Sports Medicine, and Physics, Department of Neurology, Psychosomatic Medicine, and Psychiatry, Institute of Health Promotion and Clinical Movement Science, German Sport University Cologne
Am Sportpark Müngersdorf 6, 50933 Köln
r.rein@dshs-koeln.de

Sassenberg, Uta, Dr. rer. nat. BSc. MSc., Psychologist †

Skomroch, Harald, Dipl.-Sportwiss., Graduate in Sports Science, English Studies and Educational Science, Department of Neurology, Psychosomatic Medicine, and Psychiatry, Institute of Health Promotion and Clinical Movement Science, German Sport University Cologne
Am Sportpark Müngersdorf 6, 50933 Köln
h.skomroch@dshs-koeln.de

Slöetjes, Han, Software Developer, The Language Archive, Max Planck Institute for Psycholinguistics
Wundtlaan 1, NL-6525XD Nijmegen, The Netherlands
han.sloetjes@mpi.nl

Preface

This book is a guide for empirical research on nonverbal behaviour. It focuses on investigating body movement and gesture as a reflection of cognitive, emotional, and interactive processes.

The title "Understanding body movement" is a testimonial to Martha Davis who has introduced with her bibliography of the same title a truly interdisciplinary approach to the field of movement behaviour research. Since research on movement behaviour and its relation to cognitive, emotional, and interactive processes is spread over numerous different scientific disciplines, such as medicine, psychology, linguistics, anthropology, social sciences, sports science, and dance movement therapy, the methods presented in this book are grounded on an interdisciplinary review. This included numerous discussions with colleagues from different disciplines, notably Martha Davis, Robyn Flaum Cruz, Sotaro Kita, Miriam Roskild Berger, Norbert Freedman, Georg Goldenberg, Alain Ptito, Eran Zaidel, Joachim Hermsdörfer, Cornelia Müller, Ellen Fricke, Katja Liebal, Mandana Seyfeddinipur, Marianne Eberhard-Kaechele, Peter Joraschky, Angela v. Arnim, Jörn von Wietersheim, Frank Röhricht, Lothar Stemwedel, the contributors of this book, and many other colleagues and students. Based on this broad approach, hopefully, this guide will be useful for researchers from many disciplines.

The book starts with an overview on movement behaviour analysis across different scientific disciplines. Relevant empirical findings on the relation between movement behaviour and cognitive, emotional, and interactive processes are outlined and different methodological approaches are presented. Part II introduces the NEUROGES coding system for movement behaviour and gesture as a comprehensive, objective, and reliable tool. The system is designed for basic research to explore the anatomy of movement behaviour and its relation to cognitive, emotional, and interactive processes. Part III presents the annotation tool ELAN that enables to create complex annotations on video and audio resources. Included is a step-by-step instruction for its practical application in combination with the NEUROGES coding system. Part IV provides recommendations for experimental designs to obtain data on movement behaviour. Specifically, the impact of experimental designs on movement behaviour is discussed. Part V is dedicated to the topic of interrater agreement in movement behaviour analysis. Recommendations for rater training and rating procedures in empirical research are given. Notably, a novel algorithm is presented that enables to calculate the interrater agreement not only for the annotations but also for the segmentation of the ongoing flow of movement behaviour. Part VI provides guidelines for the statistical evaluation and for the presentation of behavioural data. Included here are innovative procedures to statistically assess the between-subjects dimension of interactive partners' body movements. While most of the chapters illustrate the methods with reference to hand movements, most of the presented principles are valid for the analysis of nonverbal behaviour in general.

Finally, I wish to express my gratitude to Corinna Klabunde for proofreading and formatting the book, and for compiling innumerable references. Furthermore, I want to thank the Peter Lang Publishing Group for their patience during the long-term development of this book and the German Research Association for supporting the NEUROGES project from 1999 - 2013 (DFG: LA 1249/1-1, 1-2, 1-3).

Cologne, August 2013 Hedda Lausberg

Contents

I. An Interdisciplinary Review on Movement Behaviour Research

II. The NEUROGES Coding System

IV. Obtaining Data on Movement Behaviour

V. Establishing Interrater Agreement

VI. Evaluating Data on Movement Behaviour

I. An Interdisciplinary Review on Movement Behaviour Research

1. Movement Behaviour Research through History and in Current Scientific Disciplines

Hedda Lausberg

In the human culture, the pursuit of understanding body movement and its link to cognitive, emotional, and interactive processes can be reliably traced back to the ancient Greek. How body movement reflects and affects cognitive, emotional, and interactive processes is not only theoretically interesting but moreover, its knowledge has far-reaching practical applications such as for obtaining communicative competencies, for learning and teaching, and for diagnostics and therapy in different clinical contexts. Currently, the spreading of visual media in all cultures implies that not only the written or spoken word but moving human bodies substantially contribute to the transfer of information. Given this situation, it is becoming more and more important to build an empirically grounded knowledge of how body movement reflects and affects the individual's cognitive and emotional processes and how it promotes communication and regulates interaction.

Not surprisingly, in numerous academic disciplines the expressive and communicative potential of movement behaviour is a focus of interest, such as in psychology, health care science including medicine, linguistics, anthropology, sociology, human physical performance and recreation, media studies and communication, performing arts, cultural and ethnic studies, gender and sexuality studies, computer sciences, education, etc. In addition, many therapy forms such as dance movement therapy, body-oriented psychotherapy, or neurorehabilitation use body movement as therapeutic medium. However, as it will be exposed below, the interest in body movement and its link to cognitive, emotional, and interactive processes is not a recent phenomenon but has historically a longstanding tradition.

It is noteworthy that despite many research studies having been carried through, a common body of empirical knowledge about body movement and its link to cognitive, emotional, and interactive processes has not developed far. One reason for this is the scant scientific exchange between the currently prevailing academic disciplines and a lack of passing on knowledge from historically earlier epochs of research. Among others, differences in terminology and methodology are relevant obstacles for an interdisciplinary discourse on movement behaviour. Given this situation, this book starts with a short overview on research on expressive and communicative body movement across different scientific disciplines, currently and historically. Note that for each field of research only a selection of references can be cited here.

Beforehand, the terminology used in this book shall be clarified. As a reflection of the scientific diaspora on research on body movement, different terms are applied in the field, such as nonverbal communication (e.g. Knapp & Hall, 1992), nonverbal behaviour, body language, kinesics (Birdwhistell, 1952), expressive movement (e.g. Allport & Vernon, 1933), or movement behaviour (Davis, 1972). While the terms nonverbal communication and nonverbal behaviour are the most popular ones, they have the disadvantage that they define a topic by negation ("not verbal"). The terms body language and kinesics focus on the interactive and communicative function of body movement. In contrast, the term expressive body movement underlines that body movement reflects an individual's mental processes. The term movement behaviour has been introduced by M. Davis (1972) for her interdisciplinary bibliography to refer to "the anthropology and psychology of physical body movement." Furthermore, it includes the aspect of behaviour: "Behavior or behaviour is the range of actions and mannerisms made by organisms, systems, or artificial entities in conjunction with their environment, which includes the other systems or organisms around as well as the physical environment. It is the response of the system or organism to various stimuli or inputs, whether internal or external, conscious or subconscious, overt or covert, and voluntary or involuntary." (Web Page Wikipedia, May 21, 2013). Davis' term is adopted in this book since it is comprehensive, neutral, and suitable for an interdisciplinary approach. It is used to refer to individual, cultural, and universal patterns of expressive, communicative, and practical body movements including the classical categories gesture, self-touch, action, shift, posture, and rest position.

A first testimony of the interest to relate movement behaviour to cognitive and emotional processes dates back to the ancient Greek philosophical school of Pythagoras. In that school, the application procedure comprised an evaluation of the applicant's gait and posture to assess his qualification (Jamblichus, cited by J. B. Porta, 1593, cited by Kietz, 1952). Later, during the Roman Empire, given the important role of political speech, knowledge on mime and the gestures of oratory was elaborated. During the Renaissance, the ancient knowledge on the relation between movement behaviour and personality was re-appreciated in the idea of the physiognomonics. The opus "De humania physiognomonia" by Porta (1593, cited by Kietz, 1952) documents this approach. For further literature on this period of time see e.g. Critchley, 1939, reprint 1970; Efron, 1941; Kietz, 1952; Kendon, 2004).

In 1872, Darwin published his seminal work "The Expression of the Emotions in Man and Animals" (1872, reprint 1955) in which he investigated the universality of emotional expression in facial and bodily movements. At the beginning of the last century, Darwin's thoughts and the ideas of the Renaissance had a revival in the expression psychology (e.g. Klages, 1926; Allport & Vernon, 1933; Eisenberg, 1937; Eisenberg & Reichline, 1939; Buytendijk, 1956; Mason, 1957). Physiognomonics, facial expression, gesture, posture, gait, voice, and handwriting were interpreted as expression of affective states or personality (for a more detailed review see Asendorpf & Wallbott, 1982).

At that time, research activity also started to focus on movement behaviour in patients with mental disease and brain damage. In psychiatry, alterations of movement behaviour were reported in patients with depressive and schizophrenic disorders (e.g. Kahlbaum, 1874; Wernicke, 1900; Kleist, 1943; Kretschmer, 1921; Reiter, 1926; Leonhard, 1957). These alterations were classified into hypokinetic and hyperkinetic ones. In neurology, movement behaviour disturbances were analysed with regard to brain damage and brain disease, such as paralysis, ataxia, dystonia, etc. Of special interest for movement behaviour research are those deficits that are related to neuropsychological functions, notably apraxia, which affects practical action and gesture (e.g. Liepmann, 1907; Goldstein, 1908). In psychomotor research, methods of experimental psychology were applied (e.g. Oseretzky, 1931; Luria, 1965). Psychomotor tests, such as finger tapping, dexterity, or rhythm tasks, enable to register even fine motor deficits in patients with neurotic and psychotic disturbances (Wulfeck, 1941; King, 1954; Manschreck, 1985, 1989, 1990; Günther et al., 1991). In 1933, the psychiatrist and psychoanalyst Wilhelm Reich published his work "Charakteranalyse" in which he outlined the relation between an individual's character and body, specifically muscle tension patterns. Many of the current movement and body-oriented (psycho)therapies refer to his ideas. Dance movement therapy integrated knowledge from German expression dance and psychoanalysis (e.g. Kestenberg, 1965, 1967; Espenak, 1985; Schoop, 1981; Bartenieff, 1991). For the analysis of movement behaviour, dance movement therapists apply the Laban Movement Analysis, an elaborated descriptive dance notation (Laban, 1950, reprint 1988).

During the 1960's, reflecting the general trend toward social sciences, the focus of research shifted from the individual's expressive movement to the role of body movement in communciation and interaction and on its cultural differences (e.g. Efron, 1941; Hall, 1968; Birdwhistell, 1979; Ekman & Friesen, 1969; Davis, 1979, 1982; Kendon, 1990). Basically the same movement parameters as applied in expression psychology were then investigated with regard to their function in interactive processes: posture / position, gesture, touching behaviour / self-touch, facial expression, eye movement behaviour, personal space / territory, and vocal cues. Research on nonverbal interaction was also introduced to psychoanalysis and psychotherapy for the analysis of patient - therapist interaction (e.g. Mahl, 1968; Freedman, 1972; Krause & Luetolf, 1989). In psychosomatic medicine, with reference to the bio-psycho-social model, the patient's movement behaviour was considered as a symptom that reflects his/her psychosomatic state (e.g. Uexküll & Wesiack, 1986). A reduction of nonverbal emotional expression was found to be associated with psychosomatic disease and alexithymia (e.g. Birbaumer, 1983; Birbaumer et al., 1986; Berry & Pennebaker, 1993; von Rad, 1983).

At the end of the last century, linguists have gained interest in gesture and sign language as nonverbal means of communication, reflecting cognitive processes (e.g. McNeill, 1985, 1987, 1992; Feyereisen, 1987; Müller, 1998; Kita & Özyürek, 2003). In line with psycholinguistic research on gesture and cognition, child psychologists study gesture to understand cognitive development (e.g. Goldin-Meadow et al., 1993). Moreover, recent evolutionary theories propose that language has evolved from manual gestures (e.g. Corballis, 2002). In the developing field of neuroscience, neuropsychologists investigate where in the brain gesture and sign language are produced (e.g. Kimura, 1973; Corina et al., 1992; Corina et al., 2003; Lausberg et al., 2007). Several studies examine gesture perception with functional neuroimaging (e.g. Gallagher & Frith, 2004; MacSweeney et al., 2004; Holle et al., 2008). Most recently, artificial intelligence researchers have started to develop gesture production models for embodied agents (Kopp & Bergmann, 2012).

This short historical review reveals that expressive and communicative movement behaviour has long been subject of scientific interest. Nowadays, its impact is reflected by the fact that movement behaviour is subject of investigation in many academic disciplines. The other side of the coin is that the diaspora of movement behaviour research across different disciplines is an obstacle for developing a common body of knowledge. This entails that movement behaviour research has not become an independent scientific discipline. Davis (1972, p. 2) makes an interesting observation regarding movement behaviour researchers: "The list of those who have written about expressive movement or nonverbal communication since 1872 reads like a "Who's Who" in the behavioural sciences; yet writers still defend the relevance of such study or introduce the subject as if it were esoteric or unheard of. It is as if a great many serious behavioural scientists have shown a fleeting interest in body movement and then gone on." Since Davis has reported this observation 40 years ago, obviously, not much has changed. Thus, not only the identity of movement behaviour research as an academic discipline but also the professional identity of the individual researcher who deals with movement behaviour seems to be fragile.

A thorough analysis of the complex question why this might be the case is beyond the scope of this chapter. It shall only be indicated that this might be related to the status of the body and thus, of body movement in the Christian-occidental culture that considers the body inferior to the mind. While the materialistic-functional aspect of body is accepted, such as the effort to achieve a perfect, functional, and good-looking body, the existential aspect of the body is neglected (e.g. Dürckheim, 1981). Furthermore, in our culture, research on the expressive aspects of movement behaviour is often regarded with ambivalence. This is due to the fact that movement behaviour is often displayed implicitly, i.e., beyond the mover's awareness. This leads to the concern that the analysis of one's body movement might uncover aspects of one's personality or feelings that one might not want to uncover. This attitude explains, for example, why only few psychotherapists agree to have their movement behaviour analysed during psychotherapy sessions. The low esteem of the body and its movement becomes manifest in several domains of our culture. As an example, there is a scant regard for art forms that use body movement as a medium such as dance, while "non-body" art forms such as music or literature are more appreciated. Furthermore, despite the fact that they have an equally long tradition and are equally appreciated as effective by patients (Olbrich, 2004), movement and body-oriented (psycho)therapies are less accepted in the health care system than verbal psychoanalytic and psychotherapeutic therapies (e.g. Bühler, 1981). (Of course, this is also caused by a lack of empirical research which could demonstrate the effectivity of movement and body-oriented therapies). Likewise, for a long period of time, sign language has not been accepted by the society as a valid means of communication for the deaf community. Fortunately, possibly also promoted by the rise of research on sign language, the status of sign language in society has recently improved. The cultural attitude might explain why, thus far, despite the long tradition and the broad scientific interest research, movement behaviour has not developed as an academic discipline on its own.

The lack of a scientific identity entails that in the course of history movement behaviour research has always been substantially coined by the dominant scientific discipline. This situation renders it difficult to follow the central thread of movement behaviour research through history. As a consequence, references to historically earlier but nevertheless relevant research are rarely made, and in each historical scientific era, expressive and communicative movement behaviour seems to be discovered de novo. The lack of scientific identity of the research field is not only a longitudinal historical problem but also a horizontal interdisciplinary one. Nowadays, as exposed above, research on movement behaviour is spread over many different academic disciplines. While the common denominator of these different scientific approaches is that movement behaviour reflects and affects cognitive, emotional, and interactive processes, there is hardly an interdisciplinary exchange. This lack is a severe obstacle for scientific progress in movement behaviour research. Movement behaviour researchers are often simply not aware of the substantial body of research that has been done in other fields so far, historically and concurrently. Therefore, some researchers have been dedicated to making knowledge from other historical epochs and other academic disciplines available to their colleagues (e.g. Davis, 1972; Davis and Skupien, 1982; Asendorpf & Wallbott, 1982; Wallbott, 1982; Kendon, 2004). Hopefully, in the same vein, this book will contribute to promote interdisciplinary understanding and exchange, among others by demonstrating the effects of different methods on research findings.

However, while there are many obstacles in developing movement behaviour research as a discipline on its own and on building a common body of knowledge, the currently increasing distribution of visual media is a cultural development that is clearly in favour for promoting movement behaviour research. Through TV, internet, and video games, users are nowadays constantly confronted with moving human and avatar bodies. In contrast, in the first half of the last century, acoustic information transfer through radio and telephone was predominant. The current omnipresence of moving human and avatar bodies calls even more for a thorough basic knowledge and understanding of how movement behaviour – on the conscious and unconscious levels - reflects and affects cognitive, emotional, and interactive processes.

Finally, as stated above, another reason for the scant exchange of knowledge between the academic disciplines is differences in terminology and methodology. These differences make a comparison of the findings of different academic discipline difficult and inhibit that a common interdisciplinary corpus of knowledge grows. In fact, this problem is not only an interdisciplinary one but also an **intra**disciplinary one, as often within one discipline, researchers invent their own movement analysis systems. The results of their studies are then difficult to integrate in a common body of knowledge.

Furthermore, as it will be outlined in Chapter 3, the field of movement behaviour research suffers from a lack of effective and efficient methods. Until the 1960s, movement behaviour as a transitory phenomenon was difficult to register and to submit to research. This is illustrated by Efron 's "fourfold method" (1941, p. 66), in which he applied several techniques commonly used at his time: "(1) direct observation of gestural behaviour in natural situations, (2) sketches drawn from life by the American painter ... under the same conditions, (3) rough counting, (4) motion pictures studied by (a) observations and judgments of naive observers, and (b) graphs and charts, together with measurements and tabulations of the same." Thus, the painstaking analysis of movement behaviour might also explain Davis' observation that single researchers do not stay in the field.

However, also with regard to this aspect, the current situation characterized by an impressive technical progress is in favour for developing the scientific field of movement behaviour research. The registration of movement behaviour has become simple and qualitatively improved by using digital video. Furthermore, the availability of software for the annotation of videotaped movement behaviour substantially facilitates the analysis of movement behaviour data (see part III in this book). However, the technical progress will only entail scientific progress, if movement behaviour researchers identify entities of body movement behaviour that are relevant with regard to cognitive, emotional, and interactive processes.

References

Allport, G.W., & Vernon, P.E. (1933). *Studies in Expressive Movement.* New York: Macmillan.

Asendorpf, J., & Wallbott, H.G. (1982). Contributions of the German "Expression Psychology" to Nonverbal Communication Research. Part I: Theories and Concepts. *Journal of Nonverbal Behavior, 6*(3), 135-1.

Bartenieff, I. (1991). Tanztherapie. In E. Willke, G. Hölter & H. Petzhold (Ed.), *Tanztherapie - Theorie und Praxis* (pp. 259-88). Paderborn: Junfermann.

Berry, D.S., & Pennebaker, J.W. (1993). Nonverbal and Verbal Emotional Expression and Health. *Psychotherapy and Psychosomatics, 59*, 11-19.

Birbaumer, N. (1983). Psychophysiologische Ansätze. In H. Euler, H. Mandel (Ed.), *Emotionspsychologie* (pp.45-52). München: Urban & Schwarzenberg.

Birbaumer, N., Miltner, W., & Gerber W. D. (1986). *Verhaltensmedizin*. Berlin: Springer.

Birdwhistell, R.L. (1979). Kinesik. In K. R. Scherer, H.G. Wallbott (Ed.), *Nonverbale Kommunikation: Forschungsberichte zum Interaktionsverhalten* (pp. 192-202). Weinheim: Beltz 1979.

Bühler, C. (1981). Vorwort. In H. Petzhold (Ed.), *Psychotherapie & Körperdynamik.* Paderborn: Junfermann.

Buytendijk, F.J.J. (1956). *Allgemeine Theorie der menschlichen Haltung und Bewegung*. Berlin: Springer.

Corballis, M.C. (2002). From hand to mouth: Gesture, speech, and the evolution of right-handedness. *Behavioral and Brain Sciences, 26(2),* 199-208.

Corina, D.P., Poizner, H., Bellugi, U., Feinberg, T., Dowd, D., & O'Grady-Batch, L. (1992). Dissociation between Linguistic and Nonlinguisitic Gestural Systems: A Case for Compositionality. *Brain and Language, 43*, 414-47.
Corina, D.P., Jose-Robertson, L.S., Guellimin, A., High, J., & Braun, A.R. (2003) Language lateralisation in a bimanual language. *Journal of Cognitive Neuroscience, 15(5)*, 718-30.

Critchley, M. (1970). *The Language of Gesture*. New York: Haskell House Publishers.

Darwin, C. (1872, reissued 1955) *The Expression of the Emotions in Man and Animals*. New York: Philosophical Library.

Davis M. (1972). Understanding body movement - An annotated bibliography. *Advances in Semiotics*.

Davis, M. (1979). Laban. Analysis of Nonverbal Communication. In S. Weitz *Nonverbal Communication* 2nd ed. New York: Oxford University Press.

Davis, M., and Skupien, J. (1982). *Body Movement and Nonverbal Communication. An Annotated Bibliography, 1971-1980*: Indiana University Press.

Dürckheim, K. (1981). Vom Leib der man ist. In H. Petzhold (Ed.), *Psychotherapie & Körperdynamik* (pp.11-27). Paderborn: Junfermann.

Efron, D. (1941). *Gesture and culture*. The Hague: Mouton.

Eisenberg, P. (1937). Expressive Movement related to Feelings of Dominance. *Archives of Psychology, 211*.

Eisenberg, P., & Reichline, P. (1939). Judgements of Dominance Feelings from Motion Pictures of Gait. *Journal of Abnormal and Social Psychology, 10*.

Ekman, P., & Friesen, W. V. (1969). The repertoire of non-verbal behavior. *Semiotica, 1*, 49-98.

Espenak, L. (1985). *Tanztherapie - durch kreativen Ausdruck zur Persönlichkeitsentwicklung*. Dortmund: Sanduhr.

Feyereisen, P. (1987). Gestures and speech, interactions and separations: A reply to McNeill. *Psychological Review, 94,* 493-8.

Freedman, N. (1972). The analysis of movement behavior during the clinical interview. In A. W.Siegman, & B. Pope (Ed). *Studies in dyadic communication* (pp. 153-75). New York: Pergamon.

Gallagher, H.L., & Frith, C.D. (2004). Dissociable neural pathways for the perception and recognition of expressive and instrumental gestures. *Neuropsychologia, 42*, 1725-36.

Goldin-Meadow, S., Alibali, M.W., & Church, R.B. (1993). Transitions in concept acquisition: using the hand to read the mind. *Psychological Review, 100(2),* 279-97.

Goldstein, K. (1908). Zur Lehre von der motorischen Apraxie. *Journal für Psychologie und Neurologie, XI*, 169-187

Günther, W., Petsch, R., Steinberg, R., Moser, E., Streck, P., Heller, H., Kurtz, G., & Hippius, H. (1991). Brain dysfunction during motor activation and corpus callosum alterations in schizophrenia measured by cerebral blood flow and magnetic resonance imaging. *Biological Psychiatry, 29*, 535-55.

Hall, E.T. (1966). *The Hidden Dimension*. New York: Doubleday.

Holle, H., Gunter, T.C., Rüschemeyer, S.-A., Hennenlotter, A., & Iacoboni, M. (2008). Neural correlates of the processing of co-speech gestures. *NeuroImage, 39*, 2010-2024.

Kahlbaum, K. (1874). *Die Katatonie oder das Spannungsirresein*. Berlin: Hirschwald.

Kendon, A. (1990). *Conduction Interaction. Patterns of behavior in focused encounters*. New York: Cambridge University Press.

Kendon, A. (2004). *Gesture: Visible Action as Utterance*. Cambridge: University Press.

Kestenberg, J. (1965a). The Role of Movement Patterns in Development I. *Psychoanalytic Quarterly, 24(1),* 1-36.

Kestenberg, J. (1965b). The Role of Movement Patterns in Development II. *Psychoanalytic Quarterly, 24(4),* 515-63.

Kestenberg J. (1967). The Role of Movement Patterns in Development III. *Psychoanalytic Quarterly, 26(3),* 356-409.

Kietz, G. (1952). Der Ausdrucksgehalt des menschlichen Ganges. *Zeitschrift für angewandte Psychologie und Charakterkunde, Beiheft 93*, 2. erw. Aufl. Leipzig: Johann Ambrosius.
King, H.E. (1954). *Psychomotor Aspects of Mental Disease*. Cambridge: Havard University .

Kimura, D. (1973). Manual Activity during Speaking - 1. Right-Handers. *Neuropsychologia, 11*, 45-50.

Kita, S., & Özyürek, A. (2003). What does cross-linguistic variation in semantic coordination of speech and gesture reveal?: Evidence for an interface representation of spatial thinking and speaking. *Journal of Memory and Language, 48,* 16-32.

Klages, L. (1926). *Grundlagen der Charakterkunde*. Leipzig: J.A. Barth.

Kleist, K. (1943). Die Katatonien. *Nervenarzt, 16*, 1-10.

Knapp, M.L., & Hall J.A. (1992). *Nonverbal Communication in Human Interaction* (3rd edition). Harcourt Brace College Publishers, Orlando.

Kopp, S., & Bergmann, K. (2012). *Individualized Gesture Production in Embodied Conversational Agents*. In: M. Zacarias & J.V. de Oliveira (Eds.), Human-Computer Interaction: The Agency Perspective, 396, Studies in Computational Intelligence.Berlin/Heidelberg: Springer, 287-302.

Krause, R., & Luetolf, P. (1989). Mimische Indikatoren von Uebertragungsvorgaengen. *Zeitschrift für Klinische Psychologie,* XVIII: 55-67.

Laban, R. (1988). *The Mastery of Movement*, Neuauflage. Worcester: Northcote House.

Lausberg, H., Zaidel, E., Cruz, R.F., & Ptito, A. (2007). Speech-independent production of communicative gestures: Evidence from patients with complete callosal disconnection. *Neuropsychologia, 45*, 3092-3104.

Leonhard, K. (1957). *Aufteilung der endogenen Psychosen und ihre differenzierte Ätiologie*. Stuttgart, New York: Georg Thieme Verlag.

Liepmann, H, & Maas, O. (1907). Fall von linksseitiger Agraphie und Apraxie bei rechtsseitiger Lähmung. *Journal für Psychologie und Neurologie, X*, 214-27.

Luria, A.R. (1965). Neuropsychological analysis of focal brain lesion
In B. B. Woolman (Ed.), *Handbook of clinical psychology*. New York McGrawHill Book Company.

MacSweeney, M., Campbell, R., Woll, B., Giampietro, V., David, A.S., McGuire, P.K., Calvert, G.A., & Brammer, M.J. (2004) Dissociating linguistic and nonlinguistic gestural communication in the brain. *NeuroImage, 22,* 1605-18.

Mahl, F.G. (1968). Gestures and Body Movements in Interviews. *Research in Psychotherapy,* 3, 295-346.

Manschreck, T.C. (1989). Motor Abnormalities and the Psychopathology of Schizophrenia. In: B Kirkcaldy editor. Normalities and Abnormalities in Human Movement. *Medicine and Sport Science, 29*, 100-27.

Manschreck, T.C., Maher, B.M., Waller, N.G., Ames, D., & Latham, C.A. (1985). Deficient motor synchrony in schizophrenic disorders: clinical correlates. *Biological Psychiatry, 20*, 990-1002.

Manschreck, T.C., Keuthen, N.J., Schneyer, M.L., Celada, M.T., Laughery, J., & Collins, P. (1990). Abnormal involuntary movements and chronic schizophrenic disorders. *Biological Psychiatry, 27*, 150-8.

Mason, D.J. (1957). Judgements of Leadership based upon Physiognomonic Cues. *Journal of Abnormal and Social Psychology, 54 (2),* 273-4.

McNeill, D. (1992). *Hand and mind. What gestures reveal about thought.* Chicago, London: The University of Chicago Press.

McNeill D. (1985). So you think gestures are nonverbal? *Psychological Review, 92(3),* 350-71.

McNeill, D. (1987). So You Do Think Gestures Are Nonverbal! Reply to Feyereisen. *Psychological Review, 94(4),* 499-504.

Müller, C. (1998). *Redebegleitende Gesten - Kulturgeschichte, Theorie, Sprachvergleich.* Berlin: Berlin Verlag Arno Spitz GmbH.

Olbrich, D. (2004). Kreativtherapie in der psychosomatischen Rehabilitation. *Psychotherapeut, 49 (1),* 67-70.

Oseretzky, N. (1931). Psychomotorik. *Zeitschrift für Angewandte Psychologie, Beiheft 1*, 57.

Reich, W. (1971). *Charakteranalyse.* Bremen: Plopp.

Reiter, P.J. (1926). Extrapyramidal motor-disturbances in dementia praecox. *Acta Psychiatrica et Neurologica, 1*, 287-305.

Schoop, T. (1981). ... *komm und tanz mit mir*. Zürich: Musikhaus Pan.

Rad, M. von (1983). Alexithymie (Themenheft). *Monographien aus dem Gesamtgebiet der Psychiatrie, 30.*

Uexküll, v.,Th. & Wesiack, W. (Ed.) (1986). Psychosomatische Medizin, 3. Aufl. München: Urban & Schwarzenberg; 600-33.

Wallbott, H.G. (1982). Contributions of the German "Expression Psychology" to Nonverbal Communication Research. Part III: Gait, Gestures, and Body Movement *Journal of Nonverbal Behavior,* 7(1), 20-32.

Wernicke, C. (1900). *Grundriss der Psychiatrie in klinischen Vorlesungen.* Leipzig: Thieme.

Wulfeck, W.H. (1941). Motor Function in Mentally Disordered. *Psychological Reports, 4,* 271-323.

2. Empirical Research on Movement Behaviour and its Link to Cognitive, Emotional, and Interactive Processes

Hedda Lausberg

This chapter deals with empirical findings across academic disciplines concerning the relation between movement behaviour and cognitive, emotional, and interactive processes that are relevant for developing the methodology in movement behaviour research.

The first section of this chapter addresses the question what empirical evidence supports the paradigm that human movement behaviour is linked to cognitive, emotional, and interactive processes. The implications of these findings for movement research methodology are discussed.

Empirical evidence that movement behaviour is linked to cognitive, emotional, and interactive processes legitimates the application of movement behaviour analysis as a valid method to explore these processes. However, for this purpose numerous questionnaires are already available which are economic psychological research tools. Therefore, the second section focuses on the question what specific potential movement behaviour analysis bears for the investigation of emotional, cognitive, and interactive processes.

The third and fourth sections illustrate the profit of analyzing all movements of a part of the body and of segmenting the ongoing stream of movement behaviour into natural units as compared to pre-selecting certain types of movement for the analysis. Finally, the fifth section discusses why it is useful to distinguish between right side, left side, and bilateral movements when analyzing limb movements such as hand gestures.

2.1 Different classes of movement behaviour reflect and affect cognitive, emotional, and interactive processes

There is ample empirical evidence that body movements that are spontaneously displayed during interaction, soliloquy, or silent thinking are associated with cognitive processes such as language or spatial cognition (e.g. Lavergne & Kimura, 1987; Butterworth & Hadar, 1989; Cohen & Otterbein, 1992; Krauss et al., 1996; Sirigu et al., 1996; Feyereisen, 2006; Parsons et al., 1998; de Ruiter, 2000; De'Sperati & Stucchi, 2000; Emmorey et al., 2000; Kita, 2000; Garber & Goldin-Meadow, 2002; Kita & Özyürek, 2003; Lausberg & Kita, 2003; McNeill, 2005; Beattie & Shovelton 2006; Cook & Goldin-Meadow, 2006; Ehrlich et al., 2006; Goldin-Meadow, 2006; Lausberg et al., 2007; Beattie & Shovelton, 2009; Sassenberg et al., 2010; Wartenburger et al., 2010). Likewise it has been demonstrated that movement behaviour is related to emotional processes and psychopathology (e.g. Darwin, 1890; Krout, 1935; Sainsbury, 1954; Freedman & Hoffman, 1967; Ekman & Friesen, 1969, 1974; Freedman, 1972; Scheflen, 1974; Ulrich, 1977; Davis, 1981, 1997; Freedman & Bucci, 1981; Ulrich & Harms, 1985; Ellgring, 1986; Wallbott, 1989; Gaebel, 1992; Berry & Pennebaker, 1993; Willke, 1995; Cruz, 1995; Lausberg et al., 1996; Berger, 1999). Furthermore, movement behaviour serves to regulate interactive processes and to communicate information (e.g. Scheflen, 1973, 1974; Cohen & Otterbein, 1992; Davis, 1997; Cook & Goldin-Meadow, 2006; Feyereisen, 2006; Holle & Gunter, 2007; Holle et al., 2008, 2010).

In the following subsections, a widespread range of examples is given to illustrate the relations between movement behaviour and cognitive, emotional, and interactive functions. As pathological conditions are highly informative for exploring these relations, studies on patients with mental or neurological disease are included. The review is based upon the classes of movement behaviour that have been first introduced in the expression psychology and then pursued and extended in nonverbal communication research: posture, position, gesture, self-touch and touching behaviour[1]. Because of the differences in the use of these terms in different disciplines and by different researches - as outlined in the previous chapter -, the terms are used as defined in general dictionaries in the review below.

2.1.1 Gesture and spatial cognition

A gesture is defined as "a movement of part of the body, especially a hand or the head, to express an idea or meaning" (http://oxforddictionaries.com/definition/english/gesture?q=gesture) or as "a movement usually of the body or limbs that expresses or emphasizes an idea, sentiment, or attitude" (http://www.merriam-webster.com/dictionary/gesture). Kendon points out the problem of the concept of gesture: "'Gesture', we have suggested, is a name for visible action when it is used as an utterance or as part of an utterance. But what is 'utterance', and how are actions in this domain recognized as playing a part in it." (2010, p. 7) This statement reveals the difficulty to operationalize the concept of a gesture, as its definition implies a function. Pragmatically, in this review, the term gesture is used if the researcher chose this term.

It is well established that gestures are a suitable means of conveying spatially complex information (Beattie & Shovelton, 2006; Beattie & Shovelton, 2009; Kita & Özyürek, 2003; Lausberg & Kita, 2003). Explaining mathematical equivalence problems is more effective if the teacher's verbal explanations are accompanied by gestures (Cook & Goldin-Meadow, 2006). (This effect, however, is not limited to spatial topics. Also non-spatial topics are understood and recalled better if the verbal explanations are accompanied by gestures (Cohen &

1 Given the topic of this book, research on facial expression, eye movement behaviour, personal space, territory, and vocal cues is not reviewed here.

Otterbein, 1992; Feyereisen, 2006)). There is, however, also evidence that gestures that accompany descriptions not only improve the recipient's understanding, but also help the gesturer to think about space and to formulate spatial topics. When talking about spatial topics, more speech accompanying gestures are displayed than when talking about non-spatial topics (Lavergne & Kimura, 1987), especially when the speakers talk about their own movement in space (Emmorey et al., 2000). If speakers are prevented from producing gestures while talking about spatial topics, they speak more slowly and hesitantly than if prevented from producing gestures when talking about non-spatial topics. Pupils who gesture when explaining mathematical problems show better performances than pupils who do not gesture (Cook & Goldin-Meadow, 2006; Ehrlich et al., 2006).

Furthermore, spatial gestures reveal the cognitive strategies that an individual uses when (s)he thinks about space. In a geometrical analogy task experiment, participants with a higher level of intelligence used more spontaneous gestures during the explanation of the task than participants with an average IQ (Sassenberg et al., 2011). This applied especially to spatial gestures with an observer viewpoint as defined by McNeill (1992). The observer viewpoint reveals that the gesturer takes an allocentric perspective, e.g. index and middle finger depict someone walking along a street. In contrast, the character viewpoint reveals that the gesturer takes an egocentric view on the spatial scenery, e.g. the gesturer pantomimes swimming in a river. Thus, spatial gestures may reflect the mental perspective taken when imagining a spatial scenery. When solving a spatial task by Piaget, gesture - speech mismatches were noticed in pupils. They showed the correct response in their gestures but verbally they formulated a wrong answer (Goldin-Meadow et al., 1993). Also in adults solving a spatial task, such as the Tower of Hanoi, gestures and speech can reflect different cognitive strategies at the same time (Garber & Goldin-Meadow, 2002). Neuropsychological experiments also evidence that spatial gestures reveal the way we think about spatial problems. Decisions concerning the spatial orientation of objects are based on motor imagination of gesturing. This is evidenced by the fact that when asked to judge the spatial orientation of an object, participants rotate their hands mentally into the same spatial orientation as the object is in (Sirigu et al., 1996; Parsons et al, 1998; De'Sperati & Stucchi 2000).

The examination of gestures in patients with brain damages provides information about the different components that play a role in the conceptualization of spatial gestures. Split-brain patients neglect the left half of the gesture space in right hand gestures. In contrast, in their left hand gestures they use the whole gesture space. The findings evidence that the conceptualization of gesture space use is a specific function which is lateralized to the left hemisphere (Lausberg et al., 2003 a). Furthermore, patients with left brain damage show selective impairments in finding the target position, e.g. when transporting the hand to the mouth when pantomiming brushing the teeth (Poizner et al., 1990; Hermsdörfer et al., 1996). This selective deficit demonstrates that arriving at the target position constitutes a distinct component in the conceptualization of spatial gestures.

To summarize, the empirical findings from different disciplines evidence that gesture production and spatial cognition is tightly linked. Moreover, the results from spatial tests, which demonstrate a positive correlation between a high performance level and a high amount of gestures, suggest that gestures not only reflect but also promote spatial thinking. McNeill proposes that "... gesture, the actual motion of gesture itself, is a dimension of thinking." (2005, p. 98). In line with this proposition, Cook et al. suggest that gesturing is "an alternative, embodied way of representing new ideas" (2008, p. 1047) as it offers an analogous motor and visuo-spatial representation. It has to be noted, however, that in the spatial tests mentioned above, physical objects such as the Tower of Hanoi were always presented. Particularly, the gesture-speech mismatches could have been induced by the bimodal assignment of tasks, object presentation and verbal instruction. Therefore, it would be interesting to investigate if the proposition that different cognitive strategies may be spontaneously used at the same time (Garber & Goldin-Meadow, 2002) is still valid when spatial tasks are administered verbally. Thus, while there is ample evidence for a bidirectional link between gesturing and spatial cognition, more empirical research is needed to fully understand the processes that determine the interdependent relation.

2.1.2 Self-touch and arousal

The term self-touch is not listed in classical English dictionaries. However, in non-verbal communication research, anthropology, and neuropsychology, the term is commonly used. Self-touch is defined as any touching of the own body (e.g. Morris, 1978; Knapp & Hall, 1992; Kimura, 1973). Thus, in contrast to the term gesture, the term self-touch is purely descriptive and does not imply a function. A self-touch can be a practical action, a gesture, or a self-stimulation. In contrast, the terms 'autistic gestures' and *body-focused*[2] movements, which are used by some researchers for self-touching movements, refer only to self-stimulation. These types[3] do not include gestures with touching the own body such as self-deictics.

30-70% of all hand movements that are displayed in conversation and interviews are self-touch movements such as scratching oneself or as hand-to-hand fidgeting (Krout, 1935; Sainsbury, 1955; Mahl, 1968; Freedman, O'Hanlon, Oltman, & Witkin, 1972; Kimura, 1973 a; Sousa-Poza & Rohrberg, 1977; Souza-Poza et al., 1979; Dalby et al., 1980; Freedman & Bucci, 1981; Lausberg,

2 In this chapter, the names of movement types are only written in italics if they are defined values of a specific coding system that will be described in Chapter 3. As an example, *self-touch* is only written in italics if it designates the defined movement value of Kimura's coding system. It is not written in italics if it is used in the general sense.

3 Throughout the book, the terms (movement) type and (movement) value are used synonymously

1995; Dvoretska, 2009; Kryger, 2010; Lausberg, 2011; Lausberg & Kryger, 2011). This kind of self-touching behaviour is typically subject of investigation in empirical studies on emotional functions and psychopathology.

In psychotherapy research, since long it has been documented that 'autistic gestures' - as opposed to communicative gestures - could be reliably elicited through association experiments and during emotionally loaded issues (Sainsbury, 1955; Mahl, 1968). In several studies, Freedman's coding system was used (see Chapter 3), which opposes *body-focused* movements to *object-focused* movements, i.e., gestures. During free association in psychoanalytic sessions or in semi-structured interviews, field-dependent subjects, as defined by Witkin and Lewis (1954), showed significantly more *continuous direct body-focused* activity, especially *hand-to-hand* movements, than field-independent subjects (Freedman, O'Hanlon, Oltman, & Witkin, 1972; Sousa-Poza & Rohrberg, 1977; Freedman & Bucci, 1981). Furthermore, the *continuous direct body-focused* activity was more prominent in interviews with cold interviewers than in those with warm, empathetic interviewers (Freedman et al., 1972). Sousa-Poza and Rohrberg (1977) reported that in interviews with personal topics referring to interpersonal relationships and the worst life experience, there was significantly more *continuous body-touching* behaviour than in interviews with impersonal topics referring to a typical working day and the hometown. It is obvious that the topic of the worst life experience is likely to have elicited negative emotions. Moreover, during interference tasks, i.e., the Stroop-test, the *direct body-focused* activity was significantly stronger than in tasks requiring spatial imagination and anticipation (Barosso et al., 1978).

Clinical studies on patients with schizophrenic and depressive disorders revealed that the *body-focused* hand movement behaviour decreased as the psychiatric disorder improved (Freedman & Hoffman, 1967; Freedman, 1972). Likewise, in depressive patients the clinical improvement through anti-depressive pharmacotherapy was accompanied by a decrease of the *continuous body-focused* hand movements (Ulrich, 1977; Ulrich & Harms, 1985), especially in the left hand (Ulrich, 1977). In the same line, in the course of a successful psychotherapy, patients with depression and psychosomatic disorder showed a clear reduction of *on body* movements, as measured with the NEUROGES system (see Part II in this book) (Lausberg, 1995; Kryger, 2010; Lausberg & Kryger, 2011).

Thus, there is ample empirical evidence that direct touching of the body, especially if it occurs continuously, is associated with mental arousal during stress, (predominantly negative) emotional engagement, and depression. Freedman and Bucci (1981) suggested that *continuous* and *discrete body-focused* activity have distinct filtering functions. *Continuous body-focused* activity creates - according to the authors - a white noise situation, which helps to reduce the discrepancy between incoming information and the mover's internal state. *Discrete body-focused* movements serve as a contrasting strategy. However, as *on body* movements are not only observed in the presence of external stimulation but also in its absence, here it is proposed that *on body* movements rather serve to stabilize oneself, in most cases to care for oneself and to calm oneself and less often to activate oneself. Support for this proposition stems for neuroendocrinological and neurophysiological research. In rodents grooming behaviour induces a reduction in the dopamine response to stress (Berridge, Mitton, Clark, & Roth, 1999) as well as an increase in physical growth, growth hormon (GH) and Brain-Derived-Neurotropic-Factor (BDNF) (Schanberg & Field, 1987; Burton et al., 2007; Chatterjee et al., 2007). In humans, spontaneous (but not volitional) self-touch of the face in reaction to acoustic stress is associated with an increase in beta- und theta-activity in the EEG (Grunwald & Weiss, 2007). In premature babies a treatment with massage results in a faster weight gain and a decrease of blood cortisol (Schanberg & Field, 1987; Guzzetta et al., 2009). While Freedman and Bucci on one hand and Lausberg on the other hand emphasize different aspects regarding the function of self-touching behaviour, they agree on that self-touching behaviour not only reflects a mental state but also positively affects it.

2.1.3 Posture and mood

A posture is defined as "the position or bearing of the body whether characteristic or assumed for a special purpose <erect posture>" (http://www.merriam-webster.com/dictionary/posture) or as "a particular position of the body" (http://oxforddictionaries.com/definition/english/ posture?q=posture). The first definition reveals that the meaning of posture is two-folded: It can refer to an individual's habitual body alignment or to a temporary one. In the first case, the posture has the quality of a trait (hereafter trait-posture), in the second that of a state (hereafter state-posture). For a better distinction to rest position (see below), a *posture* is here defined as arrangement of the limbs with tensioned muscles characterized by motionlessness and muscle contraction (see Chapter 5).

In traditional psychiatry and expression psychology, the relation between the trait-posture and attitude or mood has been focused. There is long-standing knowledge that certain body postures are associated with a specific mood, attitude, or even personality (Darwin, 1890; Reich, 1933; Wallbott, 1989; Kleinsmith & Berthouze, 2007). In the clinical domain, a slumped posture has since long been documented as a symptom of depression (Kraepelin 1899, Kretschmer, 1921; Bleuler, 1949; Bader et al. 1999, Lemke et al. 2000; Michalak et al., 2009).

In the recent embodiment research, the link between state-posture and the affective valence of thought is focused on. It has been demonstrated that an upright posture induces a better recall of positive thoughts (Wilson and Peper, 2004; Casanto and Dijkstra, 2010), the experience of more pride (Stepper and Strack, 1993), and more persistence in problem solving (Riskind and Gotay, 1982). Thus, posture does not only reflect emotional states but also affects them.

2.1.4 Rest positions and quality of interaction

A position is defined as "a particular way in which someone or something is placed or arranged" (http://oxforddictionaries.com/definition/english/ position?q=position) or "a certain arrangement of bodily parts" (http://www.merriam-webster.com/dictionary/position). A *rest position* is here defined as a specific arrangement of the relaxed limbs characterized by motionlessness, absence of an anti-gravity position, and muscle relaxation (see Chapter 5).

The physical sign of the degree to which the person is open toward and vis a vis the other in her/his position is related to psychological openness and rapport (Charny, 1966; Scheflen, 1973). There is a significant relationship between the therapist's and the patient's rest position openness and accessibility (Davis, 1985). Physicians with open arm positions were judged more positively than those with a closed arm position (Harrigan & Rosenthal, 1983). This was confirmed by a later study by Harrigan, Oxman, Rosenthal (1985), in which physicians with arms in symmetrical, side-by-side positions (and uncrossed legs) were rated more positively. Adopting closed positions as compared to open positions increases negative emotions (Roosberg & Gempton, 1993).

Another perspective on rest position and interaction is taken in the structural approach, which was introduced to movement behaviour research by Birdwhistell (1952). As a researcher with the background of cultural anthropology and structural linguistics, Birdwhistell regarded any body movement as an arbitrary sign that served the maintenance and regulation of interaction. In this structural view, rest positions mark naturalistic units of behaviour and reflect the organization and structure of interaction (Scheflen, 1963, 1973). Certain rest positions in one partner co-occur with certain rest positions in the other, i.e., there are specific combinations of the interactive partners' rest positions (Scheflen, 1973; LaFrance, 1982; Davis & Hadiks, 1990) (for a more detailed discussion on body movement in interaction, see Chapter 18).

2.1.5 Summary

To summarize, the interdisciplinary review evidences that there is ample empirical evidence that movement behaviour is associated with cognitive, emotional, and interactive processes. More specifically, different classes of movement behaviour are related in various manners to within-subject cognitive and emotional processes and between-subjects interactive processes. While gestures have been linked predominantly to cognitive processes, self-touch has been investigated in the context of affective states and stress. Postures have been related to attitude, mood, and affective states, and rest positions have been analysed with regard to their function in interaction.

As cognitive, emotional, and interactive processes are all reflected in movement behaviour (Figure 1, arrows with straight line), movement behaviour can serve as a medium to explore these processes. Moreover, there is some evidence that the link between cognitive, emotional, and interactive processes and movement behaviour is bi-directional, i.e., movement behaviour, likewise, affects these processes (Figure 1, arrows with dotted line). More research is required to fully explore the complex relation between movement behaviour and cognitive, emotional, and interactive processes.

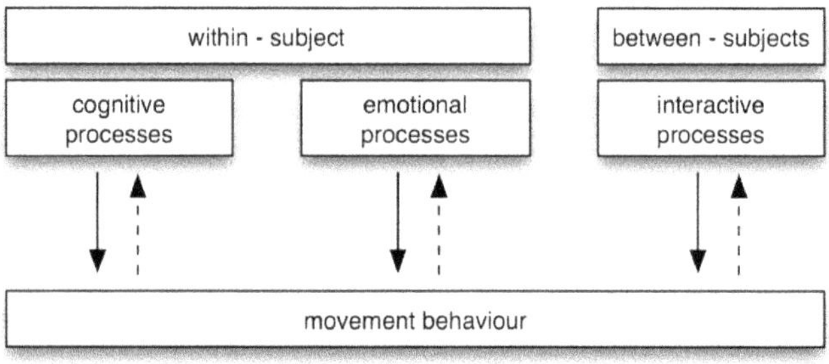

Figure 1 Bi-directional influence of movement behaviour and cognitive, emotional, and interactive processes.

2.2 Body movements are associated with implicit and explicit cognitive, emotional, and interactive processes

In the above section it has been demonstrated that movement behaviour reflects (and affects) cognitive, emotional, and interactive processes. Therefore, movement analysis can be used as a tool to explore these processes. However, its need is questionned as in psychological research many questionnaires and semi-standardized interviews are already available to examine cognitive, emotional, and interactive processes.

A commonly known advantage of movement analysis is that it is observer-based. Therefore, it is more objective than self-rating instruments such as questionnaires and then semi-standardized interviews, in which the outcome is influenced by the interviewer. Here, it shall be argued that furthermore, the specific potential of movement behaviour analysis is that it enables to investigate **implicit** cognitive, emotional, and interactive processes.

"*Explicit* knowledge refers to knowledge that is expressed as conscious experience and that people are aware that they possess; ... *Implicit* knowledge, by contrast, refers to knowledge that is revealed in task performance without any corresponding phenomenal awareness." Schacter (1992). Given this definition, many of the cognitive, emotional, and interactive processes as discussed above are implicit, such as interaction regulation (Scheflen, 1963) and the processing of emotions (Lane & Schwartz, 1987). Even cognitive strategies applied in spatial problem solving may be implicit (Cohen, 1984). This has been demonstrated in amnestic patients, who have lost their explicit memory. These patients may show over several trials a progress in solving the Tower of Hanoi Puzzle without being able to recall having practised the task or having encountered the apparatus.

In analogy to Schacter's definition, in this section, the term explicit hand movements is used for movements that the person is aware of when (s)he displays them spontaneously or on command. The term implicit movements is applied for movements that the person is not aware of when (s)he displays them spontaneously. She/he can, however, become aware of her/his movement during or immediately after the performance (compare sensory memory, e.g. Kaszniak et al., 1986).

With regard to the movement behaviour classes discussed above, there are differences in the proportions of explicit versus implicit display. While self-touches and the trait-posture are almost always displayed implicitly, gestures and rest positions may sometimes be explicit. *Emblematic* gestures, such as the Victory sign, or pointing gestures (*deictic*) are most often explicit (for the definition of the gesture values see Chapter 3). Ekman and Friesen (1969) have reported that occasionally gesturer pretended not to be aware of the fact that (s)he performed an *emblematic* gesture. Furthermore, sign language is used explicitly. Tool use actions are often performed explicitly, but patients with brain damage may perform automatized tool use actions implicitly (see below). In these explicit movements, the retrieval of the movement concept or, during learning processes, the de novo conceptualization, are intentional and conscious and the gesturer is aware of his/her performing the movement. It is plausible that the cognitive, emotional, or interactive processes that are associated with the generation of explicit body movements are partly explicit as well. As an example, the gesturer intends to show something to another person and performs a *deictic*. Or, the gesturer is aware of his anger and performs an insulting *emblem*.

A great proportion of movement behaviour, however, is displayed beyond the mover's awareness. This applies especially to self-touches and also to many idiosyncratic gestures. In this case, the retrieval of the movement concept is implicit. The movement is executed quasi automatically, and the mover is primarily not aware of the execution. The same applies to movement behaviours of continuous nature such as state-posture. As the mover is not aware of her/his state-posture or her/his fidgeting movements, it is plausible that (s)he is not aware of the underlying cognitive, emotional, or interactive process. Some examples shall be given here to illustrate the link between implicit body movements and primarily implicit cognitive, emotional, and interactive processes. An unconsciously displayed and seemingly purposeless self-touch may serve psychodynamically for self-regulation in a stressful situation. An implicitly displayed *motion presentation* gestures may reflect how the gesturer perceives the dynamics of a personal relationship, while (s)he has not deliberately reflected this impression. The opening of the rest position may reflect that the mover's attitude towards his/her interactive partner starts changing towards more sympathy. The conversion of a slumped posture into a more erect one may indicate that the mover's general mood has improved before (s)he her-/himself consciously notes of this change. Thus, the analysis of implicit body movements provides valuable insights into implicit cognitive, emotional and interactive processes.

As stated above, the primarily implicit display of a body movement does not exclude that, during the performance, the person may become aware of her/his movement or posture. As an example, during an empathetic interaction, one partner performs a self-touch of the face and the other one "automatically" tunes in but then becomes aware of his/her hand moving to the face. Catching oneself performing such an automatized behaviour is typically astonishing or even embarrassing.

The proposition that implicit body movements are associated with implicit cognitive, emotional, and interactive processes, while explicit movements are related to partly explicit processes is supported by the scientific evidence that implicit movements differ kinematically and neurobiologically from their explicit counter-parts.

In a kinematic study, the very same movement, seizing and moving a lever, was executed differently when it was displayed implicitly as compared to being done intentionally (Bock & Hagemann, 2010). As an everyday life example, stroking one's hair back while being intensely engaged in a conversation differs in terms of movement parameters from stroking one's hair back as a volitional preening behaviour to attract the partner's attention. Moreover, implicit hand movements differ in their neurobiological correlates from their explicit counterparts. Grunwald and Weiss (submitted) reported different patterns of cortical activity as measured with electroencephalography during instructed self-touches of the face as compared to spontaneous self-touches of the face, which the gesturer performed during a stress test without being aware of it. Studies in patients with brain damage provide further evidence that explicit and implicit movements rely on different neural networks. Rapcsak et al. (1993) suggested that the movement ("praxis") system in the right hemisphere is strongly biased toward the concrete and context-dependent execution of familiar, well-established routines including implicit movements, whereas the left hemisphere conceptualizes novel movements and is specialized for deliberate explicit movements. This proposition is strongly supported by patients with callosal disconnection (often split-brain patients), in whom the neural connection between the left and right hemispheres has been severed or damaged (see 2.4). These patients may be able to perform a specific movement implicitly as part of automatized routines, such as shaving when standing in front of the washbasin in the morning, while they are may not be able to perform the same movement as a deliberate action on command (Liepmann & Maas, 1907; Watson & Heilman, 1983; Buxbaum et al., 1995; Tanaka et al., 1996; Lausberg et al., 1999; Lausberg et al., 2003 b). As an example, Mr. U.H. with callosal disconnection reported not being able to take something out of his trouser pocket with his left hand when he intended to do so. The same action was performed by his left hand without hitch when he didn`t think about it (Lausberg et al., 1999). Rapcsak et al.'s proposition is further supported by the alien or autonomous hand syndrome, which also occurs particularly in patients with callosal disconnection. It is characterized by an autonomous action of the left hand, sometimes even against the will of the patient. A related syndrome is the intermanual conflict, in which the right and left hands act in a highly uncooperative manner. As an example, Mr. U.H. lifted the toilet seat with his right hand and the left hand closed it again. In clinical testing such as the Token test, his correct right hand reaction was often disturbed by incorrect left hand interference (Lausberg et al., 1999). Both syndromes, the alien/autonomous hand and the intermanual conflict, indicate that the separate right hemisphere can generate movements implicitly, i.e., independently from the motor dominant left hemisphere, which dominates the generation of explicit volitional movements (Geschwind et al, 1995; Tanaka et al., 1996; Marangolo et al., 1998).

To summarize, a great proportion of movement behaviour is displayed implicitly, i.e., beyond the mover's awareness. It is plausible that implicit body movements are associated with implicit cognitive, emotional, and interactive processes, while explicit movements are related to partly explicit processes (Figure 2). This proposition is supported by the scientific evidence that movements which are displayed beyond the mover's awareness differ kinematically and neurobiologically from their volitionally performed counter-parts. Thus, regarding the initial question of this section, movement behaviour analysis, as it includes the examination of implicit body movements, bears the special potential to investigate implicit cognitive, emotional, and interactive processes.

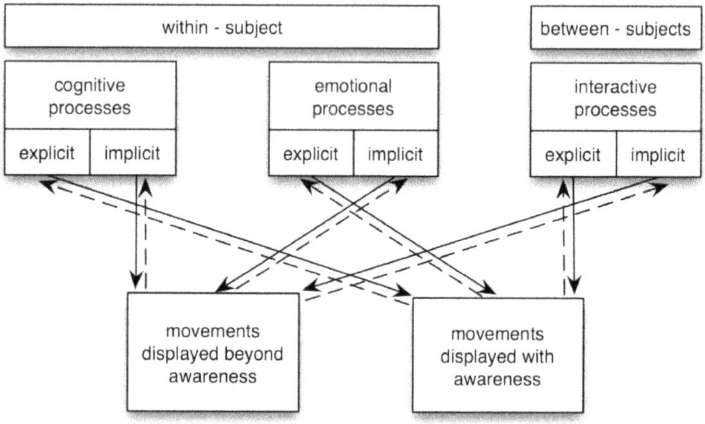

Figure 2 The link between implicit and explicit body movements and implicit and explicit cognitive, emotional, and interactive processes

2.3 Movement behaviour is organized in patterns

In movement behaviour research, many analysis systems are tailored to detect certain classes of movements in the movement behaviour and then give them value. As an example, in McNeill's coding system for hand gestures (1992), certain hand movements are identified in hand movement behaviour and then classified as *iconic, metaphoric,* or *deictic*. Few analysis systems are designed to classify all movement in a behaviour. As an example, in the kinesic analysis by Birdwhistell (1952), movement behaviour is segmented into kinemes, which are units of kinesic behaviour (for the detailed description of Birdwhistell's system see Chapter 3). As compared to the assessment of pre-selected movement units, the latter type of movement behaviour analysis opens the research options to analyze the sequences and combinations of movement units.

A pattern is "a regular and intelligible form or sequence discernible in the way in which something happens or is done" (Oxford English Dictionary). A movement pattern may be characterized by a temporal sequence consisting of several subsequent movement types, e.g. self-touch → gesture → shift → self-touch. Likewise, is may be a combination of several movement types displayed by different parts of the body at a time, e.g. crossing the legs + folding the hands + raising the head. Since long, it has been documented that the individual movement behaviour is highly reliable with regard to such sequences and combinations (Darwin, 1890; Allport & Vernon, 1933). A related well-known phenomenon is, for example, that we can recognize a person by her/his gait pattern long before we can identify her/him by her/his bodily appearance. In a study on whole body expression in dance, individuals displayed individually retest-reliable combinations of moving the body in four different improvisation tasks, e.g. small kinesphere combined with bound flow and predominant use of the upper body (Lausberg et al., 1996).

The individual movement behaviour is highly reliable just as its association with cognitive, emotional, and interactive states. As an example from the author's data, in cheerful situations, Mr. A.A. always showed a complex movement pattern in a nearly identical form: laughing → then pushing up his glasses with the left hand → then folding the arms → then pressing the knees together. Mrs. N.G. reliably performed the following pattern in depressive contexts: left shoulder shrug → then an adjustment of the left bra strap with the left hand → then a verbal statement with a depressive connotation. Note that in the two examples, neither the glasses nor the bra strap were displaced so that they would have needed to be adjusted again.

Already Darwin (1890) had described that in the process of becoming a habitual pattern, the original function of a movement could get lost. Then its only function remains to be part of a pattern. Darwin's interpretation shows some overlap with Birdwhistell's structuralist view that considered that any body movement was an arbitrary sign, which was per se meaningless and which only served as the maintenance and regulation of interaction. Thus, even body movements that seem to be purposeless have a function since they contribute to a pattern. Therefore, the proposition is here that body movements are not displayed accidentally or randomly. The exception is pathological hyperkinetic syndromes[4], the types of which are described in Chapter 3. They are mainly caused by functional or structural disorders of subcortical motor regions. With this exception in mind, it is argued here that given the expanded definition of 'function', which includes co-establishing a pattern, in healthy individuals any body movement has a function.

Patterns can consist of all classes of movement behaviour including postures and rest positions. Specific mental states and specific topics in interactions co-occur with specific rest positions (Darwin, 1890; Scheflen, 1973; LaFrance, 1982; Davis & Hadiks, 1990; Davis & Hadiks, 1994; Wallbott, 1989; Kleinsmith & Berthouze, 2007). As noted above, in psychoanalytic and psychotherapeutic sessions 'autistic gestures' could be reliably elicited through association experiments and during emotionally loaded issues (Sainsbury, 1955; Mahl, 1968). In these specific contexts, the 'autistic gestures' were displayed reliably in almost identical manners across the psychotherapy sessions. Given the reliabil-

---

4 For the moment, it shall be maintained that certain body movements displayed in neuropsychiatric disease, notably hyperkinetic syndromes, do not have a function in this sense. However, future research may reveal that even these movements have some kind of function, for example, that they serve to maintain an equilibrium within a pathological state.

ity of individual movement patterns, changes in these patterns can be used as an indicator of changes in the mental state or even in personality traits over time (Davis & Hadiks, 1990). When considered in response to therapist interventions, the patient's movement pattern changes in psychotherapy may indicate therapeutically relevant moments (Davis & Hadiks, 1994). In a case study on a doctor-patient interview, the patient's typical movement patterns were identified, such as repetitive rocking with the trunk (Lausberg, 2011). Changes in this pattern, such as interruption of the trunk rocking, co-occurred with verbal utterances that had been identified as therapeutically relevant in an independently conducted discourse analysis.

In the field of criminology, research on movement patterns coded during interviews of criminal suspects has helped to identify movement cues to deception (Davis & Hadiks, 1995). Of particular note is evidence that the cue set related to deceptive responses is distinctly different than the set of cues associated with topic stress level, suggesting that the movement patterns can distinguish what are primarily affective processes from cognitive processes such as formulating a false story while concealing information (Davis et al., 2005).

Patterns may not only occur at the intra-individual level but also at the inter-individual level. A specific movement - mental state combination in an individual may co-occur regularly with a specific movement - mental state combination in the individual's partner, and vice versa. Scheflen (1963, 1973) first identified these interaction patterns in psychotherapy sessions. He observed reliable intra-dyadic movement sequences between patient and therapist over several psychotherapy sessions. As an example, the patient assumed a certain posture by grasping the right knee with the hands → then the therapist performed a 'Bowl'-gesture → then he lighted up a pipe, etc. According to Scheflen, the 'communicational program' that is characterized by a defined sequence of both partners' movements, serves to regulate and stabilize the partners' relationship. To his opinion, the identification of such implicit movement interaction patterns is highly relevant for a successful therapy as these implicit patterns consolidate neurotic relationships.

To summarize, movement behaviour is organized in reliable within-subject and between-subjects patterns. There is ample empirical evidence that these movement patterns are associated with specific cognitive, emotional, and interactive states, such that they constitute complex movement – emotion – cognition – interaction patterns. Given that the only function of a movement can be to contribute to a pattern, with the exception of certain pathological conditions, it is argued that any body movement has a function.

The detection of movement patterns helps to explore emotional, cognitive, and interactive patterns as well as changes of these patterns. This application of movement analysis is especially relevant in fields that aim at developing personal competence, e.g. in learning contexts and psychotherapy.

2.4 The temporal dimension of movement units provides insight into the duration of the associated cognitive, emotional, and interactive processes

As outlined in the previous section, all movements in the behaviour of one part of the body or in more of them can be analyzed. A further elaboration of this method is to analyze the ongoing stream of movement behaviour in time. As in pattern detection, natural units of movement behaviour are identified but in addition, their duration in time is registered. Any moment in time is attributed to a natural unit and there is a quasi smooth coding, such that at the end of one movement unit the next unit begins. This method differs substantially from the segmentation of the stream of behaviour into standard time intervals. As an example, the ongoing behaviour is segmented into 30 seconds lasting units. This type of segmentation into time units, however, destroys natural movement units. The duration of such natural units provides insight into the temporal structure of movement behaviour. Units of different values, such as gesture units, fidgeting units, rest position units, shifts units, etc. show distinct durations. The duration of a unit with a specific value constitutes an intrinsic feature of this value. It is coined by the kinematic structure of the value and by neural and muscular factors, respectively. Furthermore, as it will be argued below, it is influenced by the duration of the associated cognitive, emotional, and interactive processes.

Thus far, little empirical research has been conducted regarding the duration of behavioural units. An approach to segmenting movement behaviour into natural units was introduced by Condon and Ogston (1967), who defined 'process units' as natural units of behaviour: "The 'process unit' is observationally defined as the initiation and sustaining of directionality of change of the body parts with each other (the *specific* directions being sustained by the individual parts may differ) across a given movement of time as contrasted with the preceding and succeeding sets of similarly sustained configurations of movement of the body parts." (p. 224). However, in their research Condon and Ogston did not focus on the duration of the single process units, but they were interested in how process units are synchronized between the parts of the body of the moving person. In fact, they demonstrated that in a healthy person the changes in the direction of moving of all parts of the body, from foot to head, are synchronized. Moreover, they demonstrated that this synchrony even expands to interactive partners. In contrast, in schizophrenic patients they observed a within-subject and between-subjects dyssynchrony (Condon & Ogston, 1966). An approach that considers the duration of natural units of behaviour was introduced by Freedman and colleagues. They measured the total time spent with different types of *body-focused* activity in seconds / 10 minutes. Their data revealed that, in clinical interviews, a substantial amount of time is spent with this movement type. As an in example, in a study on schizophrenic and depressive patients (Freedman, 1972), the paranoid patients produced a mean number of 196.8 seconds of *continuous body-focused* movements and 8.6 *discrete body-focused* movements in 10 minutes. The depressed patients displayed 203.4 second of *continuous body-focused* movements and 16.0 *discrete body-focused* movements. Concerning the subtypes of *continuous body-focused* movements (see also Chapter 3), depressed patients showed substantially more (150.6 s) *direct* movements, i.e., touching another part of the body with one hand, than paranoid patients (41.2 s). They also spent more time (36.6 s) with *indirect* movements, i.e., the manipulation of objects that are attached to the body such as clothing or accessories, than the paranoid patients (1.2 s). Paranoid patients on the other hand showed a preponderance of *hand-to-hand* movements (154.6 s) as compared to depressed patients (16.2 s). Thus, Freedman et al.'s findings show that depressive and schizophrenic patients spent different amounts of time with different subtypes of *body-focused* movements. Taking another perspective, their raw data reveal that - independent from the patients' diagnoses - about equal amounts of time are spent with *direct* and *hand-to-hand* movements, while clearly less time is spent with *indirect* movements.

The research question whether different types of hand movements show specific durations in time has been systematically investigated in a meta-analysis including 6 experimental studies using the NEUROGES system (see Part II). The mean duration of the five Structure category values *phasic, repetitive, irregular, shift* and *aborted* was examined. There were significant differences in the durations of the units of the five values. As an example, *shift* units (the hand shifts from one rest position to another one) are significantly shorter than the units of the other four values (all p = .000). The finding strongly suggests that *shift* units represent a movement entity that is distinct from the other values, as it is characterized by a distinct duration that significantly differs from the duration of the other units. In fact, this finding is line with the theoretical concept of the Structure category (5.1, Figure 1). As an example, *phasic in space* units (functionally, these are almost always gestures) have a mean duration that is significantly longer than that of *shift* units, because a *phasic in space* unit is kinematically defined by a phase structure. The hand is transported from the rest position into the central gesture space, there it performs a complex phase (in McNeill's terminology a 'stroke'), and then it is retracted again to the rest position. This phase structure, consisting of three kinematically distinct phases, entails that the mean duration of *phasic in space* movements is significantly longer than that of *shifts*, in which the hand is 'only' transported directly from one *rest position* to another. Thus, the duration of a unit is an intrinsic feature of its value.

Furthermore, it is suggested here that the duration of a unit of a specific value is coined by the duration of the associated cognitive, emotional, and interactive processes. As an example, *irregular* units last 4.3 ± 0.5 seconds (mean ± standard deviation), whereas *shift* units last 1.8 ± 0.1 seconds, and this difference in duration is statistically significant. Both types are kinematically simple, there is no phase structure, and no other movement criterion that predetermines a certain duration (in contrast, in *phasic in space* movements a lower limit of the unit duration is determined by the fact that the hand has to be transported into the gesture space and back again). Thus, it shall be argued that the difference in the duration of *irregular* and *shift* units reflects the duration of the underlying cognitive, emotional, or interactive process. As *irregular* units could - kinematically and anatomically - be as short as *shift* units, the longer duration of *irregular* units might be related to the fact that they are associated with rather 'time-consuming' self-regulatory processes. This proposition is supported by the fact that the mean durations of the *phasic, repetitive, irregular, shift* and *aborted* units are stable across different experimental settings. Following up on the above example, as *irregular* units are associated with self-regulation, they have an intrinsic duration that is independent of the experimental setting. Furthermore, the meta-analysis revealed that the mean duration of a unit of a specific value is independent of the hand that is employed to execute the movement. Thus, the influence of handedness does not override the influence of the intrinsic duration of the motor-cognitive-emotional entity.

The duration of units of a specific movement type provides insight into the temporal structure of movement behaviour as it reveals that units of different movement types have different durations. The duration of a unit of a specific movement type constitutes an intrinsic feature of this type that is determined by the kinematic structure and by neural and muscular factors, respectively, and by the associated cognitive, emotional, and interactive process. Thereby, the registration of the duration of movement units provides insight into the temporal dimension of the underlying cognitive, emotional, and interactive processes.

2.5 Laterality preferences reflect hemispheric specialization in the production of specific types of limb movements

Many movement analysis systems do not register the laterality of limb movements. This section discusses why it might be relevant to code the laterality of the limb that displays a certain movement type. Since the Laterality literature refers almost exclusively to hand movements, the following review focuses on hand movements.

2.5.1 The anatomical basis of assessing hemispheric specialization based on laterality preference

Laterality preferences for certain movement types, e.g. a right hand preference for pointing gestures or a left hand preference for self-touch, indicate hemispheric specialization in the generation of the respective movement type. The anatomical basis for inferring hemispheric specialization from laterality preferences is that the left cerebral hemisphere controls the contralateral right limbs, and vice versa, the right cerebral hemisphere the contralateral left limbs. In Figure 3, the straight lines show the contralaterally organized neural pathways for controlling the upper limbs. The neural control of feet and leg is organized analogously, i.e., the right hemisphere controls the left leg and the left hemisphere the right one.

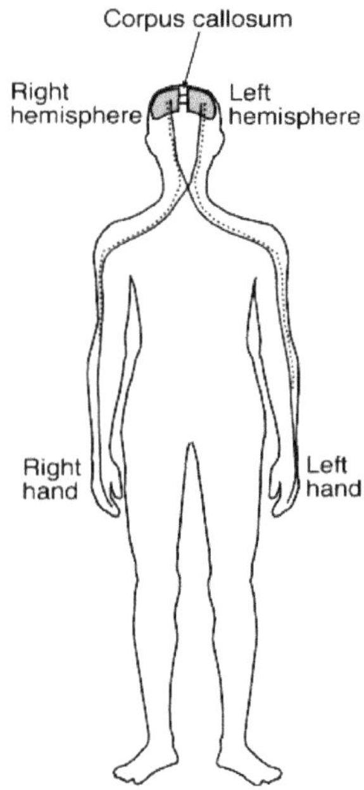

Figure 3 Contralateral (straight lines) and ipsilateral (dotted lines) neural pathways for controlling the upper limbs

The relevance of this anatomical constellation for movement behaviour research becomes most evident when examining split-brain patients. These are patients in whom the corpus callosum, which is the biggest neural fibre connection between the right and left hemispheres, has been sectioned. In most cases, the operation is undertaken because of intractable epilepsy. After callosal disconnection, each hand (and foot) can distinctly be controlled only by the contralateral hemisphere (Gazzaniga, Bogen, & Sperry 1967; Sperry 1968; Volpe et al. 1982; Trope et al. 1987; Lausberg et al. 2003 b). As a result, the movements of the right and left hands and feet reflect competence or incompetence of the contralateral hemisphere. As an example: since the left hemisphere is language dominant in most of these patients (just as in the healthy population), they cannot execute verbal commands with the left hand ("verbal apraxia" of the left hand). The verbal commands are processed in the left hemisphere, but the information cannot be transferred to the right hemisphere which controls the left hand. On the other hand, the split-brain patient's right hand performs worse than the left in copying figures ("constructional apraxia" of the right hand). The right hemisphere is specialized for visuo-spatial cognition, but the information cannot be transferred to the left hemisphere which controls the right hand (e.g. Bogen 1993; Lausberg et al. 2003 b). As a consequence, these patients spontaneously prefer the right hand for executing verbal commands, while they spontaneously choose the left hand for spatial tasks. Thus, in these patients the performance on command of the right and left hands or feet as well as the spontaneous hand or foot preferences reveal the competence and incompetence of the right and left hemispheres. In Mr. U.H., who had suffered from a callosal infarction, apraxia was severe especially with his left leg. When asked to imitate lifting the left foot as demonstrated by the investigator, he made instead a supination-pronation movement with the left hand (Lausberg et al., 1999). Thus, the examination of the split-brain patients' right and left hands and feet movements provides valuable information about the generation of specific movement types in the left and right hemispheres.

2.5.2 Laterality preferences for gesture types in split-brain patients

Split-brain patients with exclusively left hemisphere speech production reliably display the majority of gestures that spontaneously accompany speech with left hand (Lausberg et al., 2007). The spontaneous left hand preference indicates that the gestures are generated in the right hemisphere, despite the fact that the language production is localized in the patients' left hemispheres.

A more fine-grained analysis of gesture types in these patients was conducted by McNeill (1992) and by Lausberg et al. (2000, 2007). Both researchers found that patients with a complete callosal disconnection preferentially or even exclusively used the left hand to display *beats / batons*, which are gestures that emphasize prosody. In contrast, they used the right hand preferentially or even exclusively for *iconics / physiographics*, i.e. pictorial gestures, and *deictics*, i.e., pointing gestures (detailed descriptions of the gesture classification systems are provided in Chapter 3). In the study by Lausberg et al. in addition, a left side preference was found for *fall* gestures and *shoulder shrugs*. Because in these patients the right hand can only be distinctly controlled by the left hemisphere and vice versa, the left hand by the right hemisphere, their laterality preferences for specific gesture types provide strong evidence for hemispheric specializations in the generation of these gesture types. The findings by the independent researchers indicate that *physiographics* and *deictics* are predominantly generated in the left hemisphere, potentially in association with other left hemispheric processes such as language. In contrast, *batons, fall* gestures, and *shrugs* seem to be generated in the right hemisphere, potentially in association with other right hemispheric processes such as emotional processes and (emotional) prosody. Thus, gestures that accompany speech are not necessarily generated in the left hemisphere in close association with language but their production, likewise, can be associated with other cognitive processes such as emotional prosody or spatial cognition, which are lateralized to the right hemisphere (for a detailed discussion of this topic see Lausberg et al., 2000; Lausberg et al., 2007).

This proposition also provides a neuropsychological model for explaining the phenomenon of gesture-speech mismatches. Feyereisen (1987) described dissociations between verbal and gestural output in aphasia as well as during language development in children. In the same line, gesture-speech mismatches are reported during learning and problem solving (Goldin-Meadow et al., 1993; Garber & Goldin-Meadow, 2002). In split-brain patients, gesture-speech mismatches can be clearly attributed to simultaneous but not matching responses of the two hemispheres. As an example from the author's data, to Mr. U.H. a stimulus was presented in his left visual field. When he was asked if he saw a stimulus, he said 'No' but simultaneously he nodded his head in affirmation (Lausberg et al., 1999). In fact, both responses, the nonverbal one and the verbal one, were correct. In split-brain patients, a stimulus that is presented in the left visual field is processed in the contralateral right hemisphere. Therefore, Mr. U.H. recognized the stimulus with the right hemisphere and he correctly confirmed the question by nodding (since he had no language production in the right hemisphere but a limited language comprehension sufficient to understand the question). As in split-brain patients the left hemisphere processes the right visual field, Mr. U.H.'s left hemisphere did not perceive a stimulus, which was presented in the left visual field. Therefore, the left hemisphere correctly answered 'No' to the question.

An analysis of the split-brain patients' bimanual gestures revealed three subtypes: left hand dominant gestures, right hand dominant gestures, and bimanual dyssynchronous gestures (Lausberg et al., 2000; Lausberg et al., 2007). In the first two subtypes, the dominant hand performs distinct hand and finger movements and the non-dominant hand displays rough movements guided by the proximal arm muscles. As distinct distal control can only be exerted via contralateral pathways, the rough proximally guided hand movements are controlled by ipsilateral pathways. In humans, these neural pathways are only rudimentarily developed and they can control only the proximal muscles of the arm (Figure 3, dotted lines). Therefore, right hand dominant gestures are likely to be controlled by the left hemisphere, and vice versa, left hand dominant gestures by the right hemisphere. In fact, in right hand dominant gestures the same gesture types were displayed as in unimanual right hand gestures, i.e., *deictics* and *physiographs*, and in left hand dominant gestures the same type as in unimanual left hand gestures, i.e., *batons* and *fall* gestures (Lausberg et al., 2000). These findings are in line with the fact that bimanual movements with the dominance of one hand are controlled by the contralateral hemisphere.

2.5.3 Laterality preferences for different movement types in healthy individuals

In healthy subjects with normal neural connection, the corpus callosum enables to exert control also over the hand that is ipsilateral, i.e., on the same side, to the movement generating hemisphere. As an example, if a right-handed person with left hemisphere language dominance intends to write with the left hand, the command is transferred from the language competent left hemisphere via corpus callosum to the right hemisphere which controls the left hand. But, as the callosal pathway is kind of neural path detour, also healthy subjects tend to prefer the hand that is contralateral to the predominantly engaged hemisphere. In analogy to the hand preferences described above for split-brain patients, Hampson and Kimura (1984) observed in right-handed healthy subjects a shift from right hand use in verbal tasks toward greater left hand use in spatial tasks. According to their interpretation of the findings, the shift towards more left hand use reflected that the right hemisphere primarily solved the spatial task. Likewise, in behavioural laterality experiments, when resources are sufficient for both decision and response programming, there is an advantage to responding with the hand that is controlled by the same hemisphere that performs the task (Zaidel et al., 1988).

However, in healthy individuals with an intact corpus callosum this tendency can be overrun by other factors: (i) handedness: Right-handers typically prefer the right hand for movements that require dexterity and fine motor coordination and control of trajectory speed and direction, while they show a left hand preference for movements that rely on the axial musculature, involve strength and secure the accurate final position (Healey, Liedermann & Geschwind 1986; Corey, Hurley & Foundas 2001; Brown, Roy, Rohr & Bryden 2006; Wang & Sainburg 2007); (ii) a semantic purpose: When talking about the left or right of two objects, right-handers prefer the corresponding hand (Lausberg & Kita 2003); (iii) cultural conventions: As a learned behaviour, Arrente speakers in Central Australia use the left hand to refer to targets that are on the left, and vice versa, the right hand for targets that are on the right (Wilkins & de Ruiter 1999); (iv) an occupation of one hand with some other physical activity: For example, when holding a cup of coffee in the one hand, the other hand is used for gesturing. - If these factors are controlled for, in empirical studies on healthy subjects, spontaneous hand preferences are a good indicator of hemispheric specialization.

In line with the above exposed split-brain data on laterality preferences for specific gesture types (McNeill, 1992; Lausberg et al., 2000; Lausberg et al., 2007), distinct hand preferences have also been found in healthy subjects. Souza-Poza et al. (1979) reported that in right-handers a right hand preference was only significant for the representational (includes all of Efron's types except for *batons*)[5], but not for the nonrepresentational gestures (Efron's *baton*). Stephens (1983) found a significant right hand preference for iconics (Efron's *physiographic*), a non-significant right hand preference for metaphorics (overlap with Efron's *ideographic* and *physiographic*), as well as a non-significant left hand preference for beats (Efron's *baton*). In a study by Blonder et al. (1995), a right-handed control group showed a trend towards more right hand use for symbolic gestures (Efron's *emblematic*), whereas the left hand was tendencially used more often for expressive gestures (while the Blonder's term suggest otherwise, in fact expressive is equivalent to Efron's *baton*). Kita et al. (2007) reported a significant right hand preference for *deictics* (idem to Efron) and for depictive gestures (includes Efron's *ideographic* and *physiographic*), except for those depictive gestures that had a character viewpoint in a metaphor condition. Likewise, Wilkins and de Ruiter (1999) reported a right hand preference for *deictics* (idem to Efron). In Foundas et al.'s study (1995), a right-handed control group showed a significant right hand preference for content gestures (includes all of Efron's types except for *batons* and partly *ideographic*) and for emphasis gestures (Efron's *baton*) as well as a right hand trend for fillers (overlap with Efron's *ideographic*). To summarize, with the exception of Foundas et al. (1995), a trend towards more left hand use was found for *batons*. In contrast, for *physiographics* and *deictics,* there was a significant right hand preference. These findings in healthy individuals match the findings the split-brain patients. They indicate that *batons* may be generated primarily in the right hemisphere.

The laterality of self-touch movements has also been subject of investigation. Applying Kimura's coding system, several studies on right-handers reported a significant right-hand preference for *free movements* and an equal use of the right and left hands for *self-touch* (Kimura, 1973; Lavergne & Kimura, 1987; Dalby et al., 1980; Saucier & Elias, 2001). However, a review of the raw data of all four studies reveals even a non-significant trend toward more left hand use for *self-touches*. Likewise, Trevarthen (1996) observed that children between 1 and 6 months prefer left hand for self-touch and right hand for communicative gestures. More fine-grained analyses of self-touch movements show distinct patterns of hand preferences.

Applying Freedman's coding system, among the hand movements of the main value *body-focused*, Souza-Poza et al. (1979) reported a significant left-hand preference for *continuous body-focused hand-to-hand* movements, i.e., the left acted on the right one. For *discrete direct* and *continuous direct* touching of another part of the body, there was only a non-significant trend towards more left

5 The comparison of different studies on laterality preferences for gesture types is complicated by the fact that different researchers apply different gesture coding systems, the types of which show only partial conceptual overlap. To overcome this problem, Efron's coding system (1941), which is presented in Chapter 3, is used as a frame of reference here.

hand use. In the same line, a right-handed control group executed "grooming" and "fidgeting" movements more with the left hand than the right (Blonder et al., 1995). In contrast, Stephens (1983) defined self-adaptors as hand movements performed in order to change something about the body or dress, such as pushing back the hair or adjusting the glasses. She found a right-hand preference in right-handers for this type of hand movements, which she explained by the fact that she coded skilled manipulations of the body and of objects attached to the body. In the same vein, the investigation of self-touch movements in a right-handed woman revealed distinct hand preferences for the different subtypes of self-touch, as measured with the NEUROGES system. Mrs. S. used the right hand to execute *phasic on body* or *phasic on attached object* movements, such as hair preening, manipulating watch, or adjusting sleeves. In contrast, she used the left hand for *repetitive on body* and *irregular on body* movements, such as repetitive or continuous stroking or rubbing of the sternum, neck, face, and lower leg (Lausberg, 1995). This finding was confirmed in a systematic study including 37 right-handed subjects. Despite their right-handedness, the participants showed a significant left hand preference for *on body* movements, such as scratching, while they displayed a significant right hand preference for *on attached object* movements, such as manipulating the clothes (Lausberg et al., in prep.). To summarize, among the self-touch movements, the left hand preference is strongest repetitive or continuous direct touching of the body including the other hand. In contrast, for manipulations of body-attached objects, the right hand is preferred.

As outlined in 2.1.2, there is ample empirical evidence that direct self-touching of the body, especially if it occurs continuously, is associated with stress, emotional engagement, and depression (Sainsbury 1955; Freedman & Hoffman 1967; Freedman 1972; Freedman et al. 1972; Sousa-Poza & Rohrberg 1977; Ulrich 1977; Freedman & Bucci 1981; Ulrich and Harms 1985; Lausberg 1995; Lausberg & Kryger, 2011). Distress and emotional processes, especially with negative valence, are typically associated with a right hemisphere activation (Ahern & Schwarz 1979; Borod et al. 1998; Berridge et al. 1999; Grunwald & Weiss 2007; Killgore & Yurgelun-Todd 2007; Stalnaker et al. 2009). This lateralization to the right hemisphere, in turn, triggers a left hand use. Therefore, this constellation provides an explanation for the left hand preference that is observed in right-handers when they display self-touches of the body.

Finally, it shall be noted that also head movements have been related to hemispheric specialization. Kinsbourne (1972) reported distinct directions of head turning during verbal, numerical, and spatial problem solving.

2.5.4 Summary

In split-brain patients, spontaneous laterality preferences are evidenced in unilateral right limb and unilateral left limb movements but also in bilateral right dominant and bilateral left dominant movements. These laterality preferences for the execution of certain movement types reflect the generation of these movement types in the contralateral left and right hemispheres. This applies also to healthy subjects if other factors are controlled for. On this basis, studies on hand preferences in split-brain patients and healthy subjects demonstrate that the right and left hemispheres are specialized for certain types of gestures and self-touches. The left hemisphere is specialized for the generation of *physiographs, deictics*, and - with regard to self-touching behaviour - for *on attached object* manipulations. In contrast, the right hemisphere plays a dominant role in the generation of *batons* and continuous *on body* movements. The hemispheric specialization for these movement types is well compatible with the hemispheric lateralization of the hypothetically associated cognitive and emotional functions. The impressive empirical research on laterality preferences strongly suggests implementing the registration of the laterality of limb movements in movement behaviour research methods.

2.6 Conclusions for movement behaviour research methodology

The above interdisciplinary reviews have addressed several aspects that are relevant for movement behaviour research methodology. The reviews demonstrate that there is ample empirical evidence that movement behaviour is associated with cognitive, emotional, and interactive processes. Moreover, movement behaviour does not only seem to reflect these processes but also to affect them. While the reviews show that this is an exciting and promising field of research, they also evidence that more basic research is needed to fully understand the relation between the various aspects of movement behaviour and cognitive, emotional, and interactive processes.

Methodologically, in order to conduct basic research and to challenge established paradigms, a **descriptive**[6] methodological approach is required. A descriptive movement analysis enables to examine movement behaviour as a medium per se, based on the visual appearance of the movement. This is an indispensable prerequisite to explore the relation between movement behaviour and a function x, i.e., any other cognitive, emotional, and interactive function. It is further evident that the values used for movement analysis should **not** be **confounded** with values of the function x. A primary confounding of the analysis of movement behaviour with that of another function is not compatible with basic empirical research that aims at exploring the link between movement behaviour and cognitive, emotional, and interactive processes.

Applying descriptive and not confounded movement values, the following method is suitable for exploring the link between the two processes: First, the

6 The detailed explanations of methodological aspects, such as descriptive or confounding variables, are provided in Chapters 3 and 4.

movement behaviour and the function x are analysed independently from each other. Second, their relation is investigated. As an example, if the relation between speech and gesture is subject to investigation, speech and gesture are first coded independently of each other. This is highly recommended as raters who simultaneously listen to what is said and observe the gestures are influenced by the verbal content. They tend to classify gestures according to the verbal utterances, rather than vice versa. Second, based on the independent analyses of movement behaviour and speech, their relation can be explored from scratch.

The first review on movement behaviour and cognitive, emotional, and interactive processes further demonstrates that various classes of movement behaviour, such as gesture, self-touch, posture, or rest position, are differentially related to within-subject cognitive and emotional processes and to between-subjects interactive processes. Therefore, for basic research a **comprehensive** approach is required that comprises more than one movement class. At an early stage of the exploration of the relation between movement behaviour and a function x, the restriction to a specific class of movement involves the risk that other classes of body movements that might be, likewise, relevant with regard to function x, are overseen. As an example, research on cognitive functions typically neglects self-touch movements and only considers gestures, assuming that only this class of hand movements is relevant for the performance in cognitive tasks. However, it is worth considering that better performances during cognitive tasks can, likewise, be related to self-touching behaviour. As self-touching effectively serves self-regulation, it might contribute to better performances in cognitive tasks. Therefore, for basic research a comprehensive analysis system is required that comprises several classes of movement behaviour.

The review on implicitly versus explicitly displayed body movements demonstrates that **implicit** movements constitute a major component of movement behaviour. It is highly plausible that these implicit body movements are associated with implicit cognitive, emotional, and interactive processes. Such implicit processes substantially coin our thinking, feeling, and interacting, but they are difficult to investigate with research tools that are based on verbal statements. Questionnaires and semi-standardized interview rely on verbalization and thus, on conscious cognitive, emotional, and interactive processes. In contrast to these tools, movement behaviour analysis bears the specific potential that it enables to investigate implicit processes. Therefore, for basic research, movement behaviour analysis should include the registration of movements that are displayed beyond the mover's awareness.

The review on movement behaviour patterns evidences that movement behaviour is organized in intra-individually and inter-individually reliable patterns that are associated with specific cognitive, emotional, or interactive states. As such, movement patterns are the visible component of complex movement – emotion – cognition – interaction states. Pattern detection is particularly relevant in fields that aim at developing personal competence, such as in learning contexts and psychotherapy, but it has also been applied in criminology.

In order to detect such patterns, an analysis of all movements of a part of the body or of several parts at a time is required. This procedure enables to detect recurrent sequences of specific movement units including rests. Furthermore, combinations of simultaneously displayed movement types of different parts of the body can be discovered. As an example, the segmentation of the ongoing stream of hand/arm movements may reveal a recurrent sequence of shift → self-touch → gesture → rest, e.g. reflecting the gesturer's manner of gradually conceptualising thoughts.

In the course of pattern building, movements may have lost their original function. Then, while they seem to be purposeless, their new function is to be part of a pattern. With the exception of certain pathological conditions, it is argued here that in healthy individuals any body movement has a function. Thus, the above-named call for a **comprehensive** analysis is further supported, as not only various classes of movements and implicitly displayed movements, but also those movements that (only) function as part of a pattern are relevant with regard to cognitive, emotional, and interactive patterns.

An analysis of the temporal dimension of movement behaviour is achieved a segmentation of the ongoing stream of movement behaviour into natural units. This method enables to register the duration of movement units. The unit duration provides insight into the temporal dimension of certain movement types and into that of the associated cognitive, emotional, and interactive processes. Furthermore, the analysis of the durations of different values relative to each other helps to identify distinct movement entity.

Finally, the review on laterality demonstrates that a spontaneous preference for the right or left limbs for the execution of certain movement types suggests that these movement types are generated in the hemisphere that is contralateral to the moving limb. Thereby, the investigation of laterality preferences provides insight into the neuropsychology of movement types.

Neurobiological correlates of the production of spontaneous body movements are difficult to investigate, because - as outlined above - a major part of these movements are generated implicitly. In contrast, the investigation of the neurobiological correlates of explicit movements, such as pantomiming tool use, now profits from the great progress in the development of neuroimaging methods. These methods are well suited for the investigation of explicit movements as these can be generated on command, in time, and repetitively. For the same reason, spontaneously and implicitly displayed movements cannot be submitted to neuroimaging investigations. Therefore, for implicit movements, the laterality preferences in healthy individuals and in split-brain patients is a valuable method to examine where in the brain - in terms of the right and left hemispheres - they are generated (detailed discussion in Lausberg, 2013). Furthermore, as higher cognitive and emotional functions are lateralized in the brain, the laterality preference for a certain movement type gives some indications with what kind of lateralized cognitive and emotional functions the generation of that movement type may be associated. The hemispheric specialization for a certain movement type provides some indication that its generation is associated with those cognitive and emotional processes that are also lateralized to that hemisphere. Therefore, movement behaviour research should consider the **laterality** of limb movements.

To summarize, the reviews suggest that basic research on the various aspects of movement behaviour and its link to cognitive, emotional, and interactive processes is required. This should include the option to test existing paradigms. For this aim, a movement behaviour analysis method is effective that is descriptive, not confounded, and comprehensive. The method should enable to examine the ongoing stream of movement behaviour, naturally including implicit movements, as well as the laterality of limb movements.

References

Ahern, G.L., & Schwartz, G.E. (1979). Differential lateralization for positive versus negative emotion. *Neuropsychologia, 17*, 693-698.

Allport, G.W., & Vernon, P.E. (1933). *Studies in Expressive Movement.* New York: Macmillan.

Bader, J.P., Bühler, J., Endrass, J., Klipstein, A., & Hell, D. (1999). Muskelkraft und Gangcharakteristika depressiver Menschen. *Der Nervenarzt, 70*, 613-619.

Barosso, F., Freedman, N., & Grand, S. (1978). Evocation of Two Types of Hand Movements in Information Processing. *Journal of Experimental Psychology, 4*(2), 321-329.

Beattie, G. & Shovelton, H. (2006). When size really matters: how a single semantic feature is represented in the speech and gesture modalities. *Gesture 6*, 63-84.

Beattie, G. & Shovelton, H. (2009). An exploration of the other side of semantic communication. How the spontaneous movements of the human hand add crucial meaning to narrative. *Semiotica, 176.*

Berger, M.R. (1999). *Movement patterns in borderline and narcissistic personality disorders*. Dissertation Abstracts International: Section B: The Sciences and Engineering Vol. 60(9-B), Apr 2000, 4875.

Berridge, C.W., Mitton, E., Clark, W., & Roth, R.H. (1999). Engagement in a Non-Escape (Displacement) Behaviour Elicits a Selective and Lateralized Suppression of Frontal Cortical Dopaminergic Utilization in Stress. *Synapse, 32*, 187-197.

Berry, D.S. & Pennebaker, J.W. (1993). Nonverbal and Verbal Emotional Expression and Health. *Psychotherapy and Psychosomatics, 59*, 11-19.

Birdwhistell, R. (1952). *Introduction to Kinesics: An Annotation System for the Analysis of Body Motion and Gesture*. Washington, DC: Foreign Service Institute, US Department of State.

Blonder, L.X., Burns, A.F., Bowers, D., Moore, R.W., & Heilman, K.M. (1995). Spontaneous gestures following right hemisphere infarct. *Neuropsychologia, 33*, 203-213.

Bock, O., & Hagemann, A. (2010). An experimental paradigm to compare motor performence under laboratory and under everyday-like conditions. *Journal of Neuroscience Methods, 193*, 5.

Bogen, J.E. (1993). The callosal syndromes. In: K.M. Heilman, & E. Valenstein (Eds.), *Clinical Neuropsychology*, 337-408. New York, Oxford: Oxford University Press.

Bogen, J.E. (2000). Split-brain basics: Relevance for the concept of one's other mind. *The Jounal of the American Academy of Psychoanalysis, 28*, 341-369.

Borod, JC., Koff, E., Yecker, S., Santschi, C., & Schmidt, M. (1998). Facial asymmetry during emotional expression: Gender, valence, and measurement technique. *Neuropsychologia, 36(11),* 1209-1215.

Brown, S.G., Roy, E.A., Rohr, L. & Bryden, P.J. (2006) Using hand performance measures to predict handedness. *Laterality, 11(1),* 1-14.

Bryden, P.J., Pryde, K.M., & Roy, E.A. (2000). A performance measure of the degree of hand preference. *Brain and Cognition, 44*, 402-414.

Burton, C.L., Chatterjee, D., Chatterjee-Chakraborty, M., Lovic, V., Grella, S.L., Steiner M., & Fleming, A.S. (2007). Prenatal restraint stress and motherlessrearing disrupts expression of plasticity markers and stress-induced orticosterone release in adulta female Sprague-Dawley rats. *Brain Research, 1158*, 28-38.

Buxbaum, L.J., Schwartz, M.F., Coslett, B.H., & Carew T.G. (1995) Naturalistic action and praxis in callosal apraxia. *Neurocase, 1*, 3-17.

Butterworth, B., & Hadar, U. (1989). Gesture, speech, and computational stages: a reply to McNeill. *Psychological Review, 96*, 168-174.

Casanto D., & Dijkstra K. (2010) Motor Action and Emotional Memory. *Cognition, 115(1),* 179-185.

Chatterjee, D., Chatterjee-Chakraborty, M., Rees, S., Cauchi, J., de Medeiros, C.B., & Fleming, A.S. (2007). Maternal isolation alters the expression of neural proteins during development: "stroking" stimulation reverses these effects. *Brain Research, 1158*, 11-27.

Cohen, N.J. (1984). Preserved learning capacity in amnesia: Evidence for multiple memory systems. In L.R. Squire, & N. Butters (eds.), *The neuropsychology of memory* (pp.83 -103) New York: Guilford.

Cohen, R.L., & Otterbein, N. (1992). The mnemonic effect of speech gestures: Pantomimic and non-pantomimic gestures compared. *European Journal of Cognitive Psychology*, 4, 113-139.

Condon, W.S., & Ogston, W.D. (1966). Sound film analysis of normal and pathological behaviour patterns. *The Journal of Nervous and Mental Disease, 143(4),* 338-347.

Condon, W.S., & Ogston, W.D. (1967). A segmentation of behavior. *Journal of Psychiatric Research, 5*, 221-235.

Condon, W.S., & Brosin, H.W. (1969). *Micro Linguistic-Kinesic Events in Schizophrenic Behaviour*. In G. Bateson, Birdwhistell, R., Brosin, H.W., Hockett, C., & McQuown, N.A. The Natural History of an Interview. Grune & Stratton, pp. 812-837.

Cook, S.W., & Goldin-Meadow, S. (2006). The Role of Gesture in Learning: Do Children Use Their Hand to Change Their Minds? *Journal of Cognition and Development*, 7(2), 211-232.

Cook, S.W., & Mitchell, Z., & Goldin-Meadow, S. (2008). Gesturing makes learning last. *Cognition, 106*(2), 1047-1058.

Corey, D.M., Hurley, M.M., & Foundas, A.L. (2001) Right and left handedness defined: a multivariate approach using hand preference and performance. *Neuropsychiatry, Neuropsychology, Behavioural Neurology, 14(3),* 144-152.

Cruz, R.F. (1995). *An empirical investigation of the Movement Psychodiagnostic Inventory*. Dissertation Abstracts International: Section B: The Sciences and Engineering Vol. 57(2-B), 1495.

Dalby, J. Gibson, T.D., Grossi, V., & Schneider, R. (1980). Lateralized hand gesture during speech. *Journal of Motor Behaviour, 12*, 292-297.

Darwin, C.R. (1890, reissue 2009). The Expression of the Emotions in Man and Animals (2nd ed.). London: Penguin Group.

Davis, M. (1981). Movement characteristics of hospitalized psychiatric patients. *American Journal of Dance Therapy, 4(1)*, 52-71.

Davis, M. (1991, rev. 1997). *Guide to movement analysis methods*. Behavioral Measurement Database Services, P.O. Box 110287, Pittsburgh, PA, USA.

Davis, C. (1997). Eating Disorders and Hyperactivity: A Psychobiological Perspective. *Canadian Journal of Psychiatry, 42*, 168-175.

Davis, M., & Hadiks, D. (1990). Nonverbal behaviour and client state changes during psychotherapy. *Journal of Clinical Psychology, 46*(3), 340-351.

Davis, M., & Hadiks, D. (1994). Nonverbal aspects of therapist attunement. *Journal of Clinical Psychology, 50*, 393-405.

Davis, M., & Hadiks, D. (1995). Demeanor and credibility. *Semiotica, 1(2),* 5-54.

Davis, M., & Markus, K.A., Walters, S.B., Vorus, N., & Connors, B. (2005). Behavioral cues to deception vs. topic incriminating potential in criminal confessions. *Law and Human Behavior, 29 (6),* 683-704.

De Ruiter, J.P. (2000). The production of speech and gesture. In: D. McNeill (ed.), *Language and gesture* (pp. 284-311). Cambridge: Cambridge University Press.

De'Sperati, C., & Stucchi, N. (2000). Motor imagery and visual event recognition. *Experimental Brain Research, 133*, 273-278.

Dvoretska, D. (2009). *Kinetische Interaktion und Koordination.* Fachbereich Psychologie, Mathematisch-Naturwissenschaftliche Fakultät II. Berlin, Humboldt-Universität. Diploma Thesis.

Efron, D. (1941). *Gesture and culture*. The Hague: Mouton.

Ehrlich, S.B., & Levine, S.C., & Goldin-Meadow, S. (2006). The Importance of Gesture in Children's Spatial Reasoning. *Developmental Psychology, 42*(6), 1259-1268.

Ekman, P. & Friesen, W. (1974). Nonverbal behavior and psychopathology. In: R. J. Friedman, and M. M. Katz (Ed.), *The Psychology of Depression*. New York: John Wiley and Sons.

Ellgring, H. (1986). Nonverbal Expression of Psychological States in Psychiatric Patients. *European Archives of Psychiatry and Neurological Sciences, 236*, 31-34.

Emmorey, K., Tversky, B., & Taylor, H.A. (2000). Using space to describe space: Perspective in speech, sign, and gesture. *Spatial Cognition and Computation, 2*, 157-180.

Feyereisen, P. (2006). Further investigation on the mnemonic effect of gestures: Their meaning matters. *European Journal of Cognitive Psychology, 18(2),* 185-205.

Foundas, A.L., Macauley, B.L., Raymer, A.M., Mahler, L.M., Heilman, K.M. & Rothi L.J.G. (1995). Gesture laterality in aphasic and apraxic stroke patients. *Brain and Cognition, 29,* 204-213.

Freedman, N. & Hoffmann, S.P. (1967). Kinetic behaviour in altered clinical states: Approach to objective analysis of motor behaviour during clinical interviews. *Perceptual and Motor Skills, 24*, 527-539.

Freedman, N. (1972). The Analysis of Movement Behavior During the Clinical Interview. In Siegman, A. W., and Pope, B. (eds.), *Studies in Dyadic Communication* (pp. 153-175). New York: Pergamon.

Freedman, N. & Bucci, W. (1981). On kinetic filtering in associative monologue. *Semiotica, 34(3/4)*: 225-249.

Freedman, N., O'Hanlon, J., Oltman, P., & Witkin, H.A. (1972). The imprint of psychological differentiation on kinetic behaviour in varying communicative contexts. *Journal of Abnormal Psychology, 79(3),* 239-258.

Gaebel, W. (1992). Non-verbal behavioural dysfunction in schizophrenia. *British Journal of Psychiatry, 161(suppl.18)*, 65-74.

Garber, P., & Goldin-Meadow, S. (2002). Gesture offers insight into problem-solving in adults and children. *Cognitive Science, 26*, 817-831.

Gazzaniga, M.S., Bogen, J.E., & Sperry, R.W. (1967). Dyspraxia following division of the cerebral commissures. *Archives of Neurology, 16*, 606-612.

Geschwind, D.H., Iacoboni, M., Mega, M.S., Zaidel, D.W., Cloughesy, T., & Zaidel, E. (1995). Alien hand syndrome: Interhemispheric motor disconnection due to a lesion in the midbody of the corpus callosum. *Neurology, 45*, 802-808.

Goldin-Meadow, S., Alibali, M.W., & Church, R.B. (1993). Transitions in concept acquisition: using the hand to read the mind. *Psychological Review, 100(2),* 279-297.

Goldin-Meadow, S. (2006). Talking and Thinking With Our Hands. *Current Directions In Psychological Science, 15*(1), 34-39.

Grunwald, M., & Weiss, T. (2007). Emotional stress and facial self-touch gestures. Unpublished paper presented at the Lindauer Psychotherapietage.

Guzzetta, A., Baldini, S., Bancale, A., Baroncelli, L., Ciucci, F., Ghirri, P., Putignano, E., Sale, A., Viegi, A., Berardi, N., Boldrini, A., Cioni, G., & Maffei, L. (2009). Massage Accelerates Brain Development and the Maturation of Visual Function. *The Journal of Neuroscience*, *29*, 6042-6051.

Hampson, E. & Kimura, D. (1984). Hand movement asymmetries during verbal and nonverbal tasks. *Canadian Journal of Psychology, 38*, 102-125.

Harrigan, J.A., & Rosenthal, R., (1983). Physicians' Head and Body Positions as Determinants of Perceived Rapport. *Journal of Applied Social Psychology, 13 (6)*, 496-509.

Harrigan, J.A., Oxman, T.E., & Rosenthal, R. (1985). Rapport Expressed through Nonverbal Behaviour. *Journal of Nonverbal Behaviour, 9 (2),* 95-110.

Healey, J.M., Liedermann, J., & Geschwind, N. (1986). Handedness is not a unidimensional trait. *Cortex, 22(1),* 33-53.

Hermsdörfer, J., Mai, N., Spatt, J., Marquardt, C., Veltkamp, R., & Goldenberg, G. (1996). Kinematic analysis of movement imitation in apraxia. *Brain, 119*, 1575-1586.

Holle, H., & Gunter, T.C. (2007). The Role of Iconic Gestures in Speech Disambiguation: ERP Evidence. *Journal of Cognitive Neuroscience, 19(7),* 1175-1192.

Holle, H., Gunter, T.C., Rüschemeyer, S.-A., Hennenlotter, A., & Iacoboni, M. (2008). Neural correlates of the processing of co-speech gestures. *NeuroImage, 39*, 2010-2024.

Holle, H., Obleser, J., Rueschemeyer, S.A. & Gunter, T.C. (2010). Integration of iconic gestures and speech in left superior temporal areas boosts speech comprehension under adverse listening conditions. *NeuroImage, 49*, 875-884.

Hostetter, A.B., & Alibali, M.W. (2008). Visible embodiment: Gestures as simulated action. *Psychonomic Bulletin & Review,15 (3),* 495-514.

Kendon, A. (2010). *Gesture - Visible Action as Utterance*. Cambridge, U.K., Cambridge University Press.

Killgore, W.D.S., & Yurgelun-Todd, D.A. (2007). The right-hemisphere and valence hypotheses: Could they both be right (and sometimes left)? *Social Cognitive and Affective Neuroscience, 2*, 240-250.

Kimura, D. (1973a). Manual activity during speaking - I. Right-handers. *Neuropsychologia, 11,* 45-50.

Kimura D. (1973b). Manual activity during speaking - II. Left-handers. *Neuropsychologia, 11,* 51-55.

Kinsbourne, M. (1972). Eye and head turning indicates cerebral lateralization. *Science, 176*, 539-541.

Kita S. (2000). How representational gestures help speaking. In: D. McNeill (ed.), *Language and Gesture: Window into Thought and Action.* Cambridge University Press, pp. 162-85.

Kita, S. & Özyürek, A. (2003). What does cross-linguistic variation in semantic coordination of speech and gesture reveal?: Evidence for an interface representation of spatial thinking and speaking. *Journal of Memory and Language, 48*, 16-32.

Kita, S., de Condappa, O., & Mohr, C. (2007). Metaphor explanation attenuates the right-hand preference for depictive co-speech gestures that imitate actions. *Brain and Language, 101*, 185-197.

Kleinsmith, A., & Bianchi-Berthouze, N. (2007). Recognizing affective dimensions from body posture, *Proceedings of the 2nd International Conference on Affective Computing and Intelligent Interaction,* LNCS:4738, Springer-Verlag, pp. 48-58, Lisbon, Portugal.

Kraepelin, E. (1899). *Psychiatrie*, 1. Aufl.. Leipzig, Barth.

Krauss, R.M., Chen, Y. & Chawla, P. (1996). Nonverbal behavior and nonverbal communication: What do conversational hand gestures tell us? In M. Zanna (Ed.), *Advances in Experimental Social Psychology*. Tampa: Academic Press 28, 389-450.

Kretschmer, E. (1921). *Körperbau und Charakter. Untersuchungen zum Konstitutionsproblem und zur Lehre von den Temperamenten*. Berlin Springer.

Krout, M. (1935). Autistic gestures. *Psychological Monographs, 46*.

Kryger, M. (2010). *Bewegungsverhalten von Patient und Therapeut in als gut und schlecht erlebten Therapiesitzungen*. Dept. of Neurology, Psychosomatic Medicine, and Psychiatry; Institute of health promotion and clinical movement science. Cologne, German Sport University. Diploma Thesis.

Laban, R. (1988). *The Mastery of Movement*. Worcester: Billing & Sons Ltd.

La France, M. (1982). Posture Mirroring and Rapport. In M. Davis (ed.) *Interaction rhythms: Periodicity in communicative behaviour,* pp. 279-299. New York: Human Scineces Press.

Lane, R.D., & Schwartz, G.E. (1987). Levels of emotional awareness: a cognitive-developmental theory and its application to psychopathology. *American Journal of Psychiatry, 144(2),* 133-43.

Lausberg, H. (1995). Bewegungsverhalten als Prozeßparameter in einer kontrollierten Studie mit funktioneller Entspannung. Unpublished paper presented at the 42. Arbeitstagung des Deutschen Kollegiums für Psychosomatische Medizin.

Lausberg, H. (2011). Das Gespräch zwischen Arzt und Patientin: Die bewegungsanalytische Perspektive. *Balint Journal,* 12, 15-24.

Lausberg, H. (2013). Neuropsychology of gesture production. In C. Müller, Fricke, Ladewig, McNeill, Teßendorf (Ed.), *Body - Language - Communication* (pp. 164-178): de Gruyter.

Lausberg, H., & Kita, S. (2003). The content of the message influences the hand choice in co-speech gestures and in gesturing without speaking. *Brain and Language, 86,* 57-69.

Lausberg, H. & Kryger, M. (2011). Gestisches Verhalten als Indikator therapeutischer Prozesse in der verbalen Psychotherapie: Zur Funktion der Selbstberührungen und zur Repräsentation von Objektbeziehungen in gestischen Darstellungen. *Psychotherapie-Wissenschaft, 1(1),* 41-55.

Lausberg, H., Davis, M., & Rothenhäusler, A. (2000). Hemispheric specialization in spontaneous gesticulation in a patient with callosal disconnection. *Neuropsychologia, 38*, 1654-1663.

Lausberg, H., Sassenberg, U., & Holle, H. (submitted). Right-handers display distinct hand preferences for different gesture types in communicative situations: Evidence for specific right and left hemisphere contributions to implicit gesture production.

Lausberg, H., Kita, S., Zaidel, E., & Ptito, A. (2003a). Split-brain patients neglect left personal space during right-handed gestures. *Neuropsychologia, 41*, 1317-1329.

Lausberg, H., Cruz, R.F., Kita, S., Zaidel, E., & Ptito, A. (2003b). Pantomime to visual presentation of objects: Left hand dyspraxia in patients with complete callosotomy. *Brain, 126*, 343-360.

Lausberg, H., Zaidel, E., Cruz, R.F., & Ptito, A. (2007). Speech-independent production of communicative gestures: Evidence from patients with complete callosal disconnection. *Neuropsychologia, 45*, 3092-3104.

Lausberg, H., Zaidel, E., Cruz, R.F. & Ptito, A. (2007). Speech-independent production of communicative gestures: Evidence from patients with complete callosal disconnection. *Neuropsychologia, 45*, 3092-3104.

Lausberg, H., Göttert, R., Münßinger, U., Boegner, F., & Marx, P. (1999). Callosal disconnection syndrome in a left-handed patient due to infarction of the total length of the corpus callosum. *Neuropsychologia, 37*, 253-265.

Lavergne, J. & Kimura, D. (1987). Hand movement asymmetry during speech: No effect of speaking topic. *Neuropsychologia, 25* 689-93.

Lemke, M.R., Wendorff, T., Mieth, B., Buhl, K., & Linnemann, M. (2000). Spatiotemporal gait patterns during over ground locomotion in major depression compared with healthy controls. *Journal of Psychiatric Research, 34*, 277-283.

Liepmann, H., & Maas, O. (1907). Fall von linksseitiger Agraphie und Apraxie bei rechtsseitiger Lähmung. *Journal für Psychologie und Neurologie, X(4/5),* 214-227.

Mahl, F.G. (1968). Gestures and Body Movements in Interviews. *Research in Psychotherapy, 3*, 295-346.

McNeill, D. (1992). *Hand and mind. What gestures reveal about thought*. Chicago: University of Chicago.

McNeill, D. (2005). Gesture and Thought. Chicago, USA, University of Chicago Press

Marangolo, P., De Renzi, E., Di Pace, E., Ciurli, P., & Castriota-Skandenberg, A.(1998). Let not thy left hand know what thy right hand knoweth. The case of a patient with an infarct involving the callosal pathways. *Brain, 121*, 1459-1467.

Michalak, J., Troje, N.F., Fischer, J., Vollmar, P., Heidenreich, T., & Schulte, D. (2009). Embodiment of Sadness and Depression - Gait Patterns Associated With Dysphoric Mood. *Psychosomatic Medicine, 71*, 580.

Morris, D. (1978). *Der Mensch mit dem wir leben. Ein Handbuch unseres Verhaltens*. Muenchen, Zuerich: Droemer Knaur.

Parsons, L.M., Gabrieli, J.D. E., Phelps, E.A. & Gazzaniga, M.S. (1998). Cerebrally lateralized mental representations of hand shape and movement. *Journal of Neuroscience, 18*, 6539-48.

Piaget, J. (1962). Play, dreams and imitation in childhood. New York: Norton.

Poizner, H., Mack, L., Verfaellie, M., Rothi, L.J.G., & Heilman, K.M. (19990). Three-dimensional Computergraphic Analysis of Apraxia. *Brain, 113*, 85-101.

Posner, R., Krüger, R., Noll, T. & Serenari, M. (in prep.): *Berliner Lexikon der Alltagsgesten*. Berlin: Berlin-Verlag.

Rapcsak, S.Z., Ochipa, C., Beeson, P.M., & Rubens, A.B. (1993). Praxis and the right hemisphere. *Brain and Cognition, 23*, 181-202.

Reich, W. (1933, 1971). Charakteranalyse. Bremen: Plopp.

Riskind, J.H., & Gotay, C.C. (1982). Physical Posture: Could It Have Regulatory or Feedback Effects on Motivation and Emotion? *Motivation and Emotion, 6*(3), 273-298.

Rossberg-Gempton, I., & Poole, G.D. (1993). The effect of open and closed postures on pleasant and unpleasant emotions.*The Arts in Psychotherapy, Vol 20(1)*, 75-82.

Sainsbury, P. (1954). A method of measuring spontaneous movements by time-sampling motion picture. *The Journal of Mental Science, 100a*, 742-748.

Sainsbury, P. (1955). Gestural movement during psychiatric interview. *Psychosomatic Medicine, 17*, 454-469.

Saucier, D.M., & Elias, L.J. (2001). Lateral and sex differences in manual gesture during conversation. *Laterality, 6(3),* 239-45.

Sassenberg, U., Helmich, I. & Lausberg, H. (2010). *Awareness of emotions: Movement behaviour as indicator of implicit emotional processes in participants with and without alexityhmia*. Proceedings of KogWis: 10th Biannual Meeting of the German Society for Cognitive Science, Potsdam, Germany; Haack, Wiese, Abraham, Chiarcos (eds.), p. 169.

Sassenberg, U., Foth, M., Wartenburger, I. & van der Meer, E. (2011). Show your hands – are you really clever? Reasoning, gesture production, and intelligence. *Linguistics, 49(1),* 105-134.

Schacter, D.L. (1992). Implicit knowledge: New perspectives on unconscious processes. *Proceedings of the National Academy of Science of the USA, 89*, 5.

Schanberg, S.M., & Field, T.M. (1987). Sensory deprivation stress and supplemental stimulation in the rat pup and preterm human neonate. *Child Development,* 58, 1431-1447.

Scheflen, A.E. (1963). Communication and Regulation in Psychotherapy. *Psychiatry, 26.*

Scheflen, A.E. (1973). *Communicational Structure: Analysis of a psychotherapy transaction.* Bloomington: Indiana University.

Scheflen, A.E. (1974). *How Behaviour Means.* New York: Anchor / Doubleday.

Sirigu, A., Duhamel, J.R., Cohen, L., Pillon, B., Dubois, B., & Agid, Y. (1996). The Mental Representation of Hand Movements After Parietal Cortex Damage. *Science, 273*, 1564-1568.

Souza-Poza, J.F., & Rohrberg, R. (1977). Body movements in relation to type of information (person- and non-person oriented) and cognitive style (field dependence). *Human Communication Research, 4(1),* 19-29.

Souza-Posa, J.F., Rohrberg, R., & Mercure, A. (1979). Effects of type of information (abstract-concrete) and field dependence on asymmetry of hand movements during speech. *Perceptual and Motor Skills, 48*, 1323-1330.

Sperry, R.W. (1968). Hemisphere deconnection and unity in conscious awareness. *American Psychologist, 23*, 723-733.

Stalnaker, T.A., Espana, R.A., & Berridge, C.W. (2009). Coping Behaviour Causes Asymmetric Changes in Neuronal Activation in the Prefrontal Cortex and Amygdala. *Synapse, 63*, 82-85.

Stephens, D. (1983). Hemispheric language dominance and gesture hand preference. Ph.D. dissertation, Department of Behavioral Sciences, University of Chicago.

Stepper, S., & Strack, F. (1993). Proprioceptive deternminants of emotional and nonemotional feelings. *Journal of Personality and Social Psychology, 64 (2),* 211-220.

Tanaka, Y., Yoshida, A., Kawahata, N. Hashimoto, R., & Obayashi, T. (1996) Diagnostic dyspraxia - Clinical characteristics, responsible lesion and possible underlying mechanism. *Brain, 119*, 859-873.

Trevarthen, C. (1996). Lateral asymmetries in infancy: Implications for the development of the hemispheres. *Neuroscience and Biobehavioural Reviews, 20*(4), 571-586.

Trope, I., Fishman, B., Gur, R.C., Sussman, N.M., & Gur, R.E. (1987). Contralateral and ipsilateral control of fingers following callosotomy. *Neuropsychologia, 25*, 287-291.

Ulrich, G. (1977). Videoanalytische Methoden zur Erfassung averbaler Verhaltensparameter bei depressiven Syndromen. *Pharmakopsychiatrie, 10*, 176-182.

Ulrich, A., & Harms, K.A. (1985). Video Analysis of the Non-Verbal Behaviour of Depressed Patients Before and After Treatment. *Journal of Affective Disorders, 9*, 63-67.

Verfaellie, M., Bowers, D., & Heilman, K.M. (1988). Hemispheric asymmetries in mediating intention, but not selective attention. *Neuropsychologia, 26*, 521-31.

Volpe, B.T., Sidtis, J.J., Holtzman, J.D., Wilson, D.H., & Gazzaniga, M.S. (1982). Cortical mechanisms involved in praxis: Observations following partial and complete section of the corpus callosum in man. *Neurology, 32*, 645-650.

Wang, J., & Sainburg, R.L. (2007). The dominant and nondominant arms are specialized for stabilizing different features of task performance. *Experimental Brain Research, 178*, 565-570.

Wallbott, H.G. (1989). Movement quality changes in psychopathological disorders. In B. Kirkaldy (Ed.), *Normalities and abnormalities in human movement* (pp. 128-146). Basel: Karger.

Wartenburger, I., Kühn, E., Sassenberg, U., Foth, M., Franz, E.A. & van der Meer, E. (2010). On the relationship between fluid intelligence, gesture production, and brain structure. *Intelligence, 38*, 193-201.

Watson, R.T., & Heilman, K.M. (1983). Callosal apraxia. *Brain, 106*, 391-403.

Wilkins, D., & de Ruiter, J.P. (1999). Hand preference for representational gestures: A comparison of Arente and Dutch speakers. In: Verle Van Geenhoven and Natasha Warner (eds.) *Annual Report 1999*, 51-52. Nijmegen: Max Planck Institute for Psycholinguistics.

Willke, S. (1995). *Die therapeutische Beziehung in psychoanalytisch orientierten Anamnesen und Psychotherapien mit neurotischen, psychosomatischen und psychiatrischen Patienten*. DFG-Bericht Wi 1213/1-1.

Wilson, V.E., & Peper, E. (2004). The Effects of Upright and Slumped Postures on the Recall of Positive and Negative Thoughts. *Applied Psychophysiology and Biofeedback, 29*.189-195.

Witkin, H.A., & Lewis, M.B. (1954). *Personality through Perception*. New York: Wiley and Sons.

Zaidel, E., White, H., Sakurai, E., & Banks, W. (1988). Hemispheric locus of lexical congruity effects: Neuropsychological reinterpretation of psycholinguistic results. In: Christine Chiarello (Ed.), *Right Hemisphere Contributions to Lexical Semantics*, 71-88. New York: Springer.

3. Movement Behaviour Analysis across Scientific Disciplines

Hedda Lausberg

For empirical research on the relation between movement behaviour and emotional, cognitive, and interactive processes, movement analysis is applied as a research tool. The term movement analysis is used here in analogy to the general term analysis as defined by Hehlmann (1968, p. 18; translation by the author): "Analysis (Greek: Dissolution), to dissect a whole, for example an object perception, a term, a state of awareness in general, but also a character, into its single parts, structures, sides, aspects. Analysis is the basis for any type of research. Separation and dissociation must be understood as a consequence of analysis. The whole entity must be repeatedly brought to mind as its specific quality is lost through analysis....". Accordingly, movement behaviour analysis is defined here as the dissection of movement behaviour into entities that are as a stand-alone or in combination relevant with regard to cognitive, emotional, and interactive functions.

3.1 Some common shortcomings in movement behaviour analysis methodology

As outlined in Chapter 1, despite the fact that there is a long tradition and a broad scientific interest, movement behaviour research has, thus far, not been established as a scientific discipline on its own. Apart from the fact that the diaspora of movement behaviour across many different disciplines is an obstacle for developing a common body on knowledge, this situation also has negative consequences for the standard of movement behaviour research methodology. Common methodological standards have been developed only rudimentary, a condition which negatively influences the quality of research. Foremost, it is striking to find that still many researchers develop their own coding system. Often, these researchers do not have a scientific background that is related to body movement and they are not trained in movement analysis. Not surprisingly, they are not aware of the fact that the analysis of movement behaviour is just as complex as, for instance, the analysis of an electroencephalogram. A number of typical methodological shortcomings are listed below:

(i) Precipitate interpretation

A precise analysis of the movement behaviour per se based on the visual appearance of the movement is seldom conducted. Instead, researchers quickly turn to interpreting the movement behaviour with regard to the function of their research interest, e.g. emotion. However, a number of experiments on the interpretation of movement behaviour evidence that this approach is highly problematic. These interpretation experiments unanimously reveal that naïve raters may agree in their interpretations on movement behaviour, e.g. judging a person's dominance by observing his / her gait, these judgements, however, are wrong with regard to an objective measure (Eisenberg and Reichline, 1939; Mason, 1957; Wallbott, 1989). Therefore, Frijda (1965) proposed that understanding the laws of the assessment of an expression is at least as important as the laws how meaning is expressed (for a detailed discussion see Chapter 12).

(ii) Simple but not valid values

Often, movement values are chosen just because they are simple to code. Such values might show a good objectivity and reliability, but they are not valid with regard to cognitive, emotional, and interactive functions. As an example, classifying hand movements with the two types 'spread fingers' versus 'closed fingers' will show a high objectivity and interrater reliability: However, the values present entities of movement behaviour that are not particularly relevant with regard to cognitive, emotional, and interactive processes. As another example, counting the number of foot taps in a psychotherapy session is simple but the value foot tap is too unspecific and not valid with regard to psychotherapy outcome.

(iii) Broad values

The movement values are too broad. Thus, they contain different movement entities that are associated with different cognitive, emotional, and interactive functions. An example is the value *free movement,* which is defined as "any motion of the limb which did not result in touching of the body or coming to rest" (Kimura, 1973, p. 46). Recent research has demonstrated that this value comprises too many hand movements that are associated with different neuropsychological functions (Lausberg & Kita, 2003; Lausberg et al., 2007). Studies using more fine-grained values have even produced results that contradict those of the studies applying the *free movement* value. Thus, the scientific profit when conducting movement analysis with such broad values is limited.

(iv) Confounded values

Researchers who are trained in a non-movement scientific discipline typically pursue movement behaviour research more or less intensively as part of their own discipline. Accordingly, they analyze movement behaviour as a by-product of the core subject of their own scientific discipline. As a consequence, methodologically, they describe and interpret movement behaviour with the methods and terminology that they employ in their primary scientific discipline. As an example, linguists may use linguistic criteria to analyze movement behaviour. As a consequence, the specific properties of movement behaviour per se are not considered. Moreover, often the movement values these researchers design, are confounded with values of their primary scientific discipline. As an example, the factors "retardation" and "agitation" reported by Ulrich and Harms (1985) for depressive patients are confounded with psychopathological symptoms.

(v) Insufficiently operationalized values

Other researchers create more complex movement values but they operationalize them insufficiently. The imprecise definitions of the values entail an insufficient objectivity, and a lack of reliability and validity.

Furthermore, vague value definitions render it difficult to compare study results. Often it is not evident from the description given in a paper, what kind of movement had actually been coded. Hence, it is not possible to replicate the analysis and to confirm or to disapprove the results. As an example, the apparent contradictions between different research studies on the relation of aphasia and gesture are essentially caused by the fact that different researchers had investigated movement values that were termed similarly but actually included different types of movements (for an elaboration on this topic, see Lott, 1999). Controlling the quality of the value operationalization by examining interrater agreement, i.e., when two independent observers agree on the value of a movement unit, is a rather recent development in movement behaviour research, and it is still not yet fully established as a standard method.

(vi) No rater training

Researchers who do not appreciate movement analysis as a skill consequently employ naïve raters to assess movement behaviour. However, movement values that are valid with regard to complex cognitive, emotional, and interactive processes are complex, too. In other words, a simple movement value such as a foot tap is not valid with regard to a complex phenomenon such as psychotherapy outcome. Therefore, the coding of movement values that are relevant with regard to cognitive, emotional, and interactive processes requires a substantial training. It is comparable to the training that a cardiologist needs to auscultate and classify heart sounds. In fact, a rater's observation skill for the other person's movement behaviour correlates with the quality of the self-assessment of her/his own movement behaviour that, in turn, improves with her/his own movement experience (Wolff, 1932; Calvo-Merino et al., 2005; Cross et al., 2008) (for a detailed discussion of the impact of rater training, see Chapter 12).

3.2 Criteria for the review on coding systems

The fact that researchers who have no experience with movement analysis tend to develop their own coding systems has mainly negative consequences for the quality of research. Furthermore, as already discussed in Chapter 1, this trend, which leads to a multitude of different movement types, also inhibits the communication in the scientific community. The review in subsection 2.5.3 on laterality preferences for different movement types in healthy individuals reveals the difficulties that emerge when trying to compare findings of different researchers. Because of the scant interdisciplinary exchange, researchers are often not aware that a substantial number of movement analysis systems already exist. Among these, they may find a tool that suits for their purpose. While the existing systems need not to be perfect, they offer at least a methodological experience and a basis to start with.

Therefore, this chapter provides a review on behavioural movement analysis systems. The review focuses on movement analysis tools that are designed to explore the movement behaviour as a reflection of emotional and cognitive, and interactive processes. Systems that directly code the interaction, i.e., between-subjects processes such as mirroring or synchronicity, (e.g. Davis & Hadiks, 1990), are not included in the review. As demonstrated in Chapter 2, the examination of patients with mental disease and brain damage provides valuable information about the link between movement behaviour and emotional, cognitive, and interactive functions. Therefore, also coding systems are reviewed here that are designed to code alterations of movement behaviour in patients with mental disease and brain damage.

As exposed in Chapter 1, movement behaviour research is spread across scientific disciplines. Not surprisingly, the coding systems used in the diverse scientific disciplines differ substantially regarding the criteria on the grounds of which the movements are classified. In their paper "The Repertoire of Nonverbal Behaviour", Ekman and Friesen (1969) list the following criteria: (i) use of a movement: context, relation to language, consciousness and intent of the non-verbal actor, external feedback, informative, communicative, or interactive value of the movement; (ii) origin of a movement: reflex-like, universal, cultural, specific to a group, familiar, or individual; (iii) relationship between the movement and its meaning: arbitrary (there is no visible relation between the movement and its meaning, for instance, Churchill`s Victory sign), iconic (the movement is similar to its meaning, for instance, the gesture "cutting someone`s throat"), intrinsic (the movement is part of its meaning, for instance, showing the fist with anger). Many more criteria could be added to their list, such as the kinematics of the movement, the laterality of a limb movement, the psychodynamic function of a movement, etc.

In the following review, the coding systems are classified in three main groups, based on their predominant criterion for classifying body movements. This order of presenting the coding systems, instead of ordering them according to academic disciplines, also serves to overcome the borders between the scientific disciplines. It clarifies that similar approaches to movement behaviour analysis have been developed in different academic disciplines.

(i) Comprehensive descriptive coding systems

These systems are descriptive in the sense that they refer to the visually perceivable aspect of movement behaviour. They describe not only *what* type of a movement is performed, e.g. a pointing gesture, and *how* it is performed, e.g. pointing with strength. Comprehensiveness is another characteristic of these coding systems. All movements of several parts of the body or the body as a whole are coded.

(ii) Coding systems that classify movements according to function

These systems classify body movements according to specific functions, e.g. meaning or psychodynamic function. As described in section 2.1, different functions are typically attributed to different movement classes, such as cognition to gesture, psychological balance to self-touch, mood to posture, etc.. These classes are, in turn, regularly associated with different parts of the body or with the body as a whole. Therefore, the function-oriented analysis systems are often restricted to coding one part of the body, such as the hands and arms.

(iii) Coding systems that classify alterations in movement behaviour

These systems register alterations in the quality, the quantity, and the concept of body movements, as compared to their performance in the movement behaviour of healthy persons. These movement alterations are typically observed in individuals with mental disease or brain damage. Given the broad spectrum of pathological alterations, the systems vary substantially among each other.

To illustrate the practical problems that arise when ineffective coding systems are employed, this last review not only describes the coding systems but it also demonstrates the difficulties that may arise from deficient scales. That part of the review demonstrates that an ineffective methodology is not only a blemish, but that it may result in misleading or even wrong results, which in the example of a clinical context, have negative consequences for the patients' quality of life.

As concluded in Chapter 2, to fully understand movement behaviour and its link to cognitive, emotional, and interactive processes, basic empirical research is required. Therefore, the review below focuses on coding systems that are objective and reliable.

To check for objectivity, the author has studied the definitions of the values in the respective literature. Note that in the review below, the short definitions of the movement categories and values[7] that are placed in brackets can only sketch the concept of the respective category and values. For obtaining the detailed definitions, the reader should study the respective literature given in the references. A good measure for objectivity is interrater agreement.

With regard to reliability, it has to be noted that the control of interrater agreement in movement behaviour research is a rather recent standard. Accordingly, for some systems, there are no reports on interrater reliability. Even more so, studies on retest reliability are the exception, i.e., if after a certain period of time the observer gives the same value to the same movement (applies to videotaped movements). For reviewing the coding systems, another problem occurred: Those studies that report interrater agreement have used different study designs. The design of a study can facilitate or complicate the achievement of good interrater agreement. As an example, it is easier to achieve a good agreement when coding preselected units than when segmenting and coding the ongoing stream of behaviour. Furthermore, different statistical methods have been employed to measure interrater agreement. As an assessment of the equivalence of these statistical procedures is far beyond the scope of this chapter, in the review below it is only reported if interrater agreement and retest-reliability had been examined. If no reports on interrater agreement were available but the coding system had been referred to or used by several other independent researchers, it was nevertheless included in the review.

Concerning validity, it shall be noted that for none of the existing systems the validity can be judged as sufficiently established with regard to current psychometric standards. This does in no way imply that these systems would not prove validity if they were properly tested. However, the extended review of the coding system for movement psychopathology illustrates the dilemma that arises when the validity of certain values is uncritically assumed without sufficient psychometric verification.

Given the aim of this book, the following review on coding systems is not exhaustive. It is rather intended to provide an overview on the spectrum of different methodological approaches to movement behaviour analysis. The coding systems are presented and discussed concerning those factors that have been identified in Chapter 2 as being relevant for basic empirical research on movement behaviour.

---

7 Throughout the book, values are written in italics.

3.3 Comprehensive descriptive systems

Comprehensive systems for the analysis of the whole body moving in space have been developed based on the work of the dance theorist Rudolf Laban (e.g. Laban, 1950). The Labannotation / Kinetography Laban is designed to annotate dancers' movements. Its symbols note the direction and level of the movement, the part of the body doing the movement, the duration of the movement, and the dynamic quality of the movement. Comparable to notations for pieces of music, the notation system is so precise and detailed that it enables to replicate choreographies.

The Laban Movement Analysis (LMA) is an analysis system comprising four main categories: body, effort, shape, and space. As an example of this comprehensive analysis, the main category effort is described here. It refers to the movement quality, i.e., how the body concentrates its exertion (Dell, 1979). The main category effort comprises the categories flow (variations in bodily tension representing ease or restraint of movement), weight (force or pressure exerted in movement), time (compensation to outward time demands, or attitude toward duration of action), and space (attention or orientation to space, how energy is focused in action, selective versus free-floating attention). Each category contains two polar values, which can be organized in scales with 3, 5, or 7 gradations. The category flow include values from *free* to *bound*, weight from *light* to *strong*, time from *sustained* to *sudden*, and space from *indirect* to *direct*. Furthermore, the main category shape is noteworthy as it refers to the movement of the body as a whole (in contrast to coding the movements of parts of the body). It includes the categories *shape flow* ("where the body form results only from changes within the body parts", such as growing, shrinking, opening, closing), *directional movement* ("spoke-like or arc-like movement linking the body with a place in space"), and *shaping* ("where the [body] form results from the body clearly moulding itself in relation to the shape of space, whether it creates the shape of space, as in dance, or adapts to it, as in many work movements", such as spreading, enclosing) (p. 44, Dell, 1979).

The LMA values are descriptive and neutral, i.e., originally they imply no positive or negative valence. The main field of the LMA application is dance training and dance movement therapy. Depending on the therapist's theoretical orientation and her/his patient population, different aspects of the LMA have been elaborated (e.g. Bartenieff, 1991; Bernstein, 1991; North, 1991). For certain categories and values, hypotheses and theories have been set up concerning their association with personality traits, stages of child development, or mental functions. For example, the Kestenberg Movement Profile (KMP) is a developmentally oriented elaboration on Laban's concepts. The child psychoanalyst Kestenberg (1965, 1967) classified the childrens' movement behaviour according to tension flow rhythms and tension flow attributes to evaluate child development. The interrater reliability of trained raters using the KMP has been examined (Sossin, 1987). However, the validity of the KMP categories with regard to psychoanalytically oriented developmental stages in children requires more investigation.

Based on the LMA, the author has developed a coding system with operationalized scales for empirical research (BAST) (Lausberg et al., 1996). Its three main categories refer to (i) the use of the body with the categories body involvement, body-half preference, movement initiating body part, weight shift; (ii) the use of space with the categories movement area, contact with floor, floor patterns, movement level, kinesphere; and (iii) the use of efforts with the categories flow, time, weight, and space. It is suited for basic research on whole body movement in space. The BAST analysis can be applied in combination with a diagnostic movement test and with a questionnaire for the self-assessment of one's movement behaviour. The operationalized scales are available as a printed version and as a template for application with the annotation tool ELAN (http://www.latmpi.eu/tools/elan/thirdparty) (for ELAN, see Chapter 7). After a standardized training, raters show good interrater agreement (Lausberg, 1997; Lausberg, 1998; Gazzarata et al., 2010; Büning, 2011; Degener, 2013). The BAST analysis differentiates significantly between patients with psychosomatic and psychiatric diseases and healthy controls, and it is sensitive to therapy and training progress (Lausberg et al., 1988; Lausberg et al., 1996; Gazzarata et al., 2010; Marian et al. 2010; Paarmann et al., 2012; Büning, 2011; Degener, 2013).

A different approach to the analysis of whole body movement was made by Birdwhistell (1952), a researcher with the background of cultural anthropology and structural linguistics. Birdwhistell developed his system kinesics in analogy to linguistics. Body movements coded in kinemes are regarded as arbitrary signs that serve the maintenance and regulation of interaction. Given the theoretical background that body movements per se have no meaning, the system is purely descriptive. Birdwhistell developed an extensive list of kinegraphs to annotate movements of the head, face, trunk, shoulder - arm - wrist, hand - finger, hip - leg - ankle, foot, and neck. Examples for kinegraphs are *moistening lips* or *foot shuffle*. Qualitative aspects such as *norm, stress,* or *oversoft* can be annotated as well. Possibly because of the complexity of the system and the large number of kinegraphs that have to be learned for application, Birdwhistell's system has, up to now, obtained little acceptance in movement behaviour research. To the author's knowledge, there are no reports on interrater agreement.

Another comprehensive system, the Movement Signature Analysis (MSA), has been developed by the psychologist and psychotherapist Davis (1991). The MSA is a method for registering patterns of an individual's movement behaviour that appear to persist over long periods of time and in different contexts (for the relevance of movement patterns, see Section 2.3). The MSA comprises the classes facial expression, gaze direction, head movements, trunk orientation, weight shift, postural shift, trunk shape, positions, gesticulation, hand configuration, direction, reach space, path type, self touch, and instrumental actions.

Qualitative aspects, derived from the LMA, are considered in the categories dynamic intensity, directional and shaping, and pathology. To give a rough orientation, the MSA quasi combines the approaches of Birdwhistell (*what* kind of a movement a person performs) and Laban (*how* the person performs the movement). The interrater agreement is good, but somewhat lower for the categories referring to qualitative aspects (e.g. Davis et al., 2005).

The MSA involves laborious microanalysis of a few examples of the person's most complex and animated nonverbal behaviour for a detailed recording of how movement values are distinctively patterned (Davis & Dulicai, 1992; Davis, Dulicai, Hadiks, & Berger, 1992). As the MSA is a suitable method for the identification of individual and intra-dyadic movement patterns, it can be applied for the contrastive analysis (Davis & Hadiks, 1995). The contrastive analysis reveals fluctuations in the individual's movement repertoire, i.e., from her/his baseline to being minimally active or maximally complex and animated. Patterns within the behavioural stream of movements can be detected by visual scan of the movement annotations.

Possibly, the MSA could be combined with algorithms for automatize pattern detection (e.g. THEME by Magnus S. Magnusson). The contrastive analysis has been primarily applied to detect mental state changes within psychotherapy sessions or across sessions. Also THEME, in combination with other coding systems, has already been used for pattern detection in therapist-patient interaction (Spang et al., 2011).

To summarize, the LMA-based systems are designed to analyze the behaviour of the body as a whole moving in space. The Kinesic analysis and the MSA are primarily tailored for the analysis of the stationary body in communication.

These coding systems use descriptive values that refer to the visually perceivable aspect of movement behaviour. The values are not confounded with values for assess cognitive, emotional, and interactive functions. The systems are comprehensive in the sense that they comprise several classes of movement behaviour (*what*) such as positions, and the quality of movement behaviour (*how*) such as efforts. They register the movements of the body as a whole or of several parts of the body, including the laterality of the moving limb. Thereby, they enable to detect recurrent combinations of the simultaneously display of two or more movement types, e.g. head nod combined with opening of the arms. Furthermore, as all movement of a part of a body or of the body as a whole are coded in time, recurrent sequences of movement types can be detected. Thus, these systems provide a complete picture of an individual's movement behaviour. After an intensive rater training, a good reliability is achieved, but values referring to movement quality show less reliability.

To conclude, these systems are suited for basic research. However, while the comprehensiveness is the strength of these systems, it is also their weakness. Particularly, the Kinesic analysis it takes time to learn their application, as it comprises numerous kinegraphs. For all systems, the analysis is time-consuming and therefore, limited to a few minutes of an individual's movement behaviour. Furthermore, the codings of the current versions of these systems require substantial processing before they can be submitted to a quantitative statistical analysis.

3.4 Systems that classify movements according to function

Among the coding systems that classify body movements according to their function, there are many gesture coding systems. As exposed in Chapter 2, gesture is class of body movements defined by its specific function.

One of the most influential systems for hand and head gestures has been developed by the anthropologist David Efron (1941), who conducted research on traditional and assimilated Eastern Jews and South Italians. Efron combined the analysis of the function of gesture with a spatio-temporal analysis and an interlocutional analysis, which includes between-subjects phenomena. The spatio-temporal analysis refers the visual appearance of the gesture movement. It includes the categories radius, form, plane, bodily parts involved in gesticulation, and tempo. The interlocutional analysis focuses on the topographic-gestural relationships between speaker and auditor. It includes the categories familiarity with the physical person, simultaneous gesturing, conversational grouping, and gesturing with objects. The analysis of the function of the gesture refers to referential aspects: "A gestural movement may be 'meaningful' by (a) the emphasis it lends to the content of the verbal and vocal behavior it accompanies, (b) the connotation (whether deictic, pictorial, or symbolic) it possesses independently from the speech of which it may, or may not, be an adjunct. In the first case its "meaning" is of *logical* or *discursive* character, the movement being, as it were, a kind of gestural portrayal, not of the object of reference, or "thought", but of the course of the ideational process itself (i.e., a bodily reenactment of the logical pauses, intensities, inflections, etc. of the corresponding speech sequence). This type of gesture may in turn be (a) simply *baton-like,* representing a sort of "timing out" with the hand the successive stages of the referential activity, (b) *ideographic*, in the sense that it traces or sketches out in the air the "paths" and "direction" of the thought pattern. The latter variety might also be called *logico-topographic* or *logico-pictorial*. In the second case the "meaning" of the gesture is "objective", and the movement may be (a) *deictic*, referring by means of a sign to a visually present object (actual pointing), (b) *physiographic*, depicting either the form of a visual object or a spatial relationship (*iconographic* gesture), or that of a bodily action (*kinetographic* gesture), (c) *symbolic* or *emblematic*, representing either a visual or a logical object by means of a pictorial of a non-pictorial form which has no morphological relationship to the thing represented." (Efron, p. 96, 1972). To summarize, the function-oriented analysis comprises the main values *discursive* and *objective* gestures. *Discursive* gestures include the values *baton* (emphasizing the beat pattern of the speech) and *ideographic* (sketching a thought pattern). *Objective* gestures comprise the values *deictic* (pointing to a real or imagined object or indicating a direction), *physiographic* with the two subvalues *iconographic* (depicting a form) and *kinetographic* (depicting a movement), and *emblematic* gestures (conventional signs having specific linguistic translation). As Efron conducted an independent spatio-temporal analysis of gestures, his descriptions of the referential gesture values are accompanied by precise descriptions of the radius, form, plane, bodily parts involved in gesticulation, and tempo. However, his distinction between the values *physiographic* and *ideographic* is based on the analysis of the verbal statement that accompanies the gesture.

While Efron did not assess interrater agreement, he applied a fourfold method for analysing the data including direct observation, sketches by a painter, rough counting, and motion pictures studied by observation and judgments of naive observers and graphs and charts. Recent studies, applying Efron's referential values, with the exception of *ideographic* gestures, report good interrater agreement (e.g. Lausberg et al., 2000).

The psychoanalysts and psychiatrists Freedman and Hoffman (1967) designed a system to analyze the patients' hand movements in clinical interviews. The elaborated version of the coding system distinguished the two main values "*object-focused movements*, their major defining characteristic being the close linkage to the spoken word" and "*body-focused* activity which bears no apparent relation to speech" (Freedman et al., 1972, p. 240). Thus, the two main values were primarily defined by their relation to speech. Furthermore, assumptions were made about the validity of the two values: "While object-focused movement seem to function as part of the verbalizing and symbolizing process, the major function of body-focused activity appears to be self-ministration." (p. 240). However, as it will become evident below, the *body-focused* values were operationalized primarily based on the visual appearance of the movement.

Object-focused hand movements represent the content of the verbal utterance or accompany the rhythm of speech. With regard to the visual appearance, they are defined as being directed away from the gesturer's body towards the listener. *Object-focused* hand movements are subdivided into *speech primacy* and *motor primacy*, depending on whether the message is primarily given verbally or whether it is primarily conveyed through gesture. An example for *motor primacy* gestures are *emblematic* gestures (as defined by Efron), such as the Victory sign. *Emblematic* gestures convey the message independently from a verbal statement, which may be completely missing. An example for *speech primacy* gestures are *batons* (as defined by Efron). These gestures rhythmically accompany the verbal message, which is the primary medium of information transfer. *Speech primacy* gestures are further subdivided into *punctuating* and *minor qualifier*, while *motor primacy* gestures are further subdivided into *representational, concretization, speech failures,* and *pointing*.

Body-focused hand movements are touches of the own body or its adornments. The *body-focused* movements are divided into *discrete* movements that last less than three seconds, and *continuous* ones that last longer than 3 seconds. The latter value is subdivided into *hand-to-hand*, i.e., hands touching each other, *direct*, i.e., touching another part of the body with one hand, and *indirect*, i.e., the manipulation of a thing, typically articles of clothing or accessories.

In 1995, Wilke published a revised version of Freedman's Body Movement Coding System, in which some kinesically oriented terms of the hand movement values were replaced by more psychologically oriented terms. The most relevant changes were that *object-focused* hand movements were termed *narrative rhythmicities, indirect body-focused* became *instrumentals,* and *hand-to-hand body-focused* was modified to *shielding.*

Freedman`s analysis system has been used in psychiatric, psychotherapeutic and psychological research, as it registers movement entities that are sensitive to psychopathological states, clinical improvement, and personality traits. Objective definitions of the values are available (e.g Freedmann, 1972), and the interrater agreement has been investigated in all studies applying the system. However, highly arbitrary is the distinction between *discrete* and *continuous body-focused* movements based on the criterion of a duration of either less or more than 3 seconds. There is no empirical evidence why 3 seconds (and for example, not 5 seconds) represent a relevant duration in time that separates two movement entities. Kinematic criteria would be more appropriate than an arbitrary temporal criterion to distinguish movement entities.

A dichotomy as that between *object-focused* and *body-focused* movements is also fundamental to Kimura's coding system (1973), which has been used mainly for neuropsychological studies. Kimura's system is primarily descriptive, while she makes empirically based assumptions concerning the link of the two movement values to language production. The system is presented in this group, because it is more related to function-oriented gesture coding systems than to comprehensive descriptive systems.

Kimura's system comprises only the two broad values *free movements,* defined as "any motion of the limb which did not result in touching of the body or coming to rest", and *self-touch*, defined as "any act resulting in the touching of the person's own body" (p. 46). Thus, *free movements* include all gesture values described by Efron or by Freedman's value *object-focused.* The value *self-touch* corresponds to Freedman's value *body-focused,* with the exception that the value *body-focused* does not only include touching of the body but also manipulation of objects, while Kimura's value *self-touch* explicitly excludes the latter movements. Kimura's system has been applied by several researchers; most of them were interested in hand preferences. Later studies using Kimura's system reported the interrater reliability (e.g. Lavergne & Kimura, 1987).

However, recent research has demonstrated that the value *free movements* is too broad for neuropsychological research, as it collapses hand movements that are associated with different neuropsychological functions (Lausberg & Kita, 2003; Lausberg et al., 2007).

For the analysis of movement behaviour in social interaction, the psychologists Ekman and Friesen (1969) defined the main values *illustrators, emblems, adaptors*, *regulators,* and *affect display.* The definitions of these values are predominantly functional. Thus, some main values contain several movement classes, e.g. *regulators* can be position shifts but also head nods. Accordingly, there is no precise definition referring to the visual appearance of the movement.

Illustrators (equivalent to Efron's *physiographics* and *ideographics*) illustrate verbal messages and are closely linked to content and form of language statements like phrasing, contour of voice, volume, etc. Within the main value of *illustrates*, several types are distinguished that are adopted from Efron: *baton, ideograph, pictograph, spatial movements, kinetograph,* and *deictic movements*. *Emblems* are non-verbal signals which generally can be replaced by one or two words and which are known to all participants in a social group. Ekman and Friesen's definition of *emblem* is comparable but not perfectly matching Efron's definition, as they include gestures with a morphological relationship to the referent. *Affect display* is defined for facial movements (and therefore, not discussed here). *Adaptors* serve for self-regulation. There is some overlap with Freedman's *body-focused* movements. *Regulators* serve to maintain and regulate verbal interaction. The latter two main values each include various classes of movements. Particularly, the conceptualization of the system that *illustrators, emblems, adaptors*, and *affect display* may all function as *regulators* causes a methodological problem.

McNeill‘s classification system (1992), which has been primarily designed for psycholinguistic research, includes the gesture values *beats, iconics, metaphorics,* and *deictics*. *Beats* and *deictics* are equivalent to Efron's *batons* and *deictics*. *Iconics* are comparable to Efron‘s *physiographs* but only those depictive gestures are classified as *iconic* in which the concomitant verbal statement refers to a concrete content, e.g. gesturally depicting a circular form when talking about a concrete ball. In contrast, *metaphorics* are depictive gestures that are accompanied by a verbal statement that refers to abstract contents, e.g. gesturally depicting a circular form when referring to a project that is rounded off or complete. It should be emphasized that the distinction between *iconics* and *metaphorics* actually refers to the verbal message that accompanies the gesture, and not to the gesture per se.

Recent studies applying McNeill's system or expanded versions examine interrater agreement (e.g. Kita et al., 2007).

To summarize, there are several coding systems for gestures, i.e., for body movements that have a communicative or expressive function. While gestures can be head movements or foot movements, they are most often hand/arm movements. Therefore, most of the systems focus on hand movements. Some systems also include an analysis of self-touching behaviour of the hands.

Despite different scientific backgrounds and different terminologies, there is a substantial overlap between the values of the different systems. Using Efron's seminal system as a frame of reference, Table 1 provides an overview on how the gesture values of the different systems are related to each other. The main values of the respective coding systems are printed in capital letters. In anticipation of part II of this book, the Module III values of the NEUROGES system are included in the table. In addition, the class self-touch is listed.

Obviously, not all gesture values of the other systems can be clearly allocated to Efron's values. Values in the same line of the table are comparable, but they do not necessarily match perfectly. However, Table 1 may be used as a form of a translation scheme to facilitate the comparison between the research studies using the different coding systems for hand movements and gesture.

Table 1 Comparison of the values of different gesture coding systems

Efron (1941)	**Ekman & Friesen (1969)**	**Freedman (1972)**	**Kimura (1973)**	**McNeill (1992)**	**Lausberg (2009)**
DISCUR-SIVE> baton	ILLUSTRA-TOR> baton	OBJECT-FOCUSED > speech primacy >> punctuat-ing	FREE MOVE MENTS	beat	EMPHASIS > baton > super- imposed > back-toss > palm-out
DISCUR-SIVE> ideo-graphic	ILLUSTRA-TOR> ideo-graph	OBJECT-FOCUSED > motor pri-macy	FREE MOVE MENTS	meta-phoric	SPATIAL RELA-TION PRESENTA-TION > route > position
OBJECTIVE > physi-ographic> iconographic	ILLUSTRATOR > pictograph	OBJECT-FOCUSED > motor pri-macy >> represen-tational	FREE MOVE MENTS	iconic, meta-phoric	FORM PRESEN-TATION > shape > size
	ILLUSTRATOR > spatial move-ments				SPATIAL RELA-TION PRESENTA-TION > route > position

OBJECTIVE >physio-graphic>> kinetographic	ILLUSTRA-TOR> kineto-graph	OBJECT-FOCUSED > motor pri-macy >> represen-tational	FREE MOVE MENTS	iconic, meta-phoric	MOTION QUALITY PRESENTATION > manner > dynamics PANTOMIME > transitive > intransitive
OBJECTIVE > deictic	ILLUSTRA-TOR>deictic movements	OBJECT-FOCUSED > motor pri-macy >> pointing	FREE MOVE MENTS	deictic	EGOCENTRIC DEICTIC > external target > You > self > body EGOCENTRIC DIRECTION > neutral > imperative > self-related
OBJECTIVE > emblematic	EMBLEM	OBJECT-FOCUSED	FREE MOVE MENTS		EMBLEM
-	(ADAPTORS and REGULA-TORS may be self-touching movements)	BODY-FOCUSED	SELF-TOUC H	-	SUBJECT-ORIENTED AC-TION

While there are no validity studies according to psychometric standards, the fact that there is basic consensus among different - more or less independent - researchers concerning the existence of certain gesture values supports the researchers' propositions that these values constitute functional entities.

The gesture coding systems define the values by describing their function. They vary in the degree to which the visual appearance of the body movement is referred to. Kimura's system defines the two values with regard to the visual appearance. Efron supplements the functional analysis by a spatio-temporal analysis, and Freedman provides particularly for the main value body-focused movements precise descriptions of the visual appearance of the movement. However, even when values are mainly defined by their function, raters will typically be able to code the same values based on the visual appearance of the movement alone. As an example, raters can reliably identify a *deictic* (pointing gesture) or an *iconographic* gesture (depicting a form), even if they cannot listen to the speech that accompanies the gesture. Therefore, it is argued here these function-oriented coding systems partly work based on the observers' (implicit and explicit) knowledge about the meaning or the psychodynamic function that a body movement with a certain visual appearance has in a given culture. Therefore, while in the coding systems the values are primarily defined by a description of their function, they could likewise be defined by a description of their visual appearance.

Some values such as *ideographs, metaphorics,* and *iconics* are confounded with linguistic assessments. Furthermore, since the systems focus on gestures and partly on self-touch, they are clearly less comprehensive than the coding systems exposed in Section 3.3. With regard to hand / arm movements, Freedman's and Kimura's system are comprehensive insofar as they code gestures and self-touches, the latter class obviously including implicit movements. In most studies, applying Kimura's system, the laterality of the hand movement has been noted. Likewise, the laterality is reported in studies using Freedman's system (e.g. Souza-Poza et al., 1979).

While they did not conduct a segmentation of the ongoing stream of behaviour, Kimura and Freedman coded all hand movements displayed in a certain interval of time. They counted the number of *free movements* and *object-focused* movements and of *self-touches* and *discrete body-focused* movements per 5 and 10 minutes, respectively. For *continuous body-focused* activity, Freedman and colleagues also registered the time spent with this behaviour in seconds / 10 minutes (see Section 2.4).

Thus, while Kimura's system contains too broad values, Freedman's system is well suited for empirical and even quantitative research. However, it is limited to hand / arm movements. For Efron's referential coding system, some validity of the gesture values can be assumed, since - despite different terminologies - other researchers have later come to similar hypotheses concerning the meaning of certain gestures that can be identified by their visual appearance. As Efron employed a three-fold analysis, a detailed description of the visual appearance of the gesture values is provided.

3.5 Systems that register alterations in movement behaviour

3.5.1 Movement psychopathology

Several coding systems have been developed that focus especially on alterations of movement behaviour associated with mental disease. Since the beginnings of modern psychiatry, quantitative and qualitative alterations of movement behaviour have been noted in patients with psychiatric and neuropsychiatric disease. These are so prominent that the movement pathology has been considered as part of symptomology (Kraepelin, 1899, Kretschmer, 1921; Bleuler, 1949). The traditional psychiatric classification is presented here since its use is still prevalent in the clinical field. It comprises two broad values, *hypokinetic* and *hyperkinetic* forms. *Hypokinetic* disorders include *bradykinesis* (slow movement), *akinesis/hypokinesis* (absence/poverty of body movements), *amimics/hypomimics* (absence/poverty of facial expression), *catalepsy* (maintaining a fixed body position for a long time), *catatonia* (a state of immobility), *waxen flexibility, rigidity, mutism* (absence of speaking), and *retardation. Hyperkinetic* disorders include *mannerisms, habits, stereotypes, agitation, hyperactivity,* and *restlessness.*

These movement values do not form a coherent system but they unsystematically register different aspects of movement behaviour, quantitative aspects such as no or little movement (*akinesis* or *hypokinesis*), qualitative aspects such as bound flow (*waxen flexibility*), or behavioural patterns such as *stereotypes*. While most of the movement values are descriptive referring to the movement quantity or quality, some values imply hypotheses about the (absence of a) function of the movement. For example, *stereotyped* movements are defined as repetitive, rhythmic, and useless patterns of movement. However, Jones (1965) demonstrated that considering the content of the delusional belief certain *stereotypes* are psychodynamically meaningful, e.g. the repetitive performance of a praying gesture may serve to soothe delusionally visualized demons. To check the objectivity of qualitative movement values used in psychiatry, Wallbott carried out a study (1989) in which psychiatric patients' movement behaviour was judged by 20 independent raters. The interrater agreement was highest for the values that described physical aspects of movement such as tense, fast, or expansive. For values describing aspects that according to Wallbott refer to the Gestalt of the movement such as jittery, clumsy, uncontrolled or angular, the agreement was poor.

The above outlined psychiatric classification comes from a historical era in which psychiatric diseases could not yet be treated medicinally and therefore, extreme forms of the movement disorder such as *catalepsy* were displayed. Among those patients were many who would nowadays be treated in neurology, such as those with encephalitis lethargica or tertiary syphilis. Therefore, at that time, the movement values had been created to describe extreme alterations of movement behaviour including those caused by brain damage. Nowadays, due to the effective medical treatment and to the separation of psychiatric patients from neurological patients less severe movement disturbances are observed. The traditional movement values, however, are not sensitive enough to register these milder forms of movement behaviour disturbance.

Since the introduction of neuroleptics in the nineteen sixties, the psychiatric movement behaviour research has shifted to movement disorders that are due to side-effects of neuroleptic medication. In fact, these movement disturbances are severe and socially stigmatizing. They are classified as *acute dystonia* (involuntary movements such as torticollis, tongue protrusion, grimacing), *parkinsonism* (hypokinesia and rigidity), *akathesia* (restlessness with an involuntary inability to sit or stand still), and *tardive dykinesia* (involuntary movements such as chewing and sucking movements, grimacing). Contrary to the popular belief that the prevalence of the neuroleptically induced movement disorders has decreased since the introduction of the so-called atypical neuroleptics, the prevalence has doubled in the last 20 years (Halliday et al., 2002).

Several rating scales have been developed to register movement behaviour alterations that are assumed to be neuroleptically induced, such as Abnormal Involuntary Movement Scale (AIMS), Rockland Scale, Hillside Acathesia Scale, or Simpson-Angus Scale. These scales conceptually imply that the coded movement disorder is induced by neuroleptic medication. However, it is noteworthy that the descriptions of movement disorders from the pre-neuroleptic era are similar to those described today as being induced by neuroleptics (Rogers, 1985). In fact, recent research challenges the dogma that *parkinsonism* and involuntary movements such as *dystonia, dyskinesia,* and *akathesia* in schizophrenic patients are unambiguously caused to neuroleptic treatment. These studies, which are difficult to conduct as nowadays there are only few schizophrenic patients who are **not** treated with neuroleptics, indicate that the same movement disorders that can be caused by neuroleptics may occur as a symptom of the psychiatric disease per se. Using the Abnormal Involuntary Movement Scale and the Rockland Scale, Owens et al. (1982) reported involuntary movements in patients with severe chronic schizophrenic patients who had never been exposed to neuroleptic medication. Caligiuri et al. (1993) and Chatterjee et al. (1995) found *parkinsonism* in neuroleptic-naive patients. Similar alterations of movement behaviour were reported for neuroleptic-free as compared to medicated schizophrenic patients (Rogers, 1985; Bräuning, 1995). Furthermore, the descriptions of schizophrenic patients in the era before the introduction of neuroleptic medication (see above) confirm the existence of these movement disorders as part of the schizophrenic symptomatology (Kahlbaum, 1874, Wernicke, 1900; Kleist, 1943; Reiter, 1926; Leonhard, 1957). Of course, these early descriptions can only be used anecdotally because the diagnostic criteria for schizophrenic diseases have changed over time (Rogers, 1992).

As regards to the similarity of illness related movement behaviour alterations and neuroleptically induced movement behaviour alterations, it has to be considered that some of the illness related movement disorders are nowadays falsely categorized as neuroleptically induced. Brenner and Rheuban (1978) coined the term "catatonic dilemma" for the case of patient in whom it was not possible to differentiate if the *catatonic* symptoms were illness-related (then termed febrile catatonia) or medication-related (then termed malignant neuroleptic syndrome). Likewise, Krüger & Bräunig (1995) reported a deterioration of catatonic symptoms during neuroleptic therapy in 6 patients in whom it was not possible to differentiate between a non-response to medical treatment resulting in a deterioration of catatonia and a medication side effect (malignant neuroleptic syndrome). In the same line, in some neuroleptic-naïve patients *parkinsonism* and *involuntary movements* are observed (e.g. Chatterjee et al., 1995; Bräuning, 1995) that cannot be distinguished on clinical inspection from neuroleptic-induced movement disorders. Lausberg and Hellweg (1998) have pointed out that illness-related and medication-related components may interplay in a *catatonic* syndrome.

In this way, catatonic *hyper*- and *parakinesia* are similar to neuroleptically induced early and late *dyskinesia*, catatonic *hypokinesia* is similar to *parkinsonism*, and pernicious or febrile *catatonia* is similar to malignant neuroleptic syndrome (Bräunig, 1994). It is evident that to solve this "dilemma" movement categories and values are needed that suit for basic research, i.e., the categories and values need to be descriptive referring to the visual appearance of the movement, neutral with regard to hypotheses about the etiology of the movement disorder, sensitive, and comprehensive. Commonly used scales such as the Abnormal Involuntary Movement Scale (AIMS), Rockland Scale, Hillside Acathesia Scale, or Simpson-Angus Scale do not fulfil these criteria. They imply that the movement behaviour alteration observed is induced by neuroleptics (but precisely this implication is challenged by recent research). To overcome these deficits, Rogers developed the modified Rogers Scale (1985). Most of its items imply no hypotheses regarding etiology, i.e., whether the movement behaviour alteration is illness related or neuroleptically induced. To further explore the differences between illness related and neuroleptically induced movement disorders, for basic research it is useful to start with obtaining a more complete picture of the patients' movement behaviour. Thus, more comprehensive scales for movement behaviour are indicated. In this regard, the above listed scales are limited in that they focus on a narrow range of abnormal involuntary movements.

Furthermore, the prevalence data on movement disorders in studies using these scales are unacceptably diverse. In a review, Höffler (1995) reports prevalences of early dyskinesia between 2.3% - 66.7%, of Parkinson Syndrome between 8.6% - 72%, of akathisia between 5.5% - 41%, and of late dyskinesia between 8.4% - 70%. Apart from factors such as differences in patient sample, diagnosis, type and dose of medical therapy, these large ranges in prevalence suggest an insufficient reliability of scales. Accordingly, studies have been dedicated specifically to the question of reliability of the above listed rating scales for movement disorders that are assumed to be neuroleptically induced. As an example, Bergen (1988) conducted a study with three raters on the reliability of the AIMS coding. After the raters had been trained with the AIMS training tape, an AIMS examination film, and the coding of 15 training videos, their interrater agreement was good. However, the retest reliability was acceptable only for two items (item 2: facial and oral movements of lips and perioral area; item 4: facial and oral movements of the tongue) but it was poor for three items (item 1: facial and oral movements of muscles of facial expression; item 6: extremity movements: lower; item 7: trunk movements).

The most elaborate system for the detection of pathological features in psychiatric patients' movement behaviour, the Movement Psychodiagnostic Inventory, has been developed by Davis (1991). Davis originally used the Laban movement analysis to set up a list of 70 different movement features that, according to her clinical experience, were frequently found in psychiatric patients (Movement Diagnostic Scale MDS, 1978). Eight main values of movement behaviour alteration were identified: *fragmentation, spatial diffusion, exaggeration, monotony, control, limpness, reduced mobility,* and *dynamics*. In 1991, Davis published a revised version, the Movement Psychodiagnostic Inventory. The Action categories gestures, self-touch, orientation, head movement, facial expression, and position/posture are evaluated regarding *disorganisation* (fragmented and severely dyssynchronized movement behaviour), *immobility* (constriction and reduction of spontaneous movement), *low intensity* (reduction of effort qualities, see LMA), *low spatial complexity* (spatially simple movements), *perseveration / fixed-invariant* (repetition of the same movement), *flaccidity or retardation* (limpness or giving into gravity), *diffusion* (vague, formless movements), *exaggeration* (too large, too intense movements), *hyperkinesis* (rapid sequencing of movements without pause or deceleration), and *even control / suspension* (maintenance of bound flow).

The Movement Psychodiagnostic Inventory is a comprehensive and sensitive system for registering movement disorders associated with mental illness. It uses a descriptive language for the visible dynamics of movement behaviour. The interrater agreement has been examined in all empirical studies using the MPI (e.g. Davis, Cruz, & Berger, 1995; Berger, 1999; Cruz, 1995; Lausberg, 1995). A short version of the inventory was published in 2007 (Davis et al., 2007). The MPI distinguishes between patients with DSM diagnoses of schizophrenia spectrum and personality disorders (Cruz, 1995), and among the latter group between patients with narcissistic and borderline personality disorder (Berger, 1999). With regard to the "catatonic dilemma", Nichols (1985) has demonstrated that in schizophrenic patients the illness-related movement behaviour alterations can be distinguished from medication-related ones.

To summarize, the review on three very different approaches for analyzing movement behaviour alterations in patients with mental disease illustrates the necessity of an effective movement analysis system for basic research. The "catatonic dilemma" that appears when trying to distinguish between illness-related and medication-related movement behaviour alterations is, among others, caused by ineffective movement analysis tools. The traditional psychiatric values are unsystematic, not sufficiently objective, and not sensitive enough. The more recent rating scales for those movement behaviour alterations which are assumed to be induced by neuroleptic medication register only a narrow range of movement behaviour. The validity of these rating scales regarding the aetiology of the movement behaviour alterations is questioned by current empirical research, which has demonstrated that the values are not specific for medication-induced alterations of movement behaviour. The MPI may prove superior to the traditional and recent psychiatric scales because it is descriptive and assesses a broader spectrum of movement features. In fact, it is sensitive to different diagnoses of mental illness and to medication side effects.

3.5.2 Apraxia

While mental illness is accompanied by specific alterations of movement behaviour (Lausberg, forthcoming), neurological disease is associated with other forms of movement behaviour alterations. Depending on the location of the brain lesion or on the functional system that is disturbed, many different alterations of movement behaviour can be observed such as *paralysis* or *ataxia* (a deficit in coordination). Given the aim of this book, however, this section focuses on neurological disturbances of movement behaviour that are caused by impairments of higher cognitive functions. Apraxia is a selective cognitive impairment in the conceptualization of body movements. Thus, the movement behaviour alteration is not caused by paralysis, ataxia, dystonia, etc.

Apraxia is evident in the patient's spontaneous movement behaviour. However, in clinical contexts, for a standardized diagnostics, movement tasks are administered (Goldenberg, 1993; Dovern et al., 2011) (see Chapter 10). Apraxic errors are traditionally classified into two main values, *concept errors* and *execution errors* (Liepmann, 1908; Heilman und Rothi, 1993). The main value of *concept errors* refers to apraxic errors in which the patient is not able to retrieve the correct concept, i.e., for an observer the target movement is not recognizable. Among *concept errors,* the following values are classically distinguished (Liepmann, 1908; Poeck & Kerschensteiner, 1975; Poeck, 1986; Lausberg et al., 2003): *substitution* (the correct movement is replaced by another definite movement, e.g. when asked to pantomime brushing teeth, an elbow flexion / extension is displayed), *perseveration* (the correct movement is replaced by another movement that has occurred, correctly or as an error, in a previous task), *associative movement* (the correct movement is replaced by another movement that shares one feature, e.g. the idea of rotation, with the target movement, e.g. instead of pantomiming how to screw a cap on a bottle, the hand is circling around the opening of the bottle), *searching movements* (there is a clear effort to find the correct movement pattern; different movements and shapes are tried out; the movements are usually slow, hesitant, and performed under visual control). In bimanual movements, the following values of conceptual errors can be observed: *mirroring* (one hand acts like the mirror image of the other hand), *following* (the movement of one hand is immediately followed by the same movement of the other hand), and *both hands unrelated* (the actions of the two hands are spatially and temporally unrelated to each other). The main category of *execution errors* refers to minor apraxic errors in which the correct movement concept is recognizable but the execution of the movement is deficient. At least one phase of the movement needs to be conceptually correct to evaluate the execution. The following types of *execution errors* are suggested here based on categories from the Laban movement analysis (Laban, 1988; Dell, 1979), from computer based kinematic analysis (Poizner et al., 1990; Hermsdörfer et al., 1996), and from other studies that focus on the qualitative analysis of apractic errors (Haaland & Flaherty, 1984; Ochipa et al., 1994): *effort error* (the inadequate quality is chosen, e.g. pantomiming bringing a glass to the mouth with acceleration and free movement flow, i.e., the hand "shoots" to the mouth), *spatial error* (a wrong movement path, e.g. when pantomiming bringing a glass to the mouth the arm raises vertically, then makes a break, and then moves sagittally to the mouth instead of moving in a smooth curve to the mouth), *hand position er-*

ror (a wrong static position of the hand, e.g. when pantomiming brushing the teeth, the hand performs a brushing movement at the level of the forehead), and *hand shape error (*a wrong hand shape, e.g. in the screwdriver pantomime a precision grip, which is normally applied for holding a needle). While the above examples refer to hand/arm movements, apraxia is, likewise, present in the foot/leg movements. As apraxia can be observed in the right and left limbs or only in the left limbs, the laterality of the limb that displays the apraxic error is noted. Objective definitions of the *conceptual* and *execution error* types are available, and the agreement of the trained raters is reported in empirical studies (e.g. Lausberg et al., 2003).

To summarize, apraxia coding systems are descriptive containing not confounded values, but they are not comprehensive. The systems are designed to code specific alterations of movement behaviour, which are associated with neurological disorders that affect the cognitive function of conceptualizing movements. Therefore, the apraxia coding systems are not suited for basic research on the link between movement behaviour and cognitive, emotional, and interactive functions in healthy subjects. However, the apraxic error values provide valuable information about structural components of body movement, as selective deficits in movement execution indicate what components movement consist of. As an example, a selective *hand position error* indicates that the feature hand position represents a distinct element in the conceptualization of a movement. The structural components, which are identified via the selective deficits, can be used as effective criteria for describing the visual appearance of body movements in healthy subjects.

A specific limitation of apraxia coding systems is that they are mainly effective for explicit movements. In order to be able to identify a *concept error*, an observer needs to know what the correct concept would have been. As an example, if the patient spontaneously performs a vague waving movement with the hand, the observer does not know if the desired concept is not retrieved and a *substitution error* is performed, or if the patient actually intends to fan her-/himself but (s)he executes the correct concept with an *effort* error. For a reliable assessment of *concept errors*, either a command to perform a certain movement has to be given to the patient or the patient her-/himself informs the observer about the movement (s)he intended to perform (in fact, given the specific conditions of brain damage, patients with severe apraxia are rarely able to do so). For *execution errors*, the limitation to explicit movements is less prominent, as the correct concept can be recognized and therefore, the observer has a frame of reference to assess the execution. As an example, if the observer recognizes that the patient intends to pantomime brushing the teeth, there is only a limited range of possible performances.

If a frame of reference is provided, i.e., the observer knows the target movement, the apraxic error values can be applied in an objective and reliable manner. The *execution error* values can even be registered with kinematography.

3.6 Summary

The review provides an interdisciplinary overview on the spectrum of coding systems that have been designed to analyze movement behaviour as a reflection of emotional, cognitive, and interactive functions as well as their disturbances.

Many of the systems are primarily **descriptive** with regard to the visual appearance of the body movements. These are notably those of the first group, i.e., Laban Movement Analysis (LMA), Kinesic analysis, Movement Signature Analysis (MSA), but also the Movement Psychodiagnostic Inventory, some scales for 'neuroleptic-induced' alterations, and the apraxia coding systems. Among the gesture coding systems, Kimura's, Freedman's and Efron's system provide some descriptions of the visual appearance of the gestures and self-touches. While, otherwise, the gesture coding systems primarily refer to the function of the movement, it has been argued that their values could likewise be identified based on movement criteria. Some gesture values are **confounded** with linguistic values.

Comprehensiveness applies mainly to the first group and to the MPI. These comprise several classes of body movements (MSA, MPI, Kinesic analysis) and register the quality of movement (LMA, MSA, MPI). The movement of several parts of the body or of the body as a whole is coded. These systems provide a complete picture of an individual's movement repertoire. However, their application is time-consuming and therefore, the analysis is limited to movement behaviour samples of a few minutes. Among the gesture analysis systems, Freedman's system is the most comprehensive one, as it comprises the two classes gesture and self-touch, the latter including implicit movements. All movements of the hands and arms are coded. Ekman and Friesen's system is comprehensive as well but the values are not descriptive with regard to the visual appearance of the movements. The coding systems for movement psychopathology are limited to a very narrow range of movements, with the exception of the MPI. The apraxia coding systems are practically limited to explicit body movements.

Limb movement **laterality,** in terms of right, left, and both at a time, has mainly been studied with Kimura's and Freedman's systems. No coding system provides a differentiated coding of the relation between the two hands (or feet) during simultaneous movements, such as dominance of one hand in bimanual movements or the hands acting as a unit.

Movement **patterns**, i.e., recurrent combinations of different movement types displayed by different parts of the body at a time or recurrent sequences of movement types, can be detected primarily with Kinesics, MSA, and MPI. Recurrent sequences could, theoretically, also be identified with Freedman's system as all movements of the hands are coded in a given interval of time.

With the exception of Freedman's value *continuous body focused,* the duration of movement units has not been investigated. To explore the **temporal dimension** of movement behaviour a system is required that segments the ongoing stream of movement into natural units such that any moment in time is considered and attributed to a unit. The MSA and the Kinesic analysis could, theoretically, be used for this purpose, but given their limitation to a few minutes of analysis, general conclusions about the temporal dimension of movement units with a specific value cannot be drawn.

While Objectivity and Reliability have been the criteria for the coding systems to be included in the review, a final note on the **validity** shall be given. As it has been noted above, for none of the existing systems the validity can be judged as sufficiently established with regard to current psychometric standards. For Efron's referential coding system some degree of validity can be assumed, since other - more or less independent - researchers have arrived at similar assumptions about the meaning of certain gesture values that are characterized by a specific visual appearance. Other coding systems that make an explicit claim about the validity require a careful examination. This applies especially to the scales for neuroleptic side effects concerning the aetiology of the respective alterations and to the Kestenberg Movement Profile (KMP) regarding the association with developmental stages.

To conclude, the interdisciplinary review reveals that across scientific disciplines a variety of different coding systems are available. These systems have different advantages and disadvantages for application in basic empirical research.

References

Bartenieff, I. (1991). Tanztherapie. In E. Willke, G. Hölter, & H. Petzhold (Ed.), *Tanztherapie - Theorie und Praxis* (pp. 259-88). Paderborn: Junfermann.

Bergen, J.A., Carter, N.B., Craig, J., MacFarlane, D., Smith, E.F., & Beumont, P.J.V. (1988). AIMS Ratings - Repeatability. *British Journal of Psychiatry, 152*, 670-673.

Berger, M.R. (1999). Movement patterns in borderline and narcissistic personality disorders. Dissertation Abstracts International: Section B, *The Sciences & Engineering Vol. 60(9-B)*, Apr 2000, 4875.

Bernstein, P.L. (1991). Objektbeziehungen, Selbstpsychologie und Tanztherapie. In E. Willke, G. Hölter, and H. Petzhold (Ed.), *Tanztherapie, Theorie und Praxis* (pp. 217-44). Paderborn: Junfermann

Birdwhistell, R.L. (1970). *Kinesics and Context. Essays on Body Motion Communication.* Philadelphia: University of Pennsylvania Press.

Bleuler, M. (1949 (8. Aufl.), 1983 (15. Aufl.)). Lehrbuch der Psychiatrie, Berlin: Springer.

Bogen, J.E. (1993). The callosal syndromes. In: Kenneth M. Heilman and E. Valenstein (eds.), *Clinical Neuropsychology*, 337-408. New York, Oxford: Oxford University Press.

Bogen, J.E. (2000). Split-brain basics: Relevance for the concept of one's other mind. *The Jounal of the American Academy of Psychoanalysis 28*, 341-369.

Bohnemeyer, J., Enfield, N.J., & Essegbey, J. (2007): Principles of event segmentation in language: The case of motion events. *Language 83*, 495-532.

Bräunig, P. (Ed.) (1995). *Differenzierung katatoner und neuroleptika-induzierter Bewegungsstörungen.* Stuttgart, New York: Georg Thieme

Brenner, I, & Rheuban, W.J. (1978). The catatonic dilemma. *The American Journal of Psychiatry, 135 (10)*, 1242-3.

Büning, C. (2012). *Untersuchung des Bewegungsverhaltens und Körpererlebens männlicher Patienten mit Borderline-Persönlichkeitsstörung.* German Sports University, Cologne.

Caligiuri, M.P., Lohr, J.B., Panton, D., & Harris J. (1993). Extrapyramidal motor abnormalities associated with late-life psychosis. *Schizophrenia Bulletin 19*, 747-53.

Chatterjee, A., Chakos, M., Koreen, A., Geisler, S., Sheitman, B., Woerner, M., Kane, J.M., Alvir, J., & Lieberman J.A. (1995). Prevalence and clinical correlates of extrapyramidal signs and spontaneous dyskinesia in never-medicated schizophrenic patients. *The American Journal of Psychiatry 152*, 1724-9.

Cruz, R. (1996). An empirical investigation of the movement psychodiagnostic inventory. Unveröffentlichte Dissertation in Psychologie: Section B, *The Sciences & Engineering Vol. 57(2-B).* University of Arizona, Dept. of Educational Psychology, August 1996, 1495.

Davis, M. (1991, rev. 1997). *Guide to movement analysis methods.* Pittsburgh, PA. USA.: Behavioral Measurement Database Services, P.O. Box 11028.

Davis, M. (1983). An Introduction to the Davis Nonverbal Communication Analysis System. *American Journal of Dance Therapy, 6*, 49-74.

Davis, M., Markus, K. A., Walters, S. B., Vorus, N., & Connors, B. (2005). Behavioral Cues to Deception vs. Topic Incriminating Potential in Criminal Confessions *Law and Human Behavior, 29*(6), 683-704.

Davis, M., & Hadiks, D. (1990). Nonverbal behaviour and client state changes during psychotherapy. *Journal of Clinical Psychology, 46*(3), 340-351.

Davis, M., & Dulicai, D. (1992). Hitler's movement signature. *TDR The Drama Review, 36,* 152-172

Davis, M., Dulicai, D., Hadiks, D., & Berger, M.R. (1992). Body language of world leaders. Presented at the Convention of the American Psychological Association, Washington, D.C.

Davis, M., & Hadiks, D. (1994). Nonverbal aspects of therapist attunement. *Journal of Clinical Psychology, 50*(3), 393-405.

Davis, M. Cruz, R.F., & Berger, M.R. (1995). Movement and psychodiagnosis: Schizophrenia spectrum and dramatic personality disorders. Presented at the Conference of the American Psychological Association, NYC.

Davis, M. (1996). Guide to Movement Analysis Methods. Unpublished Coding Guide.Part 1, Movement Signature Analysis (MSA), Part 2, Movement Psychodiagnostic Inventory (MPI), Part 3 Nonverbal Interaction and States Analysis (NISA)

Davis, M., Lausberg, H., Cruz, R., Berger, M.R., & Dulicai, D. (2007). The Movement Psychodiagnostic Inventory (MPI). In S. C. Koch, & S. Bender (Ed.), *Movement Analysis - Bewegungsanalyse. The Legacy of Laban, Bartenieff, Lamb and Kestenberg*. Berlin: Logos Verlag.

Degener, A. (2013). *Bewegungsverhalten und Körperbild von Patientinnen mit Borderline-Persönlichkeitsstörung unter besonderer Berücksichtigung von selbstverletzendem Verhalten* Technische Universität Dortmund.

Dell, C. (1979). *A primer for movement description using effort-shape and supplementary concepts*. New York: Dance Notation Bureau Press.

Dovern, A., Fink, G.R., & Weiss, P.H. (2011). Diagnostik und Therapie der Gliedmaßenapraxie. *Fortschritte der Neurologie-Psychiatrie, 79*, 345-357.

Efron, D. (1941, 2nd ed. 1972). *Gesture and culture*. The Hague: Mouton.

Eisenberg, P., & Reichline, P. (1939). Judgements of Dominance Feelings from Motion Pictures of Gait. *Journal of Abnormal and Social Psychology 10*.

Ekman, P., & Friesen, W.V. (1969). The Repertoire of Nonverbal Behaviour: Categories, Origins, Usage and Coding. *Semiotica, 1*, 49-99.

Ekman, P., & Friesen, W. (1974). Nonverbal behavior and psychopathology. In R.J. Friedman, & M.M. Katz, (Ed.), *The Psychology of Depression* (pp.203-32). New York: John Wiley & Sons.

Ekman, P., Friesen, W., & Hager J.C. (2002). *Facial Action Coding System: The Manual on CD ROM.* Salt Lake City: A Human Face.

Freedman, N. (1972). The Analysis of Movement Behavior During the Clinical Interview. In A.W. Siegman, B. Pope (Ed.), *Studies in Dyadic Communication* (pp. 153-175). New York: Pergamon.

Freedman, N., O'Hanlon, J., Oltman, P., & Witkin, H.A. (1972). The imprint of psychological differentiation on kinetic behaviour in varying communicative contexts. *Journal of Abnormal Psychology, 79*(3), 239-258.

Frijda, N.H. (1965). Mimik und Pantomimik. In: R. Kirchhoff, Hrsg. *Handbuch der Psychologie, Band 5, Ausdruckspsychologie*. Göttingen: Hogrefe 351-422.

Gazzarata, J. (2010). *Analyse von Bewegungsmustern bei Patienten mit Depression und Schmerzstörung in stationärer Therapie. Gruppenvergleich und zeitabhängige Effekte.* Unpublished Diploma, Universität, Wien.

Golden, C.J., Hammeke, T., & Purisch, A. (1978). Diagnostic Validity of a Standardized Version of Luria's Neuropsychological Version. *Journal of Consulting and Clinical Psychology, 46*, 1258-65.

Goldenberg, G. (1993). Praxie. In D.Y. von Cramon, Mai, N., & Ziegler, W. (Ed.), *Neuropsychologische Diagnostik* (pp. 259-286). Weinheim: VCH.

Günther, W. (1980). Untersuchungen zur Wirksamkeit mentaler Trainingsverfahren bei grobmotorischen Bewegungsstörungen. Unveröffentlichte Dissertation Psychologisches Institut Tübingen.

Haaland, K.Y., & Flaherty, D. (1984). The Different Types of Limb Apraxia Errors made by Patients with Left vs. Right Hemispehre Damage. *Brain and Cognition, 3*, 370 - 384.

Hall, E.T. (1966). *The Hidden Dimension.* New York: Doubleday.

Halliday, J., Farrington, S., Macdonald, S., MacEwan, T., Sharkey, V., & McCreadie, R. (2002). Nithsdale Schizophrenia Surveys 23: movement disorders. 20 year review. *British Journal of Psychiatry, 181*, 422-427.

Hehlmann, W. (1968, 6. Aufl.). *Wörterbuch der Psychologie*, Stuttgart: Kröner

Heilman, K.M., & Rothi, L.J.G. (1993). Apraxia. In K.M. Heilman, & E. Valenstein, (Ed.), *Clinical Neuropsychology* (pp. 141-164). New York, Oxford: Oxford University Press.

Hermsdörfer, J., Mai, N., Spatt, J., Marquardt, C., Veltkamp, R., & Goldenberg, G. (1996). Kinematic analysis of movement imitation in apraxia. *Brain 119*, 1575-1586.

Höffler, J. (1995), Extrapyramidalmotorische Nebenwirkungen unter Neuroleptika – Phänomenologie und Prävalenz. In: P. Bräunig (Ed.), *Differenzierung katatoner und neuroleptika-induzierter Bewegungsstörungen* (pp. 12-17). Georg Thieme Verlag Stuttgart, New York.

Jones, I.H. (1965). Observations on Schizophrenic Stereotypies. *Comprehensive Psychiatry, 6(5),* 323-35.

Kahlbaum, K. (1874). *Die Katatonie oder das Spannungsirresein.* Berlin: Hirschwald.

Kendon, A. (1972). Some relationships between body motion and speech. In: A. Siegman and B. Pope (eds). Studies in dyadic communication, 177 - 210, Pergamon Press, New York.

Kendon, A. (2002). Some usese of the head shake. *Gesture, 2(2),* 147-182.

Kestenberg, J. (1965a). The Role of Movement Patterns in Development I. *Psychoanalytic Quarterly, 24(1),* 1-36.

Kestenberg, J. (1965b). The Role of Movement Patterns in Development II. *Psychoanalytic Quarterly, 24(4),* 515-63.

Kestenberg J. The Role of Movement Patterns in Development III. Psychoanalytic Quarterly 1967; 26(3): 356 – 409.

Kimura, D. (1973). Manual Activity during Speaking - I. Right-handers. *Neuropsychologia, 11*, 45-50.

Kita, S., de Condappa, O., & Mohr, C. (2007). Metaphor explanation attenuates the right-hand preference for depictive co-speech gestures that imitate actions. *Brain and Language* 101: 185-197.

Kleist, K. (1943). Die Katatonien. *Nervenarzt, 16*, 1-10.

Knapp, M.L., & Hall J.A. (1992). *Nonverbal Communication in Human Interaction* (3rd edition). Harcourt Brace College Publishers, Orlando.

Kraepelin, E. (1899) *Psychiatrie*. Leipzig, Barth.

Kretschmer, E. (1921). *Körperbau und Charakter. Untersuchungen zum Konstitutionsproblem und zur Lehre von den Temperamenten*. Berlin Springer.

Krüger, S., & Bräunig, P. (1995). Bipolare Erkrankungen mit katatoner Symptomaitik – periodische Katatonien. In: P. Bräunig (Ed.), *Differenzierung katatoner und neuroleptika-induzierter Bewegungsstörungen* (pp. 74-78). Georg Thieme Verlag Stuttgart, New York.

Laban, R. (1988). *The Mastery of Movement*, reprinted edition. Worcester: Northcote House.

Lausberg, H. (1995). *Bewegungsverhalten als Prozeßparameter in einer kontrollierten Therapiestudie mit funktioneller Entspannung (Movement behaviour as process parameter in a controlled therapy study with functional relaxation).* Paper presented at the 42nd Annual meeting of the Deutschen Kollegiums für Psychosomatische Medizin (German Committee of Psychosomatic Medicine).

Lausberg, H. (1997). Bewegungsdiagnosetest mit Bewertungsskalen für Diagnostik und Therapieevaluation in der Tanztherapie. *Zeitschrift für Tanztherapie, 7,* 35-42.

Lausberg, H. (1998). Does Movement Behavior Have Differential Diagnostic Potential? *American Journal of Dance Therapy 20(2)*, 85-99.

Lausberg, H. (forthcoming). *Alterations of movement behaviour associated with mental illness*. Body - Language - Communication, Vol II. C. Müller, Fricke, Ladewig, McNeill, Teßendorf. De Gruyter Berlin.

Lausberg, H. & Hellweg, R. (1998). "Catatonic dilemma". Therapy with lorazepam and clozapine. *Nervenarzt, 69(9)*, 818-22.

Lausberg, H, & Kita, S. (2003).The content of the message influences the hand choice in co-speech gestures and in gesturing without speaking. *Brain and Language, 86,* 57-69.

Lausberg, H., von Wietersheim, J., & Feiereis, H. (1996). Movement Behaviour of Patients with Eating Disorders and Inflammatory Bowel Disease. A Controlled Study. *Psychotherapy and Psychosomatics, 65(6),* 272-6.

Lausberg, H., v. Arnim, A., & Joraschky, P. (2007). Bewegungsanalyse in der Körperbild- und Körperschemadiagnostik. In G. H. P. Geißler (Ed.), *Lebensbewegungen. Zum körperlichen Geschehen in der psychoanalytischen Therapie. Ein Lehrbuch* (pp. 165-196). Wien: Springer Verlag.

Lausberg, H., von Wietersheim, J. Wilke, E., & Feiereis, H. (1989). Bewegungsbeschreibung psychosomatischer Patienten in der Tanztherapie. *Psychotherapie, Psychosomatik, Medizinische Psychologie , 38*, 259-64.

Lausberg, H., Cruz, R.F., Kita, S., Zaidel, E., & Ptito, A. (2003). Pantomime to visual presentation of objects: left hand dyspraxia in patients with complete callosotomy. *Brain, 126*, 343-360.

Lavergne, J., & Kimura, D. (1987). Hand movement asymmetry during speech: no effect of speaking topic. *Neuropsychologia, 25(4),* 689-693.

Leonhard, K. (1957). *Aufteilung der endogenen Psychosen und ihre differenzierte Ätiologie*. Stuttgart, New York: Georg Thieme Verlag.

Liepmann, H. (1908). *Drei Aufsätze aus dem Apraxiegebiet*. Berlin: Karger.

Lott, P. (1999). *Gesture and aphasia*. Bern, Peter Lang.

Marian, H., von Wietersheim, J., & Lausberg, H. (2010). *Analyse des Bewegungsverhaltens von Patientinnen mit Essstörungen und chronisch entzündlichen Darmerkrankungen: Ein Vergleich von Fremd- und Selbstwahrnehmung.* Paper presented at the Deutscher Kongress für Psychosomatik und Psychotherapie. Abstract in Psychologische Medizin, Sondernummer zur 61. Arbeitstagung des Deutschen Kollegiums für Psychosomatische Medizin (DKPM) und 18. Jahrestagung der Deutschen Gesellschaft für Psychosomatische Medizin und Ärztliche Psychotherapie (DGPM), Berlin.

McClave, E., Kim, H., Tamer, R., & Mileff, M. (2007). Head movements in the context of speech in Arabic, Bulgarian, Korean, and African-American Vernacular English. *Gesture, 7(3),* 343-390.

McNeill, D. (1992). *Hand and mind. What gestures reveal about thought.* Chicago, London: The University of Chicago Press.

Mason, D.J. (1957). Judgements of Leadership based upon Physiognomonic Cues. *Journal of Abnormal and Social Psychology 54 (2),* 273-4.

Nichols, V.L. (1985). *Effects of antipsychotic medication on the movement pathologies of chronic schizophrenic patients*. Creative Arts in Therapy Department, Hahnemann University Graduate School.

North, M. (1990). *Personality Assessment Through Movement*. Worcester: Billing & Sons.

Ochipa, C., Rothi, L.J.G., & Heilman, K.M. (1994). Conduction apraxia. *Journal of Neurology, Neurosurgery, and Psychiatry, 57*, 1241 - 1244.

Oseretzky, N. (1931). Psychomotorik. *Zeitschrift für Angewandte Psychologie, Beiheft 1*, 57.

Owens, D. G. C., & Johnstone E. C. (1982). Spontaneous involuntary disorders of movement. *Archives of General Psychiatry, 39*, 452-61.

Paarmann, C., Marian, H., von Wietersheim, J., & Lausberg, H. (2012). Junge Frauen mit Essstörungen und chronisch entzündlicher Darmerkrankung schätzen ihr Bewegungsverhalten realistischer ein als gesunde junge Frauen, die ihr Bewegungsverhalten idealisiert wahrnehmen. Unpublished paper presented at Deutscher Kongress für Psychosomatische Medizin und Psychotherapie (DKPM), 28. - 31.3.12, München

Poeck, K. (1986). The clinical examination for motor apraxia. *Neuropsychologia, 24*(1), 129-134.

Poeck, K., & Kerschensteiner, M. (1975). Analysis of the sequential motor events in oral apraxia. In K. J. Zülch, Creutzfeldt, O., Galbraith, G.C. (Ed.), *Cerebral Localization* (pp. 98-114). Berlin, Heidelberg, New York: Springer-Verlag.

Poizner, H., Mack, L., Verfaellie, M., Rothi, L.J.G., & Heilman, K.M. (1990). Three-dimensional Computergraphic Analysis of Apraxia. *Brain, 113*, 85-101.

Reiter, P.J. (1926). Extrapyramidal motor-disturbances in dementia praecox. *Acta Psychiatrica et Neurologica, 1*, 287-305.

Rogers, D. (1985). The motor disorders of severe psychiatric illness: a conflict of paradigms. *British Journal of Psychiatry, 147*, 221-32.

Sossin, K.M. (1987). Reliability of the Kestenberg Movement Profile. *Movement Studies - A journal of the Laban/Bartenieff Insitutute of Movement Studies* 2, 23-28.

Ulrich, A., & Harms, K. (1985). A Video Analysis of the Non-Verbal Behaviour of Depressed Patients Before and After Treatment. *Journal of Affective Disorders, 9*, 63-67.

Wallbott, H.G. (1989). Movement quality changes in psychopathological disorders. In: B. Kirkaldy (Ed.). *Normalities and abnormalities in human movement,* 128-146. Basel: Karger.

Wernicke, C. (1900). *Grundriss der Psychiatrie in klinischen Vorlesungen.* Leipzig: Thieme.

Wilke, S. (1995). Die therapeutische Beziehung in psychoanalytisch orientierten Anamnesen und Psychotherapien mit neurotischen, psychosomatischen und psychiatrischen Patienten. *DFG-Bericht Wi 1213/1-1.*

Zacks, J.M., Speer, N.K., Swallow, K.M., Braver, T.S., & Reynolds, J.R. (2007). Event perception: A mind-brain perspective. *Psychological Bulletin 133*, 273-293.

II. The NEUROGES Coding System

4. The Aims and the Development of the NEUROGES Coding System

Hedda Lausberg

4.1 Aims of the NEUROGES System

The previous chapters have demonstrated that there is ample evidence that movement behaviour is linked to cognitive, emotional, and interactive processes. However, thus far, these links have not yet been fully explored and established to such a degree that movement behaviour could be used as a valid measure for these processes.

Therefore, the NEUROGES system is primarily designed as a tool for basic empirical research on movement behaviour and its link to cognitive, emotional, and interactive processes. The secondary aim is to establish the validity of the movement values regarding these processes, so that NEUROGES can be used as valid instrument to measure cognitive, emotional, and interactive processes.

4.2 Application

The NEUROGES Coding system is designed for the analysis of body movement behaviour. It codes the movements of the hands/arms, the head, the trunk, and the feet/legs of the stationary, i.e., the standing, sitting, or lying body. The focus is on the analysis of expressive and communicative body movements in the context of interaction or soliloquy / silent thinking, such as during cognitive tasks. However, instrumental body movements, such as during physical exercise, and manipulating movements, such as during tool use, can be analysed as well.

4.3 Criteria for the development

Given the empirical knowledge on movement behaviour and its relation to cognitive, emotional, and interactive processes (Chapter 2), the advantages and disadvantages of the existing analysis systems (Chapter 3), and the status of movement behaviour research as a scientific discipline (Chapter 1) several demands for the development of a movement behaviour analysis system result. Their realization in the NEUROGES system is explained below.

(i) Descriptiveness

To be suitable for basic research and for the examination of existing paradigms, the values of the NEUROGES system are descriptive. They are defined with regard to the visually perceivable aspect of movement behaviour. Thus, the values can be identified in real life and video registered samples of movement behaviour without knowing the context or listening to the sound.

The movement criteria that are used to describe the body movements, such as the trajectory, the physical contact between the hands, the hand shape, etc., are reported in Chapter 5.

The NEUROGES movement values are not confounded with psychological, linguistic, or other kinds of values. They are neutral as they contain no assessment such as good or bad, correct or incorrect, pathological or healthy, etc.

(ii) Objectivity and Reliability

For empirical research, the observations on movement behaviour need to be objective and reliable. All NEUROGES categories and their values are precisely defined, as well as the criteria used for these definitions (see NEUROGES coding manual, forthcoming). The example of the NEUROGES value *emphasis* illustrates how precisely the values are operationalized (see Subsection 4.5.3).

The reliability of the values has been confirmed by repeated examinations of the interrater agreement and by kinematographic examinations (see Subsection 5.2.2 and Chapter 6). During the development of the NEUROGES system, substantial effort has been made to secure the objectivity and reliability not only for the values but also for the segmentation of the ongoing stream of behaviour. Raters do not only have to agree on the value of a unit, but they also have to agree on whether or not a motion constitutes a movement unit, and when the unit starts and when it ends. While at first glance this decision seems to be trivial, it turns out to be the most difficult one to achieve interrater agreement on. Since among the existing statistical procedures no algorithm was available to calculate the interrater agreement for the segmentation of behaviour, such a procedure has been developed in the course of the NEUROGES project. Part V of this book is entirely dedicated to the achievement and control of interrater reliability.

(iii) Comprehensiveness

It has been a basic principle for the development of the NEUROGES system to integrate the substantial existing knowledge on movement behaviour analysis. Various classes of movement behaviour, such as gesture, self-touch, posture, and rest position, have proven to be related to within-subject cognitive and emotional processes and to between-subjects interactive processes. These traditional classes of movement behaviour are all considered in NEUROGES. While most research has focused on gesture and posture, the classes self-touch and rest position are, likewise, of interest for the NEUROGES system, as they are forms of behaviour that are predominantly displayed beyond the mover's awareness. As such, they are associated with implicit cognitive, emotional, and interactive processes. As it has been pointed out in Chapter 2, in contrast to verbal diagnostic tools, movement behaviour analysis bears the specific potential that it enables to investigate implicit cognitive, emotional, and interactive processes, which substantially coin our thinking, feeling, and interacting.

The different classes are associated with different parts of the body. Gestures are performed with the hands, arms, and shoulders, with the head, and rarely with the feet and legs. Self-touching is typically executed by the hands. Posture and rest position involve the whole body. Consequently, NEUROGES enables to code the movements of different parts of the body. In this regard, limitations of the NEUROGES system are that it does not enable to code the body as a whole, i.e., the shaping of the whole body, e.g. a contraction of the body, the locomotion of the whole body in space, e.g. gait, and the static shape that the body adopts during rest or posture, e.g. a rest position with crossed legs. However, *shifts* between *rest positions / postures* and certain features of *rest positions / postures* are registered.

The NEUROGES Coding system is particularly comprehensive concerning the range of criteria on the basis of which the movement behaviour is classified. All these criteria refer to the visual appearance of the movement, such as the trajectory, the physical contact between the hands, the hand shape, etc. Based on these different criteria, seven categories have been developed: Activation[8], Structure, Focus, Contact, Formal Relation, Function, and Type. In each category, specific movement criteria are used to classify body movements (see Chapter 5). As an example, the Contact category is operationalized by the criteria 'presence/absence of physical contact between the hands (feet)' and 'quality of the contact'.

The comprehensiveness of NEUROGES implies that patterns can be detected, i.e., recurrent combinations of movement types displayed by different parts of the body at a time and recurrent sequences of movement types in the course of time. As it has been discussed in Chapter 2, these movement patterns are associated in an intra-individually and intra-dyadically reliable manner with certain emotional, cognitive, and interactive states.

8 Throughout the book, categories of the NEUROGES system are printed with a capital letter.

(iii) Registration of Laterality

It has been another basic principle for the development of the NEUROGES system to provide a differentiated analysis of the relation between the right and left limbs. In addition to the traditional values right hand, left hand, and both hands, NEUROGES provides a detailed analysis for bilateral movements. This analysis focuses on the presence and quality of physical contact, the dominance, and the symmetry.

As exposed in Chapter 2, the registration of the laterality of unilateral limb movements and of that of the dominant limb in bilateral movements enables to conclude in which hemisphere the movement is generated. If a specific movement value is preferentially performed by the right limb or the left one, the preference suggests that this type is predominantly generated in the contralateral hemisphere. Furthermore, the hemispheric specialization for a certain movement type provides some indication that its generation is associated with those cognitive and emotional processes that are also lateralized to that hemisphere.

(iv) Analysis of the ongoing stream of behaviour

It has been a further basic principle for the development of the NEUROGES system to analyse the ongoing stream of body movement behaviour including rests. The behaviour is smoothly segmented into natural units, i.e., one unit adjoins the next one. Thus, any moment in time is attributed to a unit. This procedure has several advantages.

First of all, it enables to register the duration of the units. As discussed in Chapter 2, the duration of units with a specific value constitutes an intrinsic feature of this value.

The registration of the duration of units with a specific value enables to test the validity of the value. If the mean unit duration of a specific value differs significantly from the mean unit duration of another value, this difference provides evidence that the value represents a behavioural entity that is distinct from that of the other value. Furthermore, as the duration of a unit with a specific value is determined, among others, by the duration of the associated cognitive, emotional, and interactive process, it provides insight into the temporal dimension of the underlying cognitive, emotional, and interactive processes.

Second, as it has already been noted by Freedman and colleagues (Section 2.4) for some movement values the number per time unit, e.g. per minute, is not an effective measure. This applies particularly to *continuous body-focused* activity that may last over several minutes. For this type of movement behaviour it is more effective to register its occurrence in seconds / minute (see also Chapter 17). As an example, in two 50 minutes lasting psychotherapy session, a patient spent 42.59 seconds / minute and 45.48 seconds / minute, respectively, with *irregular on body* movements (Kryger, 2011). In other terms, in each session she spent 35,49 minutes and 37.90 minutes, respectively, with *irregular on body* movements. Thus, for this value, the proportion of time spent with the specific behaviour in seconds per minute is an informative measure supplementing that of the number of units per minute, which in the example was 4,13 / minute and 5,06 / minute, respectively.

Third, the precision of the analysis is improved. The researcher is forced to thoroughly consider each motion and to attribute it to a unit. In contrast, an analysis which is not oriented along the stream of behaviour induces the rater to neglect motions that are ambiguous to code. This applies even more to those methodological approaches in which certain movements are pre-selected from the stream of movement behaviour, e.g. for a study all pointing gestures are to be selected. Movements that do not perfectly match the searched prototype at first sight are often not considered. The more ambiguous forms of the movement value might, however, provide valuable information about the movement value itself and the associated cognitive, emotional, and interactive processes.

Fourth, only the complete analysis of movement behaviour enables to understand the anatomy of movement behaviour. As any motion is identified, the complete picture of body movement behaviour emerges and the relations between the different movement types become evident.

Therefore, in NEUROGES the complete stream of movement behaviour is analysed. The technical procedure that leads to a fine-grained segmentation of behaviour is described below (see 5.5.1).

(v) User-friendly and flexible

As indicated in Chapter 3, comprehensive analysis systems are already available, but their application is time-consuming. Furthermore, the data that the current versions of these systems provide are difficult to submit to statistical analyses. Therefore, special care was taken that NEUROGES is comprehensive but remains user-friendly.

In its complete form, NEUROGES comprises the analysis of the whole body by coding six parts of the body: right hand/arm, left hand/arm, right foot/leg, left foot/leg, trunk, and head. Given the rich spectrum of movements that can be performed by the hands/arms, and accordingly, their importance in expressive and communicative nonverbal behaviour, for hand/arm movements all seven categories are assessed. Theoretically, the same seven step analysis can be conducted for the feet/ legs, but in natural data the range of foot/leg movements is much more limited than those of hand/arm movements. For head and trunk movements, the Activation, Structure, and Function categories are assessed. While this is the "full program" of the NEUROGES movement analysis, NEUROGES has been tailored for a flexible use according to the user's needs. The system has a modular structure that enables to evaluate the parts of the body as well as the categories independent of each other to a large extent. Each part of the body can be assessed individually. Therefore, the user can decide if (s)he wants to analyse all six parts of the body or only one or two of them. Furthermore, the system can be used in a flexible manner according to the researcher's needs as (s)he decide how many categories (s)he wants to analyze. Each category provides specific results and therefore, - depending on the research question - the coding of only the Activation and the Structure categories can provide valuable data.

In addition, NEUROGES is easy to learn and to apply. A detailed coding manual with many examples, an interactive training CD, and many training videos with the correct solutions (codings) are provided to learn the NEUROGES values. To facilitate the coding process, decision algorithms are provided that guide the rater through the analysis of movement behaviour, leading to a fine-grained evaluation (Chapter 5). NEUROGES training seminars are offered on a regular basis, currently in Germany at the German Sport University Cologne and in Switzerland at the University Fribourg.

Technically, the application of NEUROGES has been substantially facilitated by combining it with the annotation tool ELAN. NEUROGES is available as ready-to-use ELAN template file. Part III of this book describes in detail how the coding system is combined with the annotation tool.

Finally, the NEUROGES system is designed in such a way that its output data can be directly submitted to statistical analyses. The codings are easy to export and to transform into variables of statistical files. For SPSS users, sav template files are available in which the NEUROGES output data can be inserted. Procedures for the statistical evaluation and the presentation of the data are described in Part VI of this book.

(vi) Compatible with existing coding systems and with approaches for automatic movement recognition

Another basic principle in the development of the NEUROGES system has been its applicability across scientific disciplines.

As outlined in the previous chapters, developing a common body of knowledge in movement behaviour research has been inhibited by the fact that research is spread across many different scientific disciplines that rarely take notice of each other's findings. One reason for this lack of interdisciplinary exchange is the different terminologies and methodologies. Therefore, NEUROGES has been designed as a potentially interdisciplinary tool.

To suit this purpose NEUROGES is comprehensive and its values are purely descriptive. In particular, during the development care has been taken that NEUROGES can be combined with existing coding systems, e.g. Movement Psychodiagnostic Inventory (Davis, 1991, rev. 1997), Movement Signature (Davis, 1991, rev. 1997), Nonverbal Interaction and States Analysis (Davis, 1991, rev. 1997), Classification of head movements (Kendon, 2002; McClave et al., 2007), Modes of Representation (Müller, 1998), McNeill's gesture coding system (1992), Apraxic error classification systems (Liepmann, 1908; Heilman & Rothi, 1993; Poeck & Kerschensteiner, 1975; Poeck, 1986; Lausberg et al., 2003; Poizner et al., 1990; Hermsdörfer et al., 1996; Haaland & Flaherty, 1984; Ochipa et al., 1994). This list of systems combinable with NEUROGES is not exhaustive. Furthermore, THEME, a software for the pattern detection (Magnus

S. Magnusson, http://hbl.hi.is/), can be applied for NEUROGES. The NEUROGES coding provides no units for facial movements and therefore, it cannot be directly combined with coding systems for facial expression such as FACS (Ekman, Friesen, & Hager, 2002). However, for a comprehensive analysis of nonverbal behaviour both systems can supplement each other.

Its compatibility with other coding systems renders NEUROGES useful for interdisciplinary research. The strength of the NEUROGES system is that it provides algorithms for an objective and reliable segmentation of the ongoing flow of movement behaviour into natural units. These natural units can be used as an objective basis for further qualitative and quantitative analyses with the other coding systems. The design of the chosen system and the research question determine after which of the seven NEUROGES coding steps the chosen system can follow. As an example, McNeill's coding system for hand gestures could follow after Module II. The advantages of an analysis that is based on a segmentation of the ongoing stream of behaviour have been outlined above.

It is noteworthy that the NEUROGES analysis is suited for developing algorithms for automatized movement detection. The NEUROGES values are descriptive with reference to the visual appearance of movements and they are objectively and reliably defined by kinematic and other movement parameters. Therefore, the value definitions can be used directly for defining algorithms for automatized movement recognition. Furthermore, in Module I the right and left hands/arms and feet/legs are coded separately. This design is well compatible with the automatized approaches, in which the movements of the different parts of the body are traced. A current research project in cooperation with the Fraunhofer Heinrich Hertz Institut Berlin, granted by the Bundesministerium für Bildung und Forschung (01UG1240D), is dedicated to develop a NEUROGES-based automatized algorithm for hand/arm movement recognition (Masneri et al., 2010; http://tla.mpi.nl/projects_info/auvis/).

4.4 Methods of development

With the above listed aims and demands in mind, the NEUROGES system has been developed from 1995 to 2012 to its present version. From 1999 to 2013 the NEUROGES project was continuously granted by the German Research Association (DFG LA 1249 / 1-1, 1-2, 1-3). The methods of the development are described below in a quasi chronological order. Actually, different developmental steps occasionally were pursued simultaneously.

(i) Critical review of existing coding systems

First, a critical review was conducted of the existing coding systems and of the reseachers' reports on their experiences with these systems. The review included coding systems used in gesture research, psychology, psychosomatics, psychiatry, psychotherapy, neurology, neuropsychology, linguistics, and anthropology. The most relevant coding systems are described in Chapter 2. In addition to those, many more systems were studied (e.g. Liepmann, 1908; Krout, 1935; Laban, 1950; Sainsbury, 1954; Mahl, 1968; Kendon, 1972; Dell, 1979; Haaland & Flaherty, 1984; Le May et al., 1988; Duffy & Duffy, 1989; Poizner et al., 1990; Ochipa et al., 1994; Foundas et al., 1995; Blonder et al., 1995; Hermsdörfer et al., 1996; Müller, 1998).

While many classification systems are effective tools for specific research questions, only few systems contain values that meet the aims and demands of the NEUROGES systems (see above). From the different systems, suitable values, e.g. Efron's value *deictic,* were chosen as pilot values for the NEUROGES development.

(ii) Identification of relevant empirical findings on movement behaviour and its relation to cognitive, emotional, and interactive processes

To compile movement criteria that are potentially linked to cognitive, emotional, and interactive processes, the literature was reviewed. Included were empirical studies from gesture research, psychology, psychosomatics, psychiatry, psychotherapy, neurology, neuropsychology, psychomotor and motor control research, linguistics, and anthropology. In addition, the author's empirical research findings were considered. Chapter 2 summarizes the most relevant empirical findings for the development of the NEUROGES system.

The review helped to identify movement criteria that are relevant with regard to cognitive, emotional, and interactive functions. An example for such a movement criterion is Freedman's temporal criterion *discrete* versus *continuous*. These movement criteria were used to group movement values and thereby, to define categories.

Furthermore, new, empirically based values were identified that had, thus far, not been noted in the existing coding systems. An example for such a new value is *act as a unit.* This value was identified as a distinct behavioural unit in the author's split-brain research. Furthermore, if empirical findings strongly suggested more fine-grained distinctions of existing values, sub-values were generated. As an example, split-brain patients used their left hand for *deictics* to themselves, and their right hand for *deictics* to the external space. This finding suggested that the two forms of *deictics* are generated in different brain hemispheres, and thus, that they constitute different entities. The new values and the sub-values were added to the compilation of pilot values.

(iii) Operationalization of the pilot values and organization of the values in a system

The pilot values that had been adopted from existing coding systems were often insufficiently operationalized. Some of them were defined only by a description of their function rather than a description of the movement. Therefore, the pilot values were re-defined according to movement criteria that refer to the visual appearance of the body movements.

The newly operationalized pilot values were ordered in pilot categories. Values that were defined primarily by the same movement criteria, e.g. values referring to where the hand acts, were grouped in a category. The categories were then ordered hierarchically from simple to complex as defined by their number of movement criteria, e.g. the Structure category values (step 2) are defined by the criteria trajectory, dynamics, and phases resulting from changes in these parameters, while the Function category values (step 6) are defined by all criteria of the Structure, the Focus, the Contact, and the Formal Relation categories, as well as by the gesture/action space, the path during complex phase, the orientation, the shape, the efforts, and the body involvement.

(iv) Testing, reviewing, and re-testing of the pilot-system by the author

The pilot system was tested by the author by analyzing many video tapes with different individuals in different settings. If the classification of a movement was ambiguous, the definitions of the possible values were elaborated and made more precise and distinct from each other. If a movement could not be classified with the pilot values, a new value was created. The Structure value *aborted* is the product of such as process.

This process, i.e., the testing of the values in a large sample, the review of the values with an improvement of the operationalization, and the optimization of the system was repeated several times. Finally, a first version of the coding manual, the NGC[9] manual, was compiled.

(v) Testing of the system by independent trained raters

When the author reliably classified all movements, the next step was the testing of the system by independent raters. Several raters were trained with the NGC coding manual. They tested the system on a large sample of different individuals in different settings. The independent raters gave direct feed-back to the author concerning the intelligibility of the definitions and the user-friendliness of the system and the procedures. Discussions with the trainees of NGC / NEUROGES training workshops, which started in 2007 at the Berlin

9 The earlier version of the NEUROGES system was termed NGC system.

Gesture Center (http://www.berlingesturecenter.de/ seminare/seminare.html), further helped to improve the system.

During this process, the variety in subjective interpretation of the NEUROGES values could be successfully reduced more and more. Furthermore, the user-friendliness of the system was improved. This was achieved especially by developing coding algorithms that guide the raters through the coding process.

(vi) Development of a statistical method to calculate the interrater agreement for movement behaviour segmentation

Another source of feed-back for the system was the statistically obtained interrater agreement. As it is a specific feature of the NEUROGES coding procedure that it comprises segmentation and coding, the interrater agreement has to refer not only to the value that is given to a unit but also to the segmentation of the behaviour into units. Raters may agree on the value of a unit, but not on the segmentation of the behaviour into units, e.g. if a motion constitutes a unit, and when exactly the unit begins and when it ends and the next unit starts. Vice versa, raters may agree on that a new unit starts, but they may give different values to the unit.

In the stream of behaviour, the rater identifies a movement with a specific value and (s)he tags the beginning and the end of the movement with the specific value. This procedure implies the segmentation of the behaviour. As an example, in a one-minute lasting video-clip of hand movement behaviour, a *shift,* then a *rest position,* and then an *irregular* movement are identified. The rater then searches and tags the beginning of the *shift,* the end of *shift* - which is also the beginning of the *rest position* - , the end of the *rest position* - which is also the beginning of the *irregular* movement - , and the end of the *irregular* movement.

The perceptual process may, however, also happen the other way round. The rater first identifies changes in the behaviour, such as a change in the trajectory. Accordingly, (s)he segments the behaviour into units, and then gives values to the units.

Most likely, in coding both types of perceptual processes are ongoing.

Since not many movement behaviour researchers have segmented the ongoing stream of behaviour into natural units, until recently, no statistical procedure was available to calculate the interrater agreement concerning the segmentation of behaviour into units. A major project during the development of the NEUROGES system was, therefore, to create a statistical method that enabled to calculate the raters' agreement concerning the segmentation of behaviour. The recently developed algorithm by Holle & Rein, the modified Cohen's Kappa, is described in detail in Chapter 15.

(vii) Review of the values based on the modified Cohen's Kappa scores

After the successful development of the modified Cohen's Kappa, several studies with trained raters were conducted to further test the objectivity and the reliability of the segmentation process. The modified Cohen's Kappa score for each value helped particularly to identify those values for which it was difficult to identify their units in the stream of behaviour and to determine the beginning and end of these units. As an example, raters often had difficulties to identify the beginning and end of continuous *irregular* movement units.

The criteria for the segmentation of behaviour in each category and the operationalization of the values were improved. This process was repeated several times until a substantial agreement for segmentation and coding was achieved for many trained raters with different educational backgrounds.

(viii) Finalization of the NEUROGES coding manual

Over time, the increasing operationalization of the categories and values and the improvement of the instruction for the coding process resulted in a comprehensive coding manual. The 230 pages comprising Coding Manual is forthcoming as a book, supplemented by an interactive CD. The manual consists of seven chapters, each of which contains the coding manual for one category. The seven coding manuals for the categories Activation, Structure, Focus, Contact, Formal Relation, Function, and Type are always set up in the same way:

1. The category is defined.
2. The units or unit segments are specified that are submitted to the analysis with the respective category (i.e., not all units are further classified in all categories).
3. The criteria for the segmentation of the behaviour and for the definition of the values are defined.
4. The values are defined. After a short definition that orients the reader about the content of the value a more detailed definition of the value follows. For each criterion, the qualities are explained that may occur in the value, e.g. what kinds of hand shape may occur in a *deictic*. Furthermore, for each value examples are provided. Finally, it is reported how to distinguish the value from other values or phenomena that are similar regarding the visual appearance of the movement. NEUROGES trainees reported the latter information to be particularly helpful.
5. The technical procedure is described for coding the category with the NEUROGES-template.

4.5 Development of the modules, categories, and values, and of the hierarchy

The theoretical and empirical background of the development of the three modules, of the seven categories, and of each of the 58 values is reported in detail in the book 'The NEUROGES system' (forthcoming). Here, only a short overview can be given.

The division of the body in six parts of the body, the right hand/arm, the left hand/arm, the right foot/leg, the left foot/leg, the head, and the trunk is adopted from nonverbal behaviour research. This division is not only anatomically legitimated but it also reflects the fact that these parts of the body play different roles in nonverbal behaviour, i.e., they are associated with different movement classes.

The NEUROGES system consists of three modules that fulfil different aims and focus on different aspects of movement behaviour. The development of the modules and their ordering in a hierarchy was chronologically overlapping.

4.5.1 Module I

Module I has been developed for a very basic segmentation and classification of movement behaviour. Movement behaviour is classified with a few movement criteria only and therefore, Module I coding is compatible with automatized techniques for movement recognition. Module I consists of three categories that build up on each other: Activation, Structure, and Focus.

The development of the Activation category was influenced by the concept of 'gesture units' in gesture research (Kendon, 1972; Davis, 1991, rev. 1997; Kendon, 2010). The gesture unit definitions were taken as a basis to define *movement* units. Kendon (2010, p. 111) defines: "That is, in the case of forelimb gesturing, for instance, the articulators are moved away from some position of rest or relaxation (…) toward a region of space (or sometimes toward some location specifiable with reference to the speaker's body), and then, eventually, they are moved back again to some position of rest or relaxation. This entire *excursion*, from the moment the articulators begin to depart from a position until the moment when they finally return to one, will be referred to as a *gesture unit*." Since some individuals display very brief returns to *rest positions*, making it difficult to distinguish an interruption in gesturing from a *rest position*, Davis (1991, rev. 1997, MSA--2) proposed a time limit: "The beginning of the gesticulation is defined as the start from a 'rest' or 'home base' position in which the limbs are supported and the ending is marked by return to a 'home base' position of the upper limbs. 'Home base' positions which demarcate a gesticulation segment should be held still for at least four seconds. The exception to this rule involves sequences that start and/or end with an activity other than speech gesturing (e.g. gesticulating then lighting a cigarette)." In a pilot study, we tested Davis' four-seconds criterion. However, our data did not support the underlying assumption that four seconds constitute a critical time limit. In other words, there was no evidence that, for example, three seconds lasting *rest positions* constitute a different entity than five seconds lasting *rest positions*. In contrast, we found substantial individual differences concerning the duration of *movement* units and *rest position* units. Especially those individuals who had a high movement velocity also made very short rests. Thus, applying Davis' definition would result in missing these 'high-speed' movers' *rest position* units. Therefore, in NEU-

ROGES *rest position* units are defined by movement criteria only and not by artificially defined time limits.

The development of the Structure and Focus categories was originally inspired by Freedman's and Hoffman's hand movement classification system (Freedman & Hoffman, 1967; Freedman, 1972). Their system had been chosen because it is objective, reliable, and sensitive to different mental states (Sections 3.4. and 2.1.2). Their system consisted of two main values, *object-focused* and *body-focused* hand movements. For the latter main value, the following values were distinguished: *direct hand-to-hand, direct hand-to-body,* and *indirect* (manipulations of objects adjacent to the body). The *body-focused* movements could be either *continuous* (> 3 sec) or *discrete* (< 3 sec). *Object-focused* movements (equivalent to gestures) included the types *motor primacy* and *speech primacy* depending on whether the message was primarily conveyed via gesture or via speech (see Section 3.4).

In their conceptualization of *body-focused* movements, Freedman and Hoffman had fused two movement criteria: duration and location. However, it is proposed here - and recent studies on the validity of the Module I confirm this proposition - that these two criteria are related to different mental processes. Therefore, in the construction of Module I, these two criteria were disentangled: The Structure category was developed from the temporal dimension, i.e., *continuous* versus *discrete,* and the Focus category was developed from the spatial dimension, i.e., *object-focused* versus *body-focused.* Technically, this differentiation also improved the compatibility of Module I with automatized movement recognition techniques.

Starting with the values *continuous* and *discrete,* the Structure category was further developed. Freedman distinguished *continuous* from *discrete* by a three seconds criterion. However, three seconds is an arbitrary time limit that has not been validated. There is no empirical evidence that, for example, a two seconds lasting movement constitutes a different entity than a four seconds lasting movement. It was found that the two entities, which Freedman referred to, could actually be better defined and distinguished by the presence or absence of phases within a *movement* unit, that result from changes in the trajectory and the dynamics. Accordingly, the two values were then termed *irregular* and *phasic*. As an intermediate form, based on clinical research and motor control research, the value *repetitive* was introduced. Furthermore, inspired by Davis' Movement Signature Analysis (1991, rev. 1997) her categories weight shift, postural shift, and position change inspired the Structure values *shift,* and her descriptor "action interrupted, not completed" contributed to the definition of the Structure value *aborted.* Having added these two values to the Structure category, all movements can be classified based on their trajectory patterns. The theoretical proposition behind the Structure category is that the Structure values *irregular, repetitive,* and *phasic* reflect different levels of cognitive complexity.

The Focus category was developed from Freedman's main values *object-focused* and *body-focused,* and the values *direct* and *indirect.* These values were operationalized more precisely by the location where the hand acts (on). Based on behavioural observations on where the hand acts, a more fine-grained scale was set up with the values: *on body* (Freedman's value *direct body-focused*), *on attached object* (Freedman's value *indirect body-focused*), *on separate object, on person,* and *in space* (Freedman's value *object-focused*). Furthermore, it was found that those movements in which the hand (or foot) was not acting on anything could be further distinguished. The focus of these movements could actually be external (*in space*) or internal, i.e., on body-internal structures such as joints, muscles, or tendons (*within body*). Thus, the final NEUROGES Focus category consists of 6 values. These are ordered on an axis from body-internal to body-external. This dichotomy between was adopted from Sainsbury (1955), Mahl (1968) and Freedman et al. (1972), since it had been proven effective for psychological and clinical psychosomatic and psychiatric research. However, their systems referred only to *on body / on attached object* movements (autistic, body-focused) on one hand and *in space* movements (communicative, object-focused) on the other. The theoretical proposition behind the Focus category is that the Focus values present different locations the pre-motor attention is directed on.

4.5.2 Module II

Module II has been developed to classify bilateral limb movements in a differentiated manner. Its development is based entirely on split-brain research and on the subsequent examination of the paradigms in healthy individuals and in patients with mental disease (Lausberg et al., 1999; Lausberg et al., 2000; Lausberg & Kita, 2002; Lausberg & Kita, 2003; Lausberg et al., 2003a; Lausberg et al., 2003b; Lausberg & Cruz, 2004; Lausberg et al., 2007; Kita & Lausberg, 2008).

The study of split-brain patients revealed that they often acted with folded hands as a compensatory strategy to avoid intermanual conflict (Lausberg et al., 2000; Lausberg et al., 2007). The further exploration of the forms of physical contact between the two hands in healthy individuals led to the three values *act as a unit, act on each other,* and *act apart.* These values form the Contact category (step 4). The Contact values are associated with different levels of stability of interhemispheric cooperation.

Furthermore, with regard to the dominance of one hand in bilateral movements, the author's split-brain research revealed that there are three types of bilateral movements: right hand dominance, left hand dominance, and equal dominance movements, the latter with the subtypes synchronous and dyssynchronous. These values are each characterized by a different pattern of neural control by the two hemispheres (Lausberg et al., 2000; Lausberg et al., 2003; Lausberg et al., 2007). After exploring these values in large samples of neurologically healthy individuals and in individuals with unilateral brain damage, these values resulted in the Formal Relation category with the values *right hand dominance, left hand dominance, symmetrical,* and *asymmetrical*. The Formal Relation category reflects hemispheric dominance in bilateral movements. As it has been exposed in Section 2.5, the registration of the laterality of unilateral limb movements and of the dominant limb in bilateral movements enables to infer in which hemisphere the movement is generated.

4.5.3 Module III

Module III has been originally designed for classifying gestures. The name of the whole coding system has historically resulted from this module: NEUROGES means NEUROpsychological GEStture coding system. Since several publications by different researchers refer to this name, it has been kept, although the system is designed not only for coding gestures but for coding body movement behaviour (sometimes termed 'extended NEUROGES').

Module III consists of two categories that complement each other in coding: Function and Type. Therefore, below, the development is described for the two categories together.

Efron's seminal coding system for gestures (1941) has substantially coined the development of Module III (see Section 3.4). His system had been chosen for two reasons. First, since Efron noted gestures and words online during direct observation, i.e., without video recording, he often had difficulties in keeping track the verbal context (p. 100). Nevertheless, his classification system was perfectly effective to classify the gestures without reference to the verbal context. Thus, Efron's gesture values can be identified by the visual appearance of the movement alone. Second, for Efron's referential coding system some degree of validity can be assumed, since - more or less independent - researchers have later arrived at similar propositions about the meaning of certain gesture values that are each characterized by a specific visual appearance. Thus, in the Module III developement, there was the trend to first define the function and then operationalize the visual appearance of the movements with the specific function. In contrast, in the development of the Modules I and II, the trend was reversed. Rather, first specific movement features were identified and then their function was explored. While these were trends, all three modules shared the bidirectional development of visual appearance ⇔ function.

Table 1 below illustrates the relation between Efron's values and the NEUROGES Function values. Only the NEUROGES Function values *emotion/attitude, object-oriented action,* and *subject-oriented action*, which are not listed in Table 1, are not derived from Efron's values.

Table 1 Efron's coding system as the basis for the development of the NEUROGES Function and Type categories

Efron (1941)		NEUROGES Module III	
Main Types	**Subtypes**	**Function values**	**Type values**
discursive	*ideographic*	*spatial relation presentation*	*route* *postion*
	baton	*emphasis*	*baton* *super-imposed* *back-toss* *palm-out*
objective	*physiographic - iconographic*	*form presentation*	*shape* *size*
		spatial relation presentation	*route* *position*
	physiographic - kinetographic	*motion quality presentation*	*manner* *dynamics*
		pantomime	*transitive* *intransitive*
	deictic	*egocentric deictic*	*external target* *You* *self* *body*
		egocentric direction	*neutral* *imperative* *self-related*
	emblematic	*emblem*	

Table 1 reveals that some of Efron's values have been subdivided into two Function values. Almost all Function values have been further subdivided into more fine-grained Type values. These subdivisions were undertaken when there was empirical evidence that the subtypes represent different entities.

Efron's value *ideographic* ("*ideographic*, in the sense that it traces or sketches out in the air the "paths" and "direction" of the thought pattern. The latter variety might also be called *logico-topographic* or *logico-pictorial*."[10]) was omitted, since based on the visual appearance of the movement alone, this gesture type could not be reliably be distinguished from other gesture types that depict con-

10 This citation as well as the following ones are from Efron, 1941, republished 1972, p.96.

crete spatial relations. Instead, in NEUROGES, it is coded with the value *spatial relation presentation,* and if desired, the researcher can note that (s)he assumes that the gesture depicts a thought pattern.

Efron's value *baton* ("*baton-like,* representing a sort of "timing out" with the hand the successive stages of the referential activity") was found to share movement features and function with the types *superimposed batons* (Kendon, 1972), *tosses* (Davis, 1991). Davis' tosses were further subdivided into *back-tosses* and *palm-outs* based on differences in the visual appearance and the meaning. The grouping of the four values *batons, superimposed, back-tosses,* and *palm-outs* in the Function value *emphasis* is based on gesture research, neuropsychological research and on functional neuroimaging studies (e.g. Souza-Poza et al., 1979; Stephens, 1983; Blonder et al., 1995; McNeill, 1992; Lausberg et al., 2000; Schirmer, Alter, Kotz, and Friederici, 2001; Lausberg et al., 2007; Hubbard et al., 2006).

Efron's value *iconographic* ("depicting either the form of a visual object or a spatial relationship (*iconographic* gesture)") was subdivided into *form presentation* and *spatial relation presentation* gestures, based on neuropsychological research (e.g. Hartje & Poeck, 2002; Nichelli, 1999; see also subsection 2.1.1). Efron's value *kinetographic* ("depicting ... that of a bodily action (*kinetographic* gesture)") was subdivided into *motion quality presentation* and *pantomime.* This subdivision reflects a general concept in Module III to distinguish between the egocentric (*pantomime*) and the mento-heliocentric (*motion quality presentation*) cognitive perspectives that are reflected in gesture (see subsection 2.1.1). The *pantomime* values *transitive* and *intransitive* are based on neuropsychological apraxia research (e.g. Bartolo et al., 2001; Rapcsak et al., 1993; Dumont et al., 1999; Cubelli et al., 2000; Haaland & Flaherty, 1984; Roy et al., 2001; Heath et al., 2001). The six *presentation* Type values *shape, size, route, position, manner*, and *dynamics* specify geometric and qualitative aspects (e.g. Kita & Özyürek, 1999; Beattie & Shovelton, 2006).

Efron's value *deictic* ("*deictic*, referring by means of a sign to a visually present object (actual pointing)") was modified such that it can refer to non-visible objects as well. Furthermore, it was subdivided into *egocentric deictic* and *egocentric direction* gestures based on differences in their visual appearance and in their meaning. The values *egocentric deictic* and *egocentric direction* are opposed to *spatial relation presentation position* and *spatial relation presentation route*, as they depict spatial relations from an egocentric perspective, while the latter values depict them from a mento-heliocentric perspective. The four *egocentric deictic* values *external target, You, self,* and *body* were added with reference to the different targets. Split-brain patients performed *self-deictics* only with the left hand and external target *deictics* only with the right hand. This hand preference indicates that the two types are generated in different areas of the brain, and thus, they represent different entities. In analogy to the *egocentric deictics* values, the three *egocentric direction* Type values *neutral, imperative,* and *self-related* were defined with reference to the agent.

Efron's value *emblematic* ("*emblematic*, representing either a visual or a logical object by means of a pictorial of a non-pictorial form which has no morphological relationship to the thing represented.") was adopted. However, the NEUROGES definition is closer to the subsequent definition by Ekman & Friesen (1969), who code those conventionalized gestures as *emblems* that have a morphological relationship to the referent.

To classify expressive movements, the Function value *emotion/attitude* was introduced. The types *shrug, palming,* and *fist clenching* are inspired by Darwin's descriptions (1890, republished 2009). *Shrugs* have first been described by Bulwer (1649, cited by Darwin) and since then they have been confirmed by other researchers (e.g Johnson, Ekman, & Friesen, 1975; Davis, 1991; Lausberg et al., 2000). The values *rise, fall, opening, closing* are based on split-brain and embodiment research (e.g. Förster & Strack, 1996; Lausberg et al., 2000; Wilson & Peper, 2004; Casanto & Dijkstra, 2010, Charny, 1966; Scheflen, 1973; Davis, 1985). The Function values *object-oriented action* and *subject-oriented action* were introduced to classify the purpose of actions.

Substantial effort was made to operationalize the Function and Type values with movement criteria, because Efron's value definitions - in the stricter sense - referred primarily to the function, e.g. "..*baton-like,* representing a sort of "timing out" with the hand the successive stages of the referential activity." (Efron, p. 96, 1972).

As argued in Chapter 3, raters are typically able to classify gestures even if they can only observe movement, i.e., without information about the verbal utterance, the social context, etc.. As an example, raters can reliably identify a *baton* based on the visual appearance alone. They are able to do so because of their (partly implicit) knowledge about the function that a certain movement with a specific visual appearance has (universally or culturally). Therefore, in NEUROGES the raters are provided with precise descriptions of the visual appearance of gestures, expressive movements, and actions. The example below illustrates how precisely NEUROGES values are defined in the coding manual. The comparison between Efron's definition of a *baton* gesture (see above) and the below NEUROGES definition of an *emphasis* gesture reveals the substantial effort that has been made to operationalize the Efron-based values.

emphasis

Short definition

SETTING ACCENTS ON SPEECH

Definition

Function: Emphasis is defined as "force or intensity of expression that gives impressiveness or importance to something".

In gesture, emphasis can be produced by setting dynamic accents. These are hand/arm movements that are strong, direct, and quick. These kinesic accents point out short segments of the speech. In synchrony with prosody, they emphasize certain aspects of the verbal statement. Obviously, a sequence of accents creates a metre or a rhythm. As such *emphasis* gestures can be regarded as manual equivalents of prosody. They convey rhythmical and potentially acoustical information (if the Focus value is *on body* or *on separate object*). In the latter case, their effect is less dependent on a well visible location of the hand in the gesture/action space than that of the other gesture Function values that provide visual information.

Furthermore, emphasis can be put to speech by accompanying process of verbalizing, i.e., bringing out a concept and presenting it. By embodying a direction of movement, e.g. rotating the palm out, these emphasis gestures accompany – and thereby enforce – the process of quasi rotating out words (thoughts) and then presenting them.

Emphasis gestures may superimpose emphasis on *emotion/attitude* (only extrinsic gestures), *egocentric deictic, egocentric direction, form presentation, spatial relation presentation,* and *emblem* gestures.

Movement: *Emphasis* gestures are *repetitive* or *phasic in space* movements. They are spatially simple seesaw movements, either up-down, in-out (supination-pronation), or rarely, forth-back. All *emphasis* gestures have an endpoint accent. The up-down movements may have a downward accent or an upward accent. The supination-pronation movements may be alternating with an outward accent or they may have a static complex phase in the supination end position (in the latter case, there is an emphasis on the process of bringing (rotating) out the idea and presenting it). All *emphasis* gestures are synchronized with mouth and head movements (unless they accompany internal speech, which is not accompanied by mouth movements but often by head movements).

If *emphasis* gestures follow the static complex phase of *emotion/attitude* (only extrinsic gestures), *egocentric deictic, egocentric direction, form presentation, spatial relation presentation,* or *emblem* gestures, they have up-down / forth-back path with a downward / forward accent (superimposed *emphasis*). Once the primary gesture has come to the static complex phase, the *emphasis* gesture follows. The hand shape, the hand orientation, and the position in gesture/action space of the primary gesture are preserved during the display of the *emphasis* gesture. As an example, the fingers are shaped to V-sign and a repetitive up/forth - down/back of the hand/arm is superimposed (*emblem + emphasis*), or hand points and up-down movements are added (*egocentric deictic + emphasis).* Technically in superimposed *emphasis*, the unit adopted from Module I or II, which typically has the value *repetitive*, is split into a subunit with the primary Function value and a subunit with the Function value *emphasis*.

Types: As indicated above, the kinesic forms used to create emphasis may differ among the *emphasis* gestures. They differ with regard to the path during complex phase and to the direction towards end point accent. Accordingly, four Type values are distinguished: *baton* (up-down movements of lower arm or hand with downward accent), *superimposed* (up-down or back-forth movements with downward or forward accent that directly follow the static complex phase of another gesture type), *back-toss* (small up-down movements with an upward accent with back of hand leading), and *palm-out* (small supination-pronation movements with outward accent).

Specifications: *Emphasis* units can be further specified with the Specification category Temporal Structure.

Temporal Structure: The Specification category enables to register the temporal structure that is created by the *emphasis* gestures.

Meeting the criteria

Structure:	***repetitive*** > *phasic*
Focus:	*in space*, only in exceptional cases *on body* or *on separate object*
Laterality:	bh 0.49 ± 0.44 > lh = 0.44 ± 0.27 > rh 0.31 ± 0.16 ; lh 1.69 ± 4.74 > bh 1.63 ± 1.24 > rh 1.15 ± 1.22 units / minute
Gesture/action space:	ipsilateral hemi-space, level of trunk, middle kinesphere
Path:	**one-dimensional up-down** or **two-dimensional arch-like supination - pronation**
Hand orientation:	no distinct orientation; if superimposed to other gesture types, hand orientation of primary gesture is maintained
Hand shape:	relaxed open hand; if superimposed to other gesture types, hand shape of primary gesture is maintained
Efforts:	acceleration (quick) with change from free to bound flow to generate **end point accent**
Body involvement:	*emphasis* gestures are **synchronized with mouth and head** movements
Gaze:	not at hands
Other criteria:	in line with prosody
Frequency:	4.45 ± 4.61; 1.24 ± 0.71 units / minute
Duration:	0.98 ± 0.30 seconds / unit

Differentiate *emphasis* gestures from…

✎ *emotion/attitude*: see *emotion/attitude*

✎ gestures with a meaning-intrinsic *repetitive* Structure in general: Note that superimposed *emphasis* to a primary gesture is **not** to be confused with a *repetitive* gesture in which the repetition is an intrinsic component of the meaning. As an example, the repetitions in a *pantomime* gesture presenting tooth brushing or in a *form presentation* gesture presenting a star by tracing several sharp points are **not** *emphasis* as the repetition does not serve to reinforce a primary gesture but the repetition per se constitutes the meaning. One up-down movement in front of the mouth does not convey the meaning of tooth brushing nor does one sharp point not make up a star.

✎ *pantomime*: In *pantomime* gestures with a *repetitive* Structure the meaning is conveyed by the repetition per se, e.g. when pantomiming tooth brushing or hammering. In these cases, one up-down movement in front of the mouth or one downward movement would **not** unambiguously convey the meaning of tooth brushing or hammering, respectively. In *repetitive pantomimes* there is often a displacement of the hand, e.g. the hand moves in front of the mouth from the left side to the right side while executing the up-down movements. Furthermore, there is a distinct hand shape or hand orientation and the gaze is at the hand.

In contrast, in *emphasis* gestures there is no displacement of the hand during the forth-back movement, there is no distinct hand shape or hand orientation, and the gaze is not at the hand.

✎ *form presentation:* In *form presentation* gestures with a *repetitive* Structure the repetition serves to create a repetitive pattern, e.g. to depict a star with 5 sharps. The repetition of one segment of the form is necessary to create the whole form, e.g. six identical sharps are needed to create a star. There is a displacement of the hand, there is a distinct hand shape or hand orientation and the gaze is at the presented form.

In contrast, as the repetitive movements of *emphasis* gestures are back and forth, they cannot create a form. There is no distinct hand shape or hand orientation, and the gaze is not at the hand.

✎ *spatial relation presentation: Spatial relation presentation* gestures with a *repetitive* Structure may serve to present several independent locations or to create a route with a repetitive pattern, e.g. a zigzag course.

In contrast to *emphasis* gestures, in *spatial relation presentation* gestures there is always a distinct use of gesture/action space reflecting the mento-heliocentric perspective and thus, a displacement of the hand. The hand is typically shaped, with a distinct orientation, and the gaze is typically at the presented path.

✎ *motion quality presentation*: *Motion quality presentation* gestures and *emphasis* gesture share the *repetitive* Structure. However, *motion quality presentation* gestures typically have a repetitive within hand / wrist trajectory, a complex dynamics, and a shaped hand to present the object that is moving. Furthermore, in addition to the within hand / wrist trajectory, there is often a displacement of the hand to represent locomotion. The gaze is typically at the presented motion.

In contrast, *repetitive emphasis* gestures are spatially simple back-forth movements, with an endpoint accent and they are synchronized with the mouth and head movements.

✎ *emblems:* In *emblems* with a *repetitive* Structure the repetition is part of the conventionalization, e.g. waving the hand to say good-bye or tapping on the temple to indicate that someone is crazy. In this case, a one-way wave or one tap would not unambiguously constitute the sign and the repetition helps to clarify the message. Note, however, that *emblems* with a *phasic* Structure may be combined with a superimposed *emphasis* gestures, e.g. adopting the shape of the victory sign and then moving the V-shaped hand repetitively back and forth. In this case, the unit is split up into an *emblem* and a *emphasis* gesture.

Emphasis gestures are characterized by some degree of standardization of the kinesic form just like *emblems*. The latter, however, are perfectly standardized with regard to the kinesic form. In contrast to *emphasis* gestures, *emblems* are not a complement to a verbal utterance, but they are the message itself. Furthermore, *emblems* are displayed explicitly, i.e., within the gesturer's awareness, while *emphasis* gestures are not.

✎ *egocentric direction: Egocentric direction* gestures are used explicitly to convey the message concerning a designated direction. The information about the designated direction can be conveyed independently from the verbal utterance. As specific directions are indicated, there is a great variety in spatial direction, e.g. from down left to up right. The Structure is *phasic*.

In contrast, *emphasis* gestures are typically performed implicitly and they accompany the speech (or inner speech) process. The spatial directions of the path during main are stereotypical, i.e., up-down, in-out. The Structure is typically *repetitive*.

4.5.4 The hierarchy of the modules and categories

The three modules have been ordered in a hierarchy that constitutes the seven step coding algorithm. The categories are ordered from simple and comprehensive to complex and specialized.

In Step 1 all six parts of the body, the right hand/arm, the left hand/arm, the right foot/leg, the left foot/leg, the head, and the trunk are coded. With only three criteria, i.e., motion, anti-gravity position, and muscle contraction, the movement behaviour is segmented into two Activation values ((i) *movement*, (ii) *rest position / posture).* In contrast, in Step 7 mainly hand/arm gestures are left to be assessed. Many criteria are employed to define the values: the criteria of the Activation, Structure, Focus, Contact, and Formal Relation categories, and in addition, the criteria gesture/action space, path during complex phase, orientation, hand shape, efforts, body involvement, gaze, and - as a meta-criterion - cognitive perspective.

At each step (which represents a category), the units of the previous step are reassessed and the new criteria are added, and, if necessary, the units are segmented into subunits. Thereby, the seven step comprising segmentation and coding of movement behaviour leads to more and more fine-grained units and more and more complex values. Accordingly, NEUROGES codings look like an inverted tree. However, it is noteworthy that while the seven categories are ordered hierarchically in a decision process, each category functions on its own and - with some limitations - can be assessed independently of the others.

Given their simplicity, the Module I value definitions can be used for kinematographic investigations and for automatized movement recognition techniques. To further improve the compatibility with kinematographic and automatized methods, in this module the right and left limbs are coded independently of each other.

Module II constitutes a bridge between Module I and Module III, as it clarifies the relation between the two limbs, which in Module I have been assessed independently of each other. The Module II codings determine whether in Module III the function is assessed for both hands (feet) together, e.g. both hands together pantomime drumming, or whether it is assessed separately for the right hand (foot) and for the left hand (foot), e.g. one hand scratches the leg while the other hand points to an external location.

Module III analyses the function of limb, head, and trunk movements. Based on the Module I and Module II codings, at the stage of Module III when the assessment of complex phenomena such as the function of the movement is required, fine behavioural units are provided that are based on objective movement criteria.

References

Bartolo, A., Cubelli, R., Della Sala, S., Drei, S., & Marchetti, C. (2001). Double Dissociation between Meaningful and Meaningless Gesture Reproduction in Apraxia. *Cortex, 37*, 696-9.

Beattie, G. & Shovelton, H. (2006). When size really matters: how a single semantic feature is represented in the speech and gesture modalities. *Gesture 6*, 63-84.

Birdwhistell, R.L. (1970). *Kinesics and Context. Essays on Body Motion Communication*. Philadelphia: University of Pennsylvania Press.

Blonder, L.X., Burns, A.F., Bowers, D., Moore, R.W., & Heilman, K.M. (1995). Spontaneous Gestures Following Right Hemisphere Infarct. *Neuropsychologia, 33*(2), 203-213.

Casanto D, & Dijkstra K. (2010) Motor Action and Emotional Memory. *Cognition, 115(1),* 179-185.

Charny, E.J. (1966). Psychosomatic manifestations of rapport in psychotherapy. *Psychosomatic Medicine, 29 (4),* 305-15.

Cubelli, R., Marchetti, C., Boscolo, G., & Della Sala, S. (2000). Cognition in Action: Testing a Model of Limb Apraxia. *Brain and Cognition, 44*, 144-65.

Darwin, C.R. (1890, reissue 2009). The Expression of the Emotions in Man and Animals (2nd ed.). London: Penguin Group.

Davis, M. (1991, rev. 1997). *Guide to movement analysis methods.* Pittsburgh, PA. USA.: Behavioral Measurement Database Services, P.O. Box 11028.

Dell, C. (1979). *A primer for movement description using effort-shape and supplementary concepts*. New York: Dance Notation Bureau Press.

Duffy, R.J., & Duffy, J.R. (1989). An investigation of body part as object (BPO) responses in normal and brain-damaged adults. *Brain and Cognition, 10*, 220-236.

Dumont, C., Ska, B.,& Schiavetto, A. (1999). Selective impairment of transitive gestures: An unusual case of transitive gestures. *Neurocase, 5*, 447-58.

Efron, D. (1941, 2nd ed. 1972). *Gesture and culture*. The Hague: Mouton.

Ekman, P., & Friesen, W. (1969). The Repertoire of Nonverbal Behaviour: Categories, Origins, Usage and Coding. *Semiotica, 1*, 49-99.

Ekman, P., Friesen, W., & Hager, J.C. (2002). *Facial Action Coding System. The Manual*. Salt Lake City, A Human Face.

Förster, J., & Strack, F. (1996). Influence of overt head movements on memory for valenced words: a case of conceptual-motor compatibility. *Journal of personality and social psychology 71(3),* 421-30.

Foundas, A.L., Macauley, B.L., Raymer, A.M., Mahler, L.M., Heilman, K.M., & Rothi L.J.G. (1995). Gesture laterality in aphasic and apraxic stroke patients. *Brain and Cognition 29:* 204-213.

Freedman, N. (1972). The Analysis of Movement Behavior During the Clinical Interview. In A. W. Siegman, B. Pope (Ed.), *Studies in Dyadic Communication* (pp. 153-175). New York: Pergamon.

Freedman N., & Hoffman S.P. (1967). Kinetic Behaviour in Altered Clinical States: Approach to Objective Analysis of Motor Behaviour during Clinical Interviews. *Perceptual Motor Skills, 24*, 527-539.

Freedman, N., & Bucci, W. (1981). On kinetic filtering in associative monologue. *Semiotica*, 34(3/4), 225-249.

Haaland, K.Y., & Flaherty, D. (1984). The Different Types of Limb Apraxia Errors made by Patients with Left vs. Right Hemispehre Damage. *Brain and Cognition, 3*, 370 - 384.

Hall, E.T. (1966). *The Hidden Dimension*. New York: Doubleday.

Hartje, W., & Poeck, K. (2002). *Klinische Neuropsychologie*. Stuttgart: Georg Thieme Verlag.

Heath, M., Roy, E.A., Black, S.E., & Westwood, D.A. Intransitive Limb Gestures and Apraxia Following Unilateral Stroke. *Journal of Clinical and Experimental Neuropsychology, 23*, 628-42.

Heilman, K.M., Rothi, L.J.G. (1993). Apraxia. In K. M. Heilman, & Valenstein, E. (Ed.), *Clinical Neuropsychology* (pp. 141-164). New York, Oxford: Oxford University Press.

Hermsdörfer, J., Mai, N., Spatt, J., Marquardt, C., Veltkamp, R., & Goldenberg, G. (1996). Kinematic analysis of movement imitation in apraxia. *Brain, 119*, 1575-1586.

Hubbard, A., Callan, D., & Dapretto, M. (2006). How the Brain Sees What we say: an fMRI Study of Speech and Beat Gestures. Presented at the 12th Annual Meeting of the Organization for Human Brain Mapping, Florence.

Johnson, H.G, Ekman, P., & Friesen, W.V. (1975). Communicative body movements: American emblems. *Semiotica 15*, 335-353.

Kendon, A. (1972). *Some relationships between body motion and speech.* In A. Siegman and B. Pope (eds). Studies in dyadic communication, 177-210, Pergamon Press, New York.

Kendon, A. (2002). Some uses of the head shake. *Gesture, 2*(2), 147-182.

Kendon, A. (2010). *Gesture - Visible Action as Utterance.* : Cambridge University Press.

Kita, S., & Lausberg, H. (2008). Generation of co-speech gestures based on spatial imagery from the right-hemisphere: evidence from split-brain patients. *Cortex, 44*, 131-139.

Kita, S., & Özyürek, A. (1999). *Espressing manner and path in English and Turkish: differences in speech, gesture, and conceptualization.* Paper presented at the 21st Annual Conference of the Cognitive Science Society London.

Krout, M.(1935). Autistic gestures. *Psychological Monographs 46.*

Kryger, M. (2010). *Bewegungsverhalten von Patient und Therapeut in als gut und schlecht erlebten Therapiesitzungen*. Diploma Thesis. Dept. of Neurology, Psychosomatic Medicine, and Psychiatry; Institute of health promotion and clinical movement science. Cologne, German Sport University.

Laban, R. (1988). *The Mastery of Movement*, Neuauflage. Worcester: Northcote House.

Lausberg, H. (1998). Does Movement Behavior Have Differential Diagnostic Potential? *American Journal of Dance Therapy 20(2)*, 85-99.

Lausberg, H, & Kita S. (2003).The content of the message influences the hand choice in co-speech gestures and in gesturing without speaking. *Brain and Language, 86,* 57-69.

Lausberg, H., & Cruz, R.F. (2004). Hemispheric specialization for imitation of hand-head positions and finger configurations: a controlled study in patients with complete callosotomy. *Neuropsychologia, 42*, 320-334.

Lausberg, H., & Sloetjes, H. (2009). Coding gestural behavior with the NEUROGES-ELAN system. *Behavioral Research Methods, 41(3),* 841-849.

Lausberg, H., Davis, M., & Rothenhäusler, A. (2000). Hemispheric specialization in spontaneous gesticulation in a patient with callosal disonnection. *Neuropsychologia, 38*, 1654-1663.

Lausberg, H., v. Arnim, A., & Joraschky, P. (2007). Bewegungsanalyse in der Körperbild- und Körperschemadiagnostik. In G. H. P. Geißler (Ed.), *Lebensbewegungen. Zum körperlichen Geschehen in der psychoanalytischen Therapie. Ein Lehrbuch* (pp. 165-196). Wien: Springer Verlag.

Lausberg, H., Kita, S., Zaidel, E., & Ptito, A. (2003). Split-brain patients neglect left personal space during right-handed gestures. *Neuropsychologia 41*, 1317-1329.

Lausberg, H., Zaidel, E., Cruz, R.F., & Ptito, A. (2007). Speech-independent production of communicative gestures: Evidence from patients with complete callosal disconnection. *Neuropsychologia, 45*, 3092-3104.

Lausberg, H., Göttert, R., Münßinger, U., Boegner, F., & Marx, P. (1999). Callosal disconnection syndrome in a left-handed patient due to infarction of the total length of the corpus callosum. *Neuropsychologia, 37*(3), 253-265.

Lausberg, H., Cruz, R.F., Kita, S., Zaidel, E., & Ptito, A. (2003). Pantomime to visual presentation of objects: Left hand dyspraxia in patients with complete callosotomy. *Brain 126*, 343-360.

Lausberg, H., Cruz, R.F., Kita, S., Zaidel, E., & Ptito, A. (2003). Pantomime to visual presentation of objects: left hand dyspraxia in patients with complete callosotomy. *Brain, 126*, 343-360.

Le May, A., David, R., & Thomas, A.P. (1988). The use of spontaneous gesture by aphasic patients. *Aphasiology, 2*(2), 137-145.

Liepmann, H. (1908). *Drei Aufsätze aus dem Apraxiegebiet*. Berlin: Karger.

Mahl, F.G. (1968). Gestures and Body Movements in Interviews. *Research in Psychotherapy, 3*, 295-346.

Masneri, S. Schreer, O., Schneider, D., Tschöpel, S., Bardeli, R., Bordag, S., Auer, E., Sloetjes, H., & Wittenburg, P.: Towards Semi-Automatic Annotations for Video and Audio Corpora, *4th Workshop on Representation and Processing of Sign Languages: Corpora and Sign Language Technologies in conjunction with 7th Int. Conf. on Language Resources and Evaluation (LREC), Malta*, June 22, 2010.

McClave, E., Kim, H., Tamer, R., & Mileff, M. (2007). Head movements in the context of speech in Arabic, Bulgarian, Korean, and African-American Vernacular English. *Gesture* 7(3): 343-390.

McNeill, D. (1992). *Hand and Mind: What gestures reveal about thought*. Chicago: The University of Chicago Press.

Müller, C. (1998). *Redebegleitende Gesten - Kulturgeschichte, Theorie, Sprachvergleich*. Berlin: Berlin Verlag Arno Spitz GmbH.

Nichelli, P. (1999). Visuospatial and Imagery Disorders. In G. Denes, & Pizzamiglio, L. (Ed.), *Handbook of Clinical and Experimental Neuropsychology* (pp. 453-478). Hove, East Sussex: Psychology Press.

Ochipa, C., Rothi, L.J.G., & Heilman, K.M. (1994). Conduction apraxia. *Journal of Neurology, Neurosurgery, and Psychiatry, 57*, 1241 - 1244.

Poeck, K., & Kerschensteiner, M. (1975). Analysis of the sequential motor events in oral apraxia. In K. J. Zülch, Creutzfeldt, O., Galbraith, G.C. (Ed.), *Cerebral Localization* (pp. 98-114). Berlin, Heidelberg, New York: Springer-Verlag.

Poeck, K. (1986). The clinical examination for motor apraxia. *Neuropsychologia, 24*(1), 129-134.

Poizner, H., Mack, L., Verfaellie, M., Rothi, L.J.G., & Heilman, K.M. (1990). Three-dimensional Computergraphic Analysis of Apraxia. *Brain, 113*, 85-101.

Rapcsak, S.Z., Ochipa, C., Beeson, P.M., & Rubens, A.B. (1993). Praxis and the Right Hemisphere. *Brain and Cognition, 23*, 181-202.

Roy, E.A., Heath, M., Westwood, D., Schweizer, T.A., Dixon, M.J., Black, S. E., Kalbfleisch, L., Barbour, K., & Square, P.A. (2000). Task Demands and Limb Apraxia in Stroke. *Brain and Cognition, 44,* 253-79.

Sainsbury, P. (1954). A method of measuring spontaneous movements by time-sampling motion picture. *The Journal of Mental Science 100a*: 742-748.

Scheflen, A.E. (1973). *Communicational Structure: Analysis of a psychotherapy transaction.* Bloomington: Indiana University.

Schirmer, A., Alter, K., Kotz, S.A., & Friederici, A.D. (2001). Lateralization of prosody during language production: A lesion study. *Brain and Language, 76*, 1-17.

Souza-Posa, J.F., Rohrberg, R., & Mercure, A. (1979). Effects of type of information (abstract-concrete) and field dependence on asymmetry of hand movements during speech. *Perceptual and Motor Skills 48*, 1323-1330.

Stephens, D. (1983). Hemispheric language dominance and gesture hand preference. Ph.D. dissertation, Department of Behavioral Sciences, University of Chicago.

Wilson, V.E., & Peper, E. (2004). The Effects of Upright and Slumped Postures on the Recall of Positive and Negative Thoughts. *Applied Psychophysiology and Biofeedback, 29*, 189-195.

5. The NEUROGES Coding System: Design and Psychometric Properties

Hedda Lausberg

5.1 The NEUROGES design

5.1.1 The hierarchic structure of the NEUROGES system

The NEUROGES system analyzes the movement behaviour of the body standing, sitting, or lying in one place. For the purpose of the analysis, the body is divided in six parts: the right hand/arm, the left hand/arm, the right foot/leg, the left foot/leg, the head, and the trunk. The NEUROGES system is designed in such a way that the researcher can decide if (s)he wants to code all six parts or select certain parts, e.g. to code only hand/arm movements.

In Module I, these six parts are coded independently of each other. In the Modules II and III, the movements of the right and left limbs are related to each other. While the four systems head, trunk, hands/arms, and feet/legs are coded independently of each other throughout the whole system, the movements of the different systems can be related to each other in a concatenation procedure at the end of the coding process. This procedure delivers complex head - trunk - hands/arms - feet/legs units, e.g. simultaneous turning of head and trunk turn to the right pointing with right hand to the right. These complex units can be used for pattern detection.

The NEUROGES system comprises seven categories that build up on each other. The categories are ordered hierarchically from simple / comprehensive to complex / specialized. The degree of complexity of a category is defined by the number of movement criteria that are relevant for segmentation and coding in that category. At each step (category), the units of the previous step are reassessed and the new criteria are added. It is a specific feature of the NEUROGES system that coding and segmentation constitute an interdependent process, i.e., a behavioural unit is assessed, and if within this unit, the behaviour changes from one value to another one the unit is segmented into two or more subunits. These (sub)units are then used in the next coding step.

As an example, if in Step 2 (Structure category) it becomes evident that the *movement* unit that was adopted from Step 1 (Activation category) contains *irregular* and *phasic* movements, the unit is segmented into two Structure units, an *irregular* unit and a *phasic* one. These two units are then taken as the basis for Step 3 (Focus category). If in Step 3 it turns out that the adopted *phasic* unit contains *on body* and *in space* movements, the unit is further subdivided into two Focus units, etc.

As this principle of (sub)unit generation applies to all coding steps, the multi-stage evaluation process results in more and more fine-grained behavioural units. Accordingly, NEUROGES codings look like an inverted tree. Thus, at the stage of Module III when the assessment of complex phenomena such as the function of the movement is required, fine behavioural units are provided that are based on a step-wise segmentation of behaviour and on repeated assessments of the units with different movement criteria.

The seven categories are grouped into three modules that build up on each other. The categories Activation, Structure, and Focus constitute Module I, the categories Contact and Formal Relation Module II, and the categories Function and Types Module III.

Module I analyses all six parts of the body: the right hand/arm, the left hand/arm, the right foot/leg, the left foot/leg, the head, and the trunk. The Activation category (Step 1) segments the ongoing stream of movement behaviour into *movement* units and *no movement* units. In Step 2 (Structure category), the *movement* units are assessed regarding their Structure, which is defined by the movement trajectory and dynamics, and classified with five Structure values.

Since the limbs have a larger range of movement abilities than the head and the trunk, they are further analyzed with the Focus category (Step 3). With reference to the Structure value of the limb movement unit, the Focus of the limb movement is assessed and classified with six Focus values. To finalize the Module I evaluation of the limb units, the Structure values and the Focus values are concatenated.

Thus, in Module I, the movement behaviour is segmented and classified according to a few movement criteria, some of which match kinematic parameters. Furthermore, the right and left limbs are assessed separately. (Therefore, Module I is particularly suited for kinematographic investigations and for automatized movement recognition techniques.)

Module II analyzes limb movements only. Based on the right and left limb StructureFocus units, bilateral and unilateral units are generated. Bilateral units are those units, in which the right hand/arm (foot/leg) and the left one move simultaneously. Unilateral movement units are those units in which only one hand/arm (foot/leg) moves, while the other hand/arm (foot/leg) rests.

Module II then classifies the bilateral limb movements. In the Contact category (Step 4), the relation between the two hands (feet) is analyzed regarding the physical contact and the bilateral units are classified with three Contact values. After the assessment the Contact values are concatenated with the StructureFocus values. Thus, for bilateral units there are StructureFocusContact values available that contain complex information about the unit.

After this step, only units with a *phasic* or *repetitive* Structure are further assessed (i.e., hereafter the NEUROGES assessment only refers to conceptual units, see below).

In the Formal Relation category (Step 5), the relation between the two hands (feet) is assessed regarding symmetry and dominance, and the adopted Contact units with a *phasic* or *repetitive* Structure are classified with four Formal Relation values. The Formal Relation value of a bilateral unit determines whether in Module III the Function of the unit is assessed for both hands (feet) together or separately for the right and left hand (foot). Thus, Module II constitutes a bridge between Module I and Module III, as it describes the relation between the two limbs, which in Module I have been assessed independently of each other.

Module III analyses the Function of limb, head, and trunk movements (with a *phasic* or *repetitive* Structure). The Function category (Step 6) refers to the emotional, cognitive, instrumental, and practical functions of body movements. To define such complex phenomena, many movement criteria are needed. These are the values of the Activation, Structure, Focus, Contact, and Formal Relation categories, as well as the criteria body-external space, path during stroke, orientation, hand shape, efforts, body involvement, and gaze. Based on these criteria, eleven Function values are defined. Most of these Function values are further specified with Type values.

The system can be used in a flexible manner according to the researcher's needs, as each category provides specific discrete results valid independent of the findings in other categories. Therefore, the researcher can decide until which step (category) (s)he wants to analyze the behaviour. As an example, the coding of only the Activation and the Structure categories will provide valuable data that can be interpreted with regard to the level of cognitive complexity.

In the following subsections, the modules, categories, and values are described. When reading the sections below, it is important to keep in mind that the descriptions of the theoretical background of the categories and values, which is subject of ongoing validation, should not be confused with the objective definitions of the categories and values. The precise operationalizations of the values refer only to the visual appearance of the movements. They are not confounded with the hypotheses about their validity.

5.1.2 Module I

Figure 1 gives an overview on the coding algorithm for Module I.

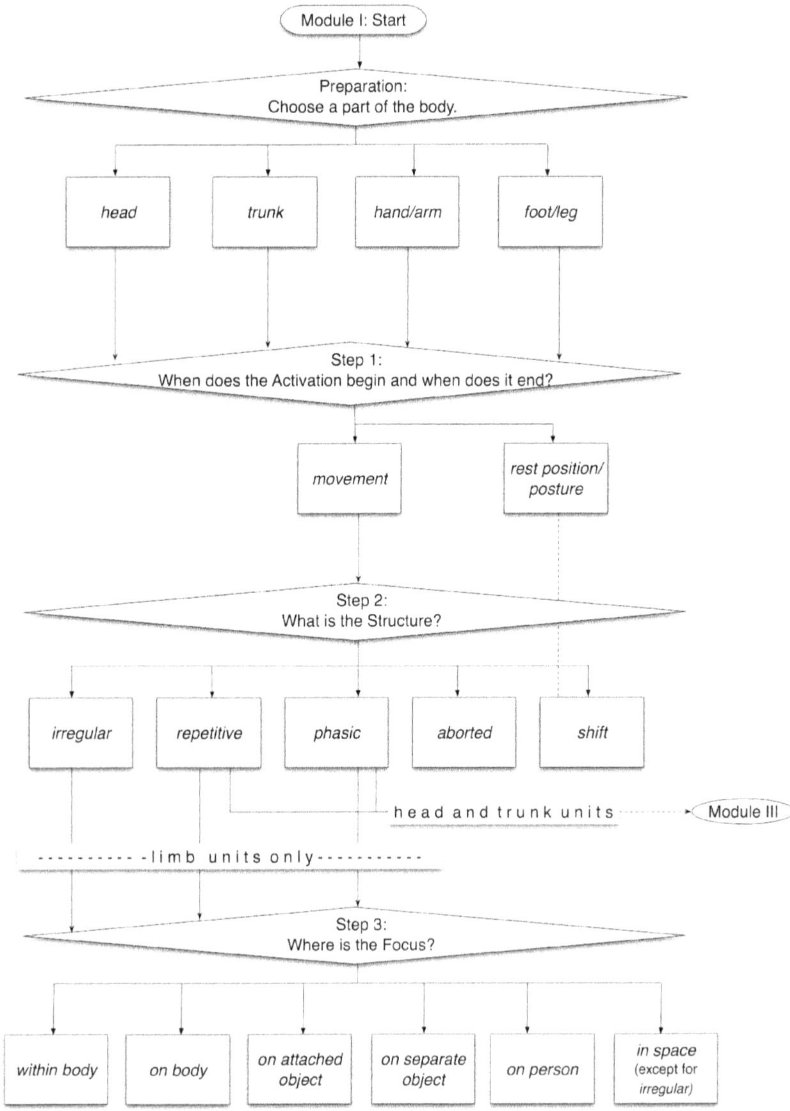

Figure 1 Coding algorithm for Module I

As a preparatory step for Module I coding, the researcher chooses the systems of the body (s)he wants to analyze (Figure 1, Preparation). This may be just one or two systems or all of them, i.e., the hands/arm, the feet/legs, the head, and the trunk.

5.1.2.1 The Activation category

In the first evaluation step, the stream of movement behaviour is segmented into Activation units (Figure 1, Step 1). Based on the movement criteria motion, anti-gravity position, and muscle contraction, two Activation values are distinguished: (i) *movement*, (ii) *no movement.* The short definitions of the two values according to these criteria are given in Table 1.

Table 1 Short definitions of the Activation values

Activation value	Short definition
movement	limb, head, or trunk in motion, potentially including transient motionless phases in anti-gravity position
no movement	limb, head, or trunk in *rest position* or in *posture;* *rest position:* specific arrangement of the relaxed limbs, defined by motionlessness, absence of an anti-gravity position, and muscle relaxation; *posture:* specific static arrangement of the limbs with tensioned muscles, defined by motionlessness and muscle contraction of the whole body, at least the hand/arm/shoulder, trunk, and head.

According to the above definition, the value *no movement* can likewise be termed *rest position / posture*.

The Activation category provides a general impression of an individual's level of motor activity. As indicated by the dotted line in Figure 1, the value *rest position / posture* is linked with the value *shift* as both values constitute the rest position - posture system.

If desired, *rest positions* of the hands/arms and feet/legs can be further classified with the Focus values *on body*, *on attached object*, *on separate object*, *on person*, and *in space,* as well as with the Contact values (*rest) act as a unit* and (*rest*) *act apart*, and with the Formal Relation values *symmetrical* and *asymmetrical.* However, for a better clarity these options are not indicated in the algorithms shown in the Figures 1 - 2.

5.1.2.2 The Structure category

The *movement* units as identified in Step 1 are further classified according to the Structure category (Figure 1, Step 2). The Structure of a *movement* unit is the 'construction' of the movement. It is primarily defined by the trajectory, the displacement, and the velocity. Therefore, the Structure values can be used in kinematographic investigations (Chapter 6). In addition to these criteria, human raters consider the presence/absence of efforts (Laban, 1988) and for hand movements, the presence/absence of hand shaping.

There are specific combinations of trajectory, displacement, and velocity. Based on some of these combinations, for certain *movement* units, specific phases can be identified, e.g. a one-dimensional trajectory with an increase in velocity and typically a centrifugal path characterizes a transport phase. Basically, three phases can be identified by the specific trajectory - displacement - velocity combinations: transport phase, complex phase with the subtypes motion complex phase and static[11] complex phase, and retraction phase. In NEUROGES, *movement* units that show these phases are termed "units with a phase structure". Given their defined structure, it is evident that these *movement* units are discrete in time. Those *movement* units that do not show at least a complex phase are termed "units with no phase structure". They can be potentially continuous in time.

Five Structure values are distinguished: (i) *irregular*, (ii) *repetitive*, (iii) *phasic,* (iv) *aborted*, and (v) *shift*. Short definitions of the Structure values are given in Table 2. The kinematographic descriptions in Chapter 6 further illustrate the characteristic patterns of trajectory, displacement, and velocity for each Structure value.

Table 2 Short definitions of the Structure values

Structure value	Short definition
irregular	movement with no phase structure; trajectory with short paths in various directions; practically no displacement between beginning and end of unit; potentially continuous in time
repetitive	movement with a phase structure; a motion complex phase in which the same movement path is used repetitively; discrete in time
phasic	movement with a phase structure; a static complex phase, in which there is transient motionlessness in an anti-gravity position, or a motion complex phase, in which the movement path is one-way; discrete in time
aborted	transport and retraction phase only; discrete in time; often no displacement
shift	displacement of the hand from a *rest position / posture* to another one; the trajectory basically equals the displacement; discrete in time

11 The term static (stroke) is adopted from Mandana Seyfeddinipur (personal communication).

Phasic and *repetitive* units are characterized by a phase structure, i.e., they typically contain a preparation phase, a complex phase, and a retraction phase. The preparation phase evidences that (implicit or explicit) planning processes are ongoing. In this phase the realization of the complex phase is prepared by moving the part of the body to a specific location where the complex phase is executed. Thereby it is evidenced that the complex phase is "something" that has been planned. In line with propositions from gesture research concerning the stroke phase in gesture (e.g. Kendon, 1972; McNeill, 1992; Seyfeddinipur, 2006), it is proposed here that the complex phase is the realization of a concept (however, in NEUROGES the identification of phases not only refers to gestures, but also to self-touches, actions, and expressive motions). "*Concept* may be tentatively defined as a representation formed in the mind by generalizing from particulars, and *conceptual thinking* as the process of performing the operations required to form and handle concepts." (Vignolo, 1999). Based on this definition, it is proposed here that *phasic* and *repetitive* units are associated with conceptual thinking. These units can be displayed explicitly or implicitly. Fine-grained movement analysis as well as neurobiological and neuropsychological investigations can distinguish between the explicit and implicit display.

However, *phasic* and *repetitive* units seem to differ with regard to cognitive complexity. Some evidence for this proposition is provided by motor control research and by clinical observation. Applying approximately comparable values, motor control research demonstrates that "single" movements are associated with more complex cognitive processes than repetitive movements, in which the part of the body moves back and forth on the same path. The latter are reported to partly rely on routine processes (Mourik & Beek, 2004; Spencer et al., 2003; Schaal et al., 2004; Huys et al., 2008). Thus, *phasic* units may rely on novel conceptualizations, while *repetitive* units seem to be associated with routine concepts.

In contrast to *phasic* and *repetitive* movements, *irregular* movements have no phase structure. In *irregular* movements the respective part of the body is not moved to a specific location to execute a complex phase, but it starts moving where it happens to be. These movements are not based on conceptual thinking but they are non-conceptual sensory-motor activations. By moving the part of the body they provide - potentially ongoing - motorsensory stimulation. It is proposed here that, thereby, they serve to regulate arousal. Arousal is the degree of activation of the central nervous system ranging from hyper- to hypoarousal. *Irregular* movements are displayed beyond the mover's awareness. As *irregular* units lack a phase structure, from the observer perspective their beginning, duration, and ending is unpredictable. In some individuals, *irregular* movements are continuously ongoing in a given context, being only interrupted by conceptual movements or by *shifts*.

On this background, the three values *irregular, repetitive,* and *phasic* are ordered with regard to the level of cognitive complexity on an axis from non-conceptual to complex conceptual.

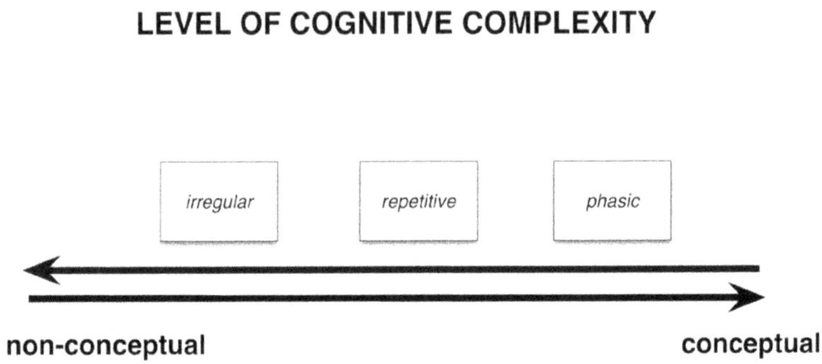

Figure 2 Structure values and level of cognitive complexity

A *shift* is a direct transition between two *rest positions / postures.* As exposed in Section 2.1, *rest-positions* and *postures* reflect emotional-cognitive-interactive states. Accordingly, *shifts* evidence changes of these states. *Shifts* are typically displayed implicitly. It is proposed here that a particularly high frequency of *shifts* between *rest positions* reflects that the individual does not find a position to rest in for a longer time. With regard to emotional, cognitive, and interactive processes, it might indicate that the individual does not find a state to stay in. Likewise, a particularly low frequency of *shifts* reflects that the individual does not leave the position.

Aborted units occur most often in bimanual units. The *aborted* unit in one limb then co-occurs with a complete *phasic* or *repetitive* unit in the other limb. This constellation reflects a lack of suppression of ipsilateral motor pathways controlling the non-dominant hand (Zülch & Müller, 1980; Lausberg et al., 2000; Zijdewind & Kernell, 2001; Westenberg et al., 2004; Lausberg et al, 2007). While the concept is to be executed unimanually by the dominant hand, the other hand, which displays the *aborted* unit, is co-activated (despite the concept) and then stopped. Unimanual *aborted* units are typically disruptions of movements that would have potentially developed to a *phasic* and *repetitive* unit. Seyfeddinipur (2006), who uses comparable values for gestures, reported in her analysis on speech-gesture coordination that, among others, these values co-occurred with speech disfluencies, and, more specifically, indicated an abandonment of the original speech plan (Seyfeddinipur, personal communication, 2011). Thus, *aborted* units reflect a disruption of concept realization. However, also shift movements can be *aborted.* In this case, there is a disruption in the process of adopting a new *rest position* or *posture.*

To summarize, *irregular, repetitive,* and *phasic* units are proposed to rely on processes with different levels of cognitive complexity ranging from non-conceptual via automatic conceptual to novel conceptual. *Shifts* are transitions between two *rest positions / postures. Aborted* units comprise different forms of disruptions in the execution of conceptual and shift movements.

After the Structure category coding, the assessment of the head and trunk movements stops for the time being. In Module III, the head and trunk Structure units that have a *phasic* or *repetitive* Structure are further assessed (indicated in Figure 1 by the right bar above the Step 3 rhombus). The Focus category as well as the subsequent Module II Contact and Formal Relation categories only serve for the further analysis of limb movements.

5.1.2.3 The Focus category

The *phasic, repetitive,* and *irregular* limb units that have been identified in Step 2 are further classified with the Focus category (Figure 1, Step 3).

The Focus category refers to the presence or absence of something/someone that the hand (or foot) acts on. If the hand (or foot) dynamically acts on something/someone, this object/subject is further specified. The Focus category is operationalized by four criteria: the presence/absence of physical contact with something/someone, the quality of that physical contact (dynamic vs. static), the object/subject of dynamic contact, and the orientation. According to these criteria, six Focus values are distinguished: (i) *within body*, (ii) *on body*, (iii) *on attached object*, (iv) *on separate object*, (v) *on person*, and (vi) *in space* (Table 3).

Table 3 Short definitions of the Focus values

Focus value	Short definition
within body	acting on body-internal structures, i.e., muscles, tendons, joints, by moving and without touching them, e.g. rolling the shoulders
on body	acting on the body surface
on attached object	acting on an object that is attached to the body
on separate object	acting on an object that is separate from the body
on person	acting on another person's body
in space	acting in space without touching anything

The values *on body*, *on attached object*, *on separate object*, and *on person* refer to transitive movements. The value *within body* shares with the transitive values that the moving part of the body acts **on** something. The value *in space* is distinct from the other values, as it does not refer to **what/where** the hand/foot acts **on** but **where** it acts **in**[12]. Thus, it is intransitive.

In *phasic* and *repetitive* units, the Focus assessment refers to the complex phase only. In *irregular* units, it refers to the whole unit.

12 The very rare cases of acting "on air" are practical actions focussing on the air as a physical entity, e.g. to fan oneself. They are coded with the *in space* value.

The theoretical background of the Focus category is compatible with the premotor theory of attention (Rizzolatti et al., 1994). According to this theory, spatial attention is strictly related to the preparation of a movement toward the object/subject of interest. At least for eye movements it has been demonstrated that it is not possible to move the eyes without an attentional shift (Shepard et al., 1986; Chelazzi et al., 1996; Schneider & Deubel, 1996).

Accordingly, the transitive Focus values indicate where to the mover shifts (part of) her/his attention. It is evident that in the case of implicit body movements this refers to primarily implicit attentional processes. The mover may shift (part of) her/his attention to the muscles, tendons, and joints (*within body*), to the body surface (*on body*), to objects that are attached to the body (*on attached object)*, to objects that are separate from the body (*on separate object*), or to another person's body (*on person*). For the intransitive *in space* movements, which are movements that are traditionally functionally defined as gestures, the spatial attention during the transport phase is directed to the space that is visually shared by the gesturer and the recipient. However, more research is needed on spatial attention during the preparation of gestures with no transport phase and for expressive motions.

In NEUROGES, the six values are ordered on an axis from body-internal to body-external: *within body*, *on body*, *on attached object*, *on separate object*, *on person,* and *in space* (Figure 3). Transitive and quasi-transitive values (acting on) are placed above the arrows. *On separate object* and *on person* represent different entities in the body-external space. The specific position of the *in space* value indicates that it is an intransitive value and that the quality of spatial attention differs from those of the transitive values.

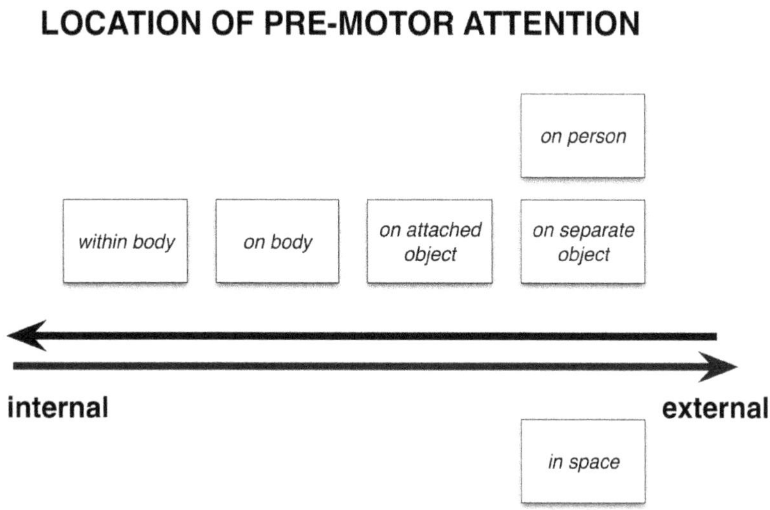

Figure 3 Focus values and location of pre-motor spatial attention

It is evident that it is of interest why an individual directs pre-motor attention to a certain location. For all transitive values, there can be physical and practical reasons, e.g. the muscles ache, the skin tickles, the (attached) watch does not function, the pen is used for writing, or the other person needs help. On the other hand, there can be mental reasons. As an example, the person is stressed, anxious, or overwhelmed and engages in jiggling the foot, in scratching her/himself, or in fidgeting with a necklace or a pen. The consideration of the Structure value of the respective Focus unit helps to distinguish between physical - practical and mental reasons (this body-mind dichotomy is useful of research but in fact a psychosomatic continuum has to be assumed).

5.1.2.4 Concatenation of the values of the Structure and Focus units

As the final evaluation step in Module I, the limb Structure units and the Focus units are concatenated (Figure 4). This procedure produces units with Structure-Focus values.

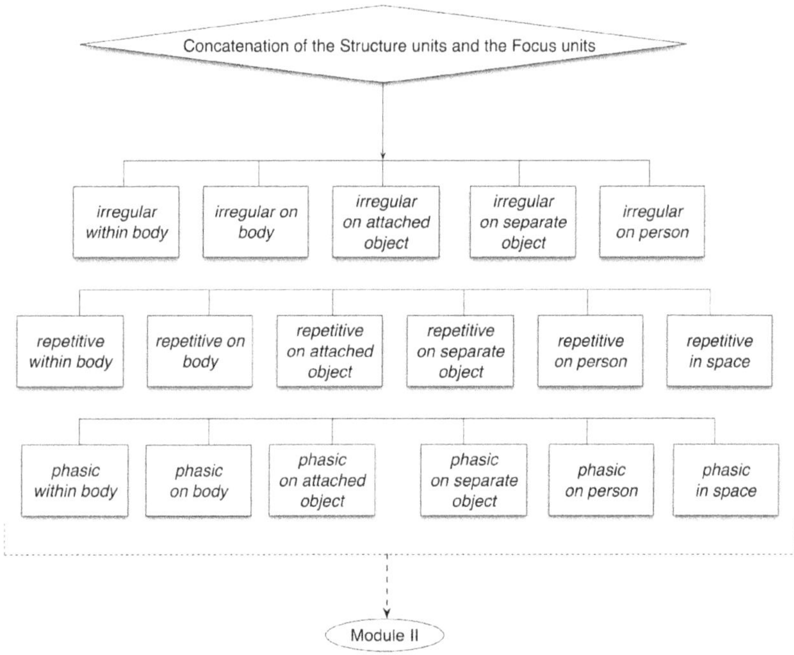

Figure 4 Concatenation of the Structure units and the Focus units

The StructureFocus values provide complex information for each unit about the combination of a certain level of cognitive complexity with a certain location of pre-motor attention.

For all StructureFocus units with an *irregular* Structure it is proposed here that they generally serve for arousal regulation. This can be either the regulation of hyper-arousal or of hypo-arousal. Based on the Focus values different subtypes of *irregular* units are distinguished.

In Subsection 2.1.2 ample empirical evidence has been provided that direct touching of the body, especially if it occurs continuously, is associated with stress, (predominantly negative) emotional engagement, and depression. This type of direct and continuous self-touching basically matches the StructureFocus value *irregular on body*. Freedman and Bucci (1981) suggested that *continuous body-focused* activity creates a white noise situation, which helps to reduce the discrepancy between incoming information and the mover's internal state. However, the author H.L. has argued that as *on body* movements are not only observed in the presence of external stimulation but also in its absence. Therefore, she has proposed that *irregular on body* movements serve to regulate hyper- or hypoarousal. Support for this proposition stems from neuroendocrinological research. In rodents grooming behaviour induces a reduction in the dopamine response to stress (Berridge, Mitton, Clark, & Roth, 1999) as well as an increase in physical growth, growth hormon (GH) and Brain-Derived-Neurotropic-Factor (BDNF) (Schanberg & Field, 1987; Burton et al., 2007; Chatterjee et al., 2007). - It is tentatively suggested here that *irregular within body* are less effective for arousal regulation than *irregular on body movements,* since there is no tactile stimulation but only a proprioceptive one. Furthermore, it is suggested that *irregular on attached object* and *irregular on separate object* movements are socially more accepted forms of *irregular* activity than the other two values. However, they are also less effective for arousal regulation than *on body* movements, since they lack the tactile stimulation of the part of the body that is acted on.

For StructureFocus units with a *phasic and repetitive* Structure and a transitive Focus value more movement criteria are needed to distinguish between physical/practical and mental reasons. These criteria are applied in Module III.

Intransitive *phasic* and *repetitive in space* units are movements that are traditionally functionally defined as gestures. In Subsection 2.1.1 it has been outlined in detail that gestures, i.e., *in space* movements, reflect and affect cognitive processes. The Focus model emphasizes the aspect that *in space* movements are externalizations of conceptual thinking. Few of these *in space* movements are immediate embodiments of emotions. Thus, from a Focus perspective *in space* movements are externalizations of thoughts and emotions.

5.1.3 Module II

Module II applies to limb movements only. While in Module I the right and left limbs have been coded independently from each other, in Module II the relation between the two hands (or feet) is assessed. Figure 5 shows the coding algorithm for Module II.

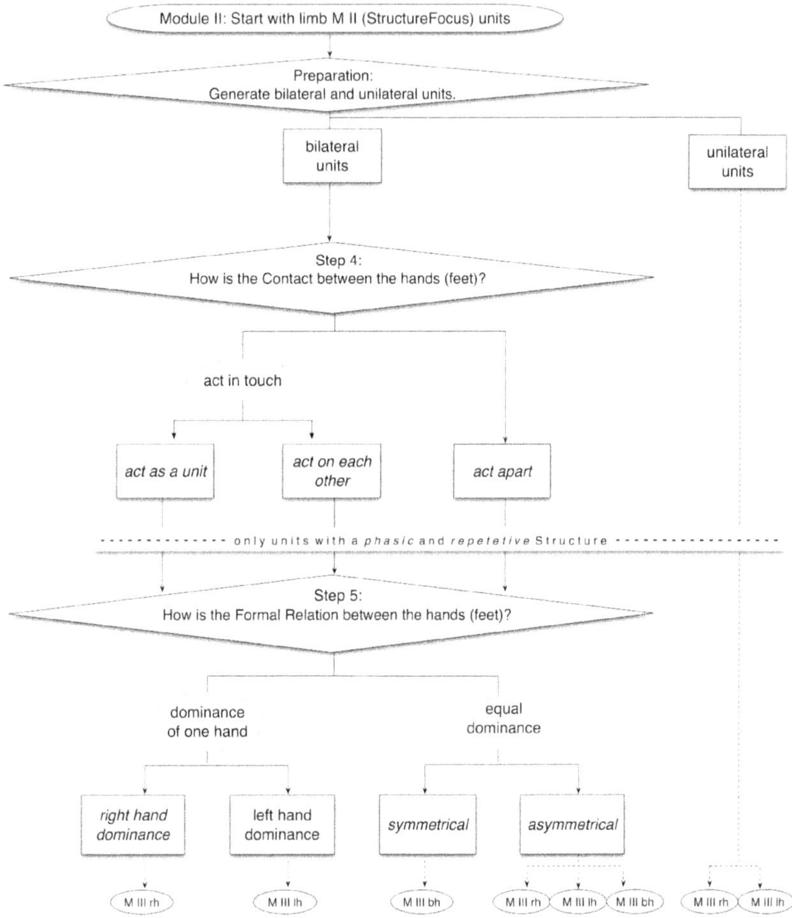
Module II: Start with limb M II (StructureFocus) units
Preparation:
Generate bilateral and unilateral units.
bilateral units
unilateral units
Step 4:
How is the Contact between the hands (feet)?
act in touch
act as a unit
act on each other
act apart
only units with a phasic and repetetive Structure
Step 5:
How is the Formal Relation between the hands (feet)?
dominance of one hand
equal dominance
right hand dominance
left hand dominance
symmetrical
asymmetrical
M III rh
M III lh
M III bh
M III rh
M III lh
M III bh
M III rh
M III lh

Figure 5 Coding algorithm for Module II

As the preparatory step in Module II (Figure 5, Preparation), bilateral and unilateral limb units are generated from the Module I right and left StructureFocus units. Unilateral limb units are units in which one limb moves while the other limb rests. The bilateral units are units in which both hands (or feet) move simultaneously. They are submitted to the Module II analysis.

5.1.3.1 The Contact category

The Contact category evaluates the physical contact between the two hands (feet)[13]. (Figure 5, Step 4). It is operationalized by the presence/absence of physical contact between the hands and the quality of that contact (dynamic versus static). According to these criteria, three Contact values are defined: (i) *act as a unit*, (ii) *act on each other*, and (iii) *act apart* (Table 4). In *phasic* and *repetitive* units, the Contact assessment refers to the complex phase only. In *irregular* units, it refers to the whole unit.

Table 4 Short definitions of the Contact values

Contact value	Short definition
act on each other	the hands dynamically touch each other
act as a unit	the two hands are in touch with a fixed configuration and they take a joint action
act apart	both hands move simultaneously without touching each other

The Contact values *act apart* and act in touch (*act as a unit, act on each other*) are associated with different levels of stability of the neural control of the bilateral movements.

Split-brain research evidences that bimanual *act apart* movements are instable with regard to neural control. *Act apart* units may evidence concept errors such as mirroring (Zülch and Müller, 1969; Preilowsky, 1975; Lausberg et al., 2003), following (Tanaka et al., 1996; Lausberg et al., 2003), unrelated movements (Akelaitis, 1945; Bogen, 1993; Tanaka et al., 1996), and to execution errors such as dyssynchronous movements (Lausberg et al., 2000; Lausberg et al., 2007). Dyssynchronous movements indicate a disturbance of the interhemispheric cooperation that is necessary to achieve a fine distal attunement of the movements of the two hands. Also in schizophrenic patients a right - left dyssynchrony has been documented (Condon, 1969; Davis 1978). In certain bilateral motor tasks, right - left incongruences can also be provoked in neurologically healthy individuals (e.g. Mechsner et al., 2001).

Split-brain research further revealed that these patients often gestured with folded hands. The patients employed these *act as a unit* movements as a compensatory strategy to avoid the manifestation of disturbances in the intermanual cooperation and coordination (Lausberg et al., 2000; Lausberg et al., 2007). In healthy individuals *act as a unit* movements are often observed in situations when mental concentration is aimed at, e.g. holding the tips of the fingers pressed against each other while displaying *batons*.

---

13 Since researchers most often code hand/arm movements with Module II, for convenience, in the definitions below, the term hand will be used instead of hand (foot) but the definitions apply likewise to foot movements.

Another type of act in touch units is *act on each other* units. These movements provide a strong sensori-motor stimulation, as each hand moves, feels, and is felt.

5.1.3.2 Concatenation of the values of the StructureFocus and Contact units

After the Contact category assessment, the StructureFocus units and the Contact units are concatenated. The StructureFocusContact units provide complex information about the bilateral units. Thereby, the interpretation of the behaviour becomes even more specific.

The combined values can be interpreted with regard to the level of cognitive complexity, the location of pre-motor attention, and the stability of neural control of the bilateral movements. As an example, *irregular on body act on each other* movements may be specifically effective to regulate arousal since they provide very strong sensory-motor stimulation. Or, *phasic in space act apart* units offer a particularly large range of movement options in the externalization of thoughts.

5.1.3.3 The Formal Relation category

Starting with Step 5 (Formal Relation category), the NEUROGES assessment applies only to movements with a *phasic* or a *repetitive* Structure, i.e., to conceptual movements (see Figure 5, horizontal bar above Step 5). The Formal Relation category and the subsequent Module III Function and Type categories primarily refer to the cognitive concepts that are evidenced in the body movements.

The Contact units that have a *phasic* or *repetitive* Structure are further evaluated concerning the Formal Relation (Figure 5, Step 5). This category compares the movements of the two hands regarding the distinctness of the movement during the complex phase and regarding the trajectories. It is operationalized by the criteria presence/absence of dominance and symmetry. Four Formal Relation values are distinguished: (i) *right hand dominance*, (i) *left hand dominance*, (iii) *symmetrical*, and (vi) *asymmetrical* (Table 5). The Formal Relation assessment refers to the complex phase only.

Table 5 Short definitions of the Formal Relation values

Formal Relation value	Short definition
right hand dominance	the right hand is dominant
left hand dominance	the left hand is dominant
symmetrical	both hands are equally dominant and move on symmetrical trajectories
asymmetrical	both hands are equally dominant and move on asymmetrical trajectories

The Formal Relation category primarily serves to prepare bilateral units with a *phasic* and *repetitive* Structure for the Module III Function and Type assessment. The four Formal Relation values determine whether the Function is assessed only for the right hand in the bilateral movement (see also Subsection 2.5.2 for the empirical background of this assessment rule), only for the left hand in the bilateral movement, for both hands together, e.g. both hands together pantomime drumming, or separately for the right hand and for the left hand, e.g. the left hand makes a rolling movement while the right hand points to an external location (Figure 5, bottom row).

Furthermore, the Formal Relation values with dominance of one hand, i.e., *right hand dominance* and *left hand dominance*, respectively, enable to make predictions about hemispheric specialization in the generation of the bilateral unit. As exposed in Subsection 2.5.2, bilateral movements with *right hand dominance* and *left hand dominance*, respectively, indicate that the movement is predominantly generated in the contralateral hemisphere. The Formal Relation values with equal dominance of the hands, i.e., *symmetrical* and *asymmetrical,* are suited to follow up the question of cognitive complexity that has been addressed with the Structure category. *Asymmetrical* movements rely on more complex cognitive processes than *symmetrical* movements (e.g. Rothwell, 1994; Preilowsky, 1975; Zaidel & Sperry, 1977; Lausberg et al., 2003).

5.1.4. Module III

The Module III assessment applies to units of the hands/arms, the feet/legs, the head, and the trunk that have a *phasic* or *repetitive* Structure (Figure 6, on top). Thus, Module III refers to conceptual movements only.

In contrast to the sequencing of the previous categories (Steps 1 - 5), the Function category (Step 6) and the Type category (Step 7) do not strictly constitute subsequent coding steps but rather the two categories can be coded interdependently (as indicated by the bi-directional arrows).

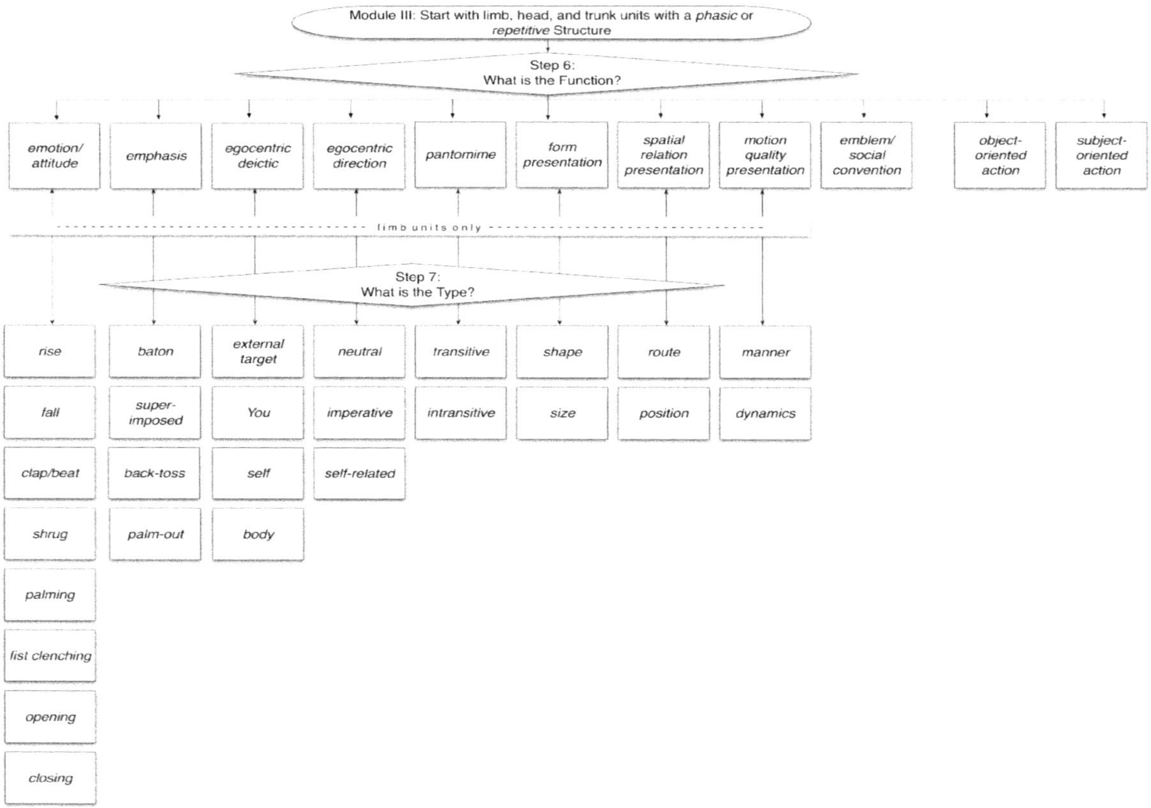

Figure 6 Coding algorithm for Module III

5.1.4.1 The Function category

The units that are submitted to the Function category assessment are the head and trunk Structure units, the bilateral limb Formal Relation units, and the unilateral limb StructureFocus units, which have been generated in the Module II preparatory step.

The Function category registers groups of movements that share certain combinations of movement features and that have the same function (as outlined in the Subsection 4.5.3, the development of Module III differed from those of the Modules I and II, as not only the visual appearance of a movement but obligatorily also function of the movement was relevant for the development of the values).

As argued in Sections 2.1 - 2.2, body movements do not only reflect cognitive, emotional, and interactive processes but they also affect these processes. Furthermore, it has been exposed (Section 2.3) that any body movement has a function and that - with the exception of some hyperkinetic syndromes in neuropsychiatric diseases - body movements are not displayed accidentally or randomly. The within-subject function of a body movement can be to promote the processing of emotional experience, to promote speech outflow, to promote cognitive processing, to change the external physical world, or to change the mover's psychosomatic state. Thus, the Function category refers to groups of movements that have specific emotional, cognitive, physical, or practical functions and that share certain features in their visual appearance. It is evident that the same movements may also have between-subjects functions. However, the Function values refer to within-subject functions. The between-subject dimension of the same movements is assessed with a specific evaluation procedure, which is introduced in Chapter 18.

Based on the function and on the combination of certain movement features (see below), eleven Function values are defined: *emotion/attitude, emphasis, egocentric deictic, egocentric direction, pantomime, form presentation, spatial relation presentation, motion quality presentation, emblem, object-oriented action,* and *subject-oriented action.* Hand movements cover all eleven values, while foot movements are typically *emotion/attitude, pantomime, object-oriented action,* and *subject-oriented action.* Head movements are typically *emotion/attitude, emphasis, egocentric deictic, egocentric direction, pantomime, emblem, object-oriented action,* and *subject-oriented action.* Trunk movements are often due to postural involvement during hand/arm gestures, e.g. moving the trunk forward when intensively pointing to an object that is in front of the gesturer. However, in this case the trunk movement would **not** be coded with the value *egocentric deictic.* The function of trunk movements is only coded if the trunk movement has a function per se such as *emotion/attitude, pantomime, object-oriented action,* and *subject-oriented action.*

In order to describe the visual appearance of a group of movements that have the same function, a high number of movement criteria are needed. Therefore, the Function values are operationalized by several criteria. These are the Activation, Structure, Focus, and Laterality (Contact and Formal Relation) values, and in addition, the criteria gesture/action space, path during complex phase, orientation, hand shape, efforts, body involvement, and gaze. In other words, all previous assessments are considered and supplemented by further movement criteria. Obviously, for foot, head, and trunk not all criteria can be used. Table 6 provides the short definitions of the Function values. For lack of space, only the definitions of the Function values for hand/arm movements are given.

Table 6 Short definitions of the Function values for hand/arm movements

Function value	Short definition
emotion/attitude	displaying exclusively an emotion or an attitude • Structure: *phasic.* • Focus: *within body, in space, on body.* • Laterality*: bh > rh > lh. • Gesture/action space: often ipsilateral hemi-space. • Path: **one- or two-dimensional.** • Hand orientation: the **hand orientation is in line with the direction of the hand/arm and trunk movement**, i.e., the hand does not adopt an orientation independently from the rest of the body e.g. when opening the arms, the palms are oriented toward the addressee. • Hand shape: the **hand shaping is in line with the whole body shaping**, e.g. contracting. • Efforts: **very distinct use of efforts.** • Body involvement: **obligatorily accompanied by a postural-facial expression**; there is strong involvement of the trunk, head, and face in gestures and postures . • Gaze: not at hands.
emphasis	setting accents on speech • Structure: ***repetitive*** > *phasic.* • Focus: *in space*, only in exceptional cases *on body* or *on separate object.* • Laterality: bh > lh > rh. • Gesture/action space: ipsilateral hemi-space, level of trunk, middle kinesphere. • Path: **one-dimensional up-down** or **two-dimensional arch-like supination – pronation.**

	• Hand orientation: no distinct orientation; if superimposed to other gesture types, hand orientation of primary gesture is maintained. • Hand shape: relaxed open hand; if superimposed to other gesture types, hand shape of primary gesture is maintained. • Efforts: acceleration (quick) with change from free to bound flow to generate **end point accent.** • Body involvement: *emphasis* gestures are **synchronized with mouth and head** movements • Gaze: not at hands. • Other criteria: in line with prosody.
egocentric deictic	indicating a location by using an egocentric frame of reference • Structure: ***phasic*** >> *repetitive.* • Focus: *in space > on body > on attached object, on separate object, on person.* • Laterality: rh > lh > bh. • Gesture/action space: variable use, determined by the designated location. • Path: one- or two-dimensional, **spoke-** or arch-**like** path. • Hand orientation: **tip of fingers oriented toward designated location.** • Hand shape: distinct hand shape: **flat hand,** or **extended index** or thumb. The thumb may be preferred when pointing to a location behind the gesturer's back. In rare cases if the hand is inhibited, the pointing might also be executed with the elbow or the shoulder. • Effort: **direct space**, often end point accent; rather bound flow. • Gaze: The gesturer looks at the designated location he/she is pointing at, except for when he/she is referring to him/herself. • Body involvement: An *egocentric deictic* gesture may be accompanied by a head movement that indicates the direction toward the designated location. • Other criteria: The pointing gesture can be accompanied by words "here", "there", "I", etc..

egocentric direction	indicating a direction or a route by using an egocentric frame of reference • Structure: *phasic.* • Focus: *in space.* • Laterality: rh > bh > lh. • Gesture/action space: **variable use, determined by the designated direction.** • Path: one- or two-dimensional, spoke- or arch-like. • Hand orientation: (i) direction: **in line with the designated direction line:** in intransitive gestures, the longitudinal hand axis (wrist - finger tips) in line with the designated direction line; in transitive gestures, the sagittal hand axis (palm - back of hand) in line with the designated direction line; (ii) route: fingers tips trace route. • Hand shape: **relaxed flat hand;** in route indications, the index may be extended. • Effort: (i) direction: **free flow, hand is often "thrown" in the direction,** emphasis on end-point of gesture; (ii) route: bound flow. • Body involvement: proximal arm muscles are often involved. • Gaze: gesturer looks into the designated direction. • Other criteria: *egocentric direction* gestures can be accompanied by words such as "towards", "upwards", "backwards", "forwards", "sidewards", "to the right", etc..
pantomime	pretending to perform an action • Structure: *phasic, repetitive.* • Focus: *in space >> on body > on separate object, on attached object*, e.g. pantomiming combing hair. • Laterality: rh > bh > lh. • Gesture/action space: variable use, **determined by the action space of the action that is subject to the pantomime.** • Path: distinct, depends on the pantomimed action. • Hand orientation: The hand adopts a specific orientation, which enables to execute the motor action and in which **the hand keeps its natural orientation as a part of gesturer's body** (exceptions: in *pantomime - transitive hand-as-object* Tech-

	nique of tool Presentation; *pantomime - intransitive* with object). • Hand shape: distinct, depends on the shape of the imaginary counterpart or the shape of the imaginary tool. • Efforts: distinct, variation in the Effort qualities, depends on the pantomimed action. • Body involvement: **involvement of head and trunk or even whole body.** • Gaze: on the hands. •
form presentation	presenting a specific form (what) • Structure: *phasic > repetitive;* a repetitive *Structure* is found when presenting a form with repetitive features such as a star. • Focus: *in space*; only in exceptional cases *on body* or *on separate object*, e.g. the form of an object is traced on a table or on the thigh. • Laterality: bh > rh > lh. • Gesture/action space: typically display of *form presentation* in the **body midline space** (body midline sagittal plane, middle kinesphere, level of upper trunk). • Path: depends on the Technique of Presentation: in *hand-as-object* and *enclosure* Techniques, there is a static complex phase, i.e., no path; in *tracing*, the path is often closed and the starting point and the end point match each other, e.g. to establish the contour of a circle. • Hand orientation: depends on the Technique of Presentation; in bimanual *form presentation* gestures, the palms of the hands are typically oriented to each other, i.e., towards the center of the imaginary form. • Hand shape: **variable**, depends on the form that is subject to the presentation gesture and on the Technique of Presentation. • Efforts: **invariant**, typically bound flow, direct space, no time, no weight. • Body involvement: isolated use of hands/arms. • Gaze: When referring to concrete objects (Referent: *material*), the gesturer often looks at the hand or at the imaginary object, respectively.

spatial relation presentation	presenting a spatial relation in a mento-heliocentric frame of reference (where or where along on an imaginary map) • Structure: *phasic*, typically only in bimanual units; *repetitive*, in bimanual but also in unimanual units. In the latter case, there is a sequential presentation of the two locations ("here… and there"). • Focus: *in space*; only in exceptional cases *on body* or *on separate object*, e.g. the position is marked on the thigh or on the table. • Laterality: rh > bh > lh. • Gesture/action space: very variable, **distinct and creative use of space**, i.e., the complex phases are displayed at specific locations in the gesture/action space, e.g. right upper gesture/action space. • Path: depends on the Type value of the *spatial relation presentation:* in *space - position*, there is a static complex phase; in *space - route*, there is a path during complex phase. • Hand orientation: The hand orientation reflects the mento-heliocentric perspective. As the map is typically projected to the horizontal plane, the **longitudinal hand axis** (wrist - middle finger tip) is **in line with the vertical axis** and the fingertips are oriented downwards. Only if the map is projected to the frontal plane, the longitudinal hand axis is in line with the sagittal axis and the fingertips are oriented forward. • Hand shape: depends on the Technique of Presentation. • Efforts: bound flow, direct space, no time, no weight, no variation in the effort factors. • Body involvement: - • Gaze: When referring to concrete spatial locations (Referent: *material*), the gesturer looks at the hand(s), i.e., more specifically, at the designated position or route on the imaginary spatial map. •

motion quality presentation	presenting a specific quality of movement in a mento-heliocentric frame of reference (how) • Structure: *phasic*, *repetitive*. A *repetitive* Structure is present when a manner of movement is represented. • Focus: *in space*; only in exceptional cases *on body* or *on separate object*. • Laterality: bh > rh > lh. • Gesture/action space: If the gesture includes additional space information about where to or where along the object or subject moves, there is a distinct and creative use of space. • Path: The path during complex phase is an obligatory feature of *motion quality presentations*. There is **never a static complex phase**. • Hand orientation: If the *motion quality* gesture includes additional spatial relation information on where the object or subject moves, a specific hand orientation is adopted. • Hand shape: If the *motion quality* gesture includes additional form information about the object or subject that or who moves, a specific hand shape is adopted. • Efforts: The **variation of effort factors** is the most prominent kinesic feature of *motion quality presentation*. The only exception is the intentional representation of monotonous motion, e.g. when representing gear transmission. In this case, special emphasis is put on the monotony and the invariance of the effort factors. • Body involvement: - • Gaze: If representing an actual motion quality, i.e., a concrete object displaying a concrete motion (Referent: *material*), the gaze is directed at the hand.
emblem / social convention	signing all kinds of information / performing a socially conventionalized action • Structure: *phasic, repetitive.* • Focus: *in space, on body, on attached object, on person.* • Laterality: bh > rh = lh • Gesture/action space: specific for each *emblem.*

	• Path: specific for each *emblem.* • Hand orientation: distinct orientation, specific for each *emblem.* • Hand shape: distinct shape, specific for each *emblem.* • Effort: specific for each *emblem.* • Body involvement: - • Gaze: often to addressee.
object-oriented action	changing the external physical world • Structure: *phasic*, *repetitive*, *shifts.* • Focus: ***on separate object***, *on attached object*, *on person,* rarely *in space.* • Laterality: lh > bh = rh • Gesture/action space: mobile target objects are typically manipulated in front of the body midline; otherwise, the use of the body-external space is determined by the location of the target object. • Path: distinct path during complex phase, specified for each action. • Hand orientation: depends on the object and the action. • Hand shape: depends on the object that is manipulated. • Efforts: variation of the effort factors. • Body involvement: often involvement of other parts of the body. • Gaze: **typically at the hand**, in order to control the execution of the action.
subject-oriented action	changing the own physical (and secondarily psychosomatic) state • Structure: *phasic, repetitive, shift.* • Focus: *on body, within body, on attached object, on separate object,* (very rarely) *in space.* • Laterality: lh > bh > rh. • Gesture/action space: variable, determined by the action. • Path: distinct path during complex phase, depends on the action. • Hand orientation: depends on the action and if it applies, on the object that is manipulated.

	• Hand shape: depends on the action and if it applies, on the object that is manipulated. • Efforts: variation of the effort factors. • Body involvement: possible. • Gaze: depends on the trigger or motive; typically **no gaze at hand** if the subject-oriented action serves mental arousal regulation.

As described in detail in Subsection 4.5.3, the Function values *emphasis, egocentric deictic, egocentric direction, pantomime, form presentation, spatial relation presentation, motion quality presentation,* and *emblem* have been developed based on Efron's system. More or less independent researchers have later arrived at similar propositions as Efron about the meaning of certain gesture values that are each characterized by a specific visual appearance. Therefore, validity can be assumed for Efron's basic values (Section 3.4). As it will become evident in the following paragraphs, starting from Efron's definitions the theoretical background of the NEUROGES Function values has been elaborated.

Emphasis: Emphasis is defined as "force or intensity of expression that gives impressiveness or importance to something"[15].

In gesture, emphasis can be produced by setting dynamic accents. These are movements that are strong, direct, and quick. These motor accents point out short segments of the speech. In synchrony with prosody, these gestures emphasize certain aspects of the verbal statement. Obviously, a sequence of accents creates a metre or a rhythm. As such, *emphasis* gestures can be regarded as manual equivalents of prosody. They convey rhythmical and potentially acoustical information (if the Focus value is *on body* or *on separate object*). In the latter case, their effect is less dependent on a well visible location of the hand in the gesture/action space than the effect of the other gesture Function values that provide visual information.

Furthermore, emphasis can be put to speech by accompanying the process of verbalizing, i.e., bringing out a concept and presenting it. By embodying a direction of movement, e.g. rotating the palm out, these *emphasis* gestures accompany – and thereby enforce – the process of quasi rotating out words (thoughts) and then presenting them.

Emphasis gestures may superimpose emphasis on *egocentric deictic, egocentric direction, form presentation, spatial relation presentation,* and *emblem* gestures.

15 http://www.merriam-webster.com/dictionary, July 23, 2013

Egocentric deictic: An *egocentric deictic* indicates where something is located by using an egocentric frame of reference.

A gesturer who provides information about spatial relations, motions, or actions may choose the egocentric or the mento-heliocentric perspective. In the egocentric perspective, the gesturer is the point of reference. The term "mento-heliocentric" (heliocentric = the sun is at the centre of the solar system) is introduced here to convey the concept that the gesturer mentally takes the perspective of the sun. Thus, his/her view on spatial relations, motions, and actions differs from the view that is obtained in an egocentric perspective.

With an *egocentric deictic* the gesturer displays spatial information from an egocentric perspective. She/he her-/himself constitutes the point of spatial reference that the other points in space are related to: "I am here and it is there." If the target is not in front of the gesturer, (s)he typically rotates the head and as a tendency also the trunk to be vis-à-vis with the target. Furthermore, the hand axis is oriented centrifugally from the body midline. As an example, if the target is on the gesturer's right, (s)he rotates the head and upper trunk to the right and then points to the target. Note that the gesturer may project him-/herself into an imaginary space while keeping the egocentric frame of reference, e.g. "In my old apartment, if I entered it, the bathroom was on my right." Here, the egocentric frame is projected into a mental imagery space.

The indication of a location may be an indirect reference to an object/subject, i.e., the pointing primarily designates an actual object/subject that/who is identified by its/his/her location. As an example, the gesturer points to the location of the chair to designate the chair.

The target may be visible ("There is the table") or invisible ("The basket is under the table"). However, for those targets that are invisible because they are far away, *egocentric direction* gestures (see below) are preferred.

Egocentric deictics are typically displayed explicitly, i.e., the gesturer is aware of displaying the gesture.

Egocentric direction: The *egocentric direction* gesture indicates where to, from where to where, or where along something/-one moves by using an egocentric frame of reference: "I am here and it is along that way." The gesturer's body is the spatial point of reference for defining the direction or the route[16].

(i) direction: A direction is defined as "a line leading to a place or point"[17]. "Direction is the information contained in the relative position of one point with respect to another without the distance information"[18]. In accordance with these definitions, one function of the *egocentric direction* gesture is to indicate a direction (towards where) without distance information. As the frame of reference is egocentric, the point of reference, which the other point is spatially related to,

16 Since in the egocentric perspective, there are more often indications of directions than of routes, the value was termed *egocentric direction*.

17 http://www.merriam-webster.com/dictionary, July 23, 2013

18 http://en.wikipedia.org/wiki , July 23, 2013

is the gesturer's body. Thus, the *egocentric direction* gesture projects a line from the gesturer to another location in the external space, e.g.: "From my perspective, Paris is in that direction". As a direction does not contain distance information, *egocentric directions* are preferred to *egocentric deictics* for indicating locations that are far away and invisible.

(ii) route: A route is defined as "a way or course taken in getting from a starting point to a destination"[19], or as "an established line of travel or access"[17]. Thus, the depiction of a route implies the indication of a start point and an end point. In an *egocentric direction* gesture that indicate a route, the emphasis may be on the change of position with an accent on the start point and the end point (from where to where) or on the path between the start and end positions (where along). These gestures may not only indicate the path from the gesturer to an external location ("...from me to there"), or the path from an external location to the gesturer ("...from there to me"), but also the route between two or more locations in the external space ("... from there to over there"). Especially in the latter case it is important that there is an egocentric frame of reference ("[I am here] and it is from there to there"). Otherwise, the correct Function value is *spatial relation*.

The *egocentric direction* gestures may be used transitively. In this case, hand indicates towards where, from where to where, or where along something/someone is moved. The moved or to be moved entity may be the addressee (parts of his/her body or his/her mental state), an object, or the gesturer her/himself (his/her body or his/her mental state). As examples, the gesturer may indicate to the addressee to move to the left, to cheer up, or to move something away. Or, the gesturer may mentally rehearse the direction his/her body shall take during a performance, or in self-suggestion indicate to her-/himself to calm down.

Just like *egocentric deictics, egocentric direction* gestures may be based on a mental translation of the gesturer into an imaginary space. The gesturer projects him-/herself into an imaginary space while keeping the egocentric frame of reference: "In Paris, if I stood in front of the Eiffel Tower, it would be in that direction". Thus, the egocentric frame is projected into the imagery space and then the *egocentric direction* gesture is performed.

Just like *egocentric deictics, egocentric direction* gestures are typically displayed explicitly, i.e., the gesturer is aware of displaying the gesture.

Pantomime: The gesturer pretends ("as if") to perform a motor action. For the definition of action see the below paragraph on *object-oriented action*.

The Function value *pantomime* refers to the intentional demonstration of such actions ("as if") but not to their actual execution. Examples for *pantomimes* are pretending to brush the teeth with an imaginary toothbrush, pretending to climb up a mountain, moving the arms as if marching, or pretending that an external

19 http://oxforddictionaries.com/ July 23, 2013

object hits the gesturer. Note that if the gesturer would actually brush the teeth, this would be coded as *subject-oriented action*, or if (s)he would move a chair aside, this would be coded as *object-oriented action.*

It is an essential criterion for the Function value *pantomime* that the cognitive perspective is egocentric. The gesturer is the actor in the pretended action. The egocentric perspective is reflected in movement by the fact that the hands keep their natural orientation as parts of the gesturer's body relative to the other parts of the body. As in real actions, the hand and head positions are coordinated such that the actions of the hands can be visually controlled, the same arrangement of parts of the body is found in *pantomime*. Therefore, in *pantomime*, there is typically an involvement of the head and upper trunk in coordination with the hand/arm movement. As an example, in the *pantomime* of hammering the hand, the arm, the head, and the trunk are spatially and dynamically coordinated.

Not coded with the value *pantomime* are "as if" demonstrations of non-action movements such as emotional expressions and gestures. As an example, a gesturer who narrates a movie in which the main character performs an *egocentric deictic* may behave as if he were the main character and as if he performed an *egocentric deictic*. In this case, the Function value *egocentric deictic* is given. Only "as if" presentations of actions are coded as *pantomime.*

In special experimental settings, a *pantomime* may be performed with an actual tool held in the hand and an actual counter-part, e.g. holding an actual hammer in the hand and pretending to hammer (but not really doing it) on an actual nail.

Presentation: The three Function values *form presentation, spatial relation presentation,* and *motion quality presentation* have in common that they present something. This might be a form, a spatial relation, or a motion quality.

The term ***presentation*** is used in delimitation to the term re-presentation. The term *presentation* indicates that the three Function values register what can actually be seen in the body movement. As examples, the hand is formed to a round shape and thereby presents a round shape, the two hands are placed at different positions in the gesture/action space and thereby a spatial relation emerges between the two hands, or the hand opens and closes with strength and thereby a motion quality is presented. In contrast, the term re-presentation refers to the assumed referent, e.g. the hand re-presents a ball, the two hands show the distance between two churches in a city, or the hand re-presents the movement of hand-bellows.

In *form presentation* and *spatial relation presentation* gestures, the form or the spatial relation may be presented in a static complex phase. As examples, the hand adopts a certain shape that is held for a while, or the two hands present a spatial relation by adopting static positions. Thus, the information is conveyed by a static visual image, i.e., a photo could capture the relevant information. However, likewise, in *form presentation, spatial relation presentation,* and *motion quality presentation* gestures, the information can be conveyed in a motion complex phase. As examples, the image of a form is created by tracing in the air a shape (Technique of Presentation value *tracing),* or the image of a form is created by stroking along the imaginary object (Technique of Presentation value *palpating).* For images that are generated in motion complex phases, such as in *tracing* or *palpating* a form, in establishing a spatial relation by sequential gestures, or in depicting a motion quality, the term **motion image** is introduced here in delimitation to a **static visual image**. It is suggested here that the cognitive process that underlies a motion image is that a mental image of an object is projected into the gesture/action space and then, the hand traces or palpates along this projection. The mental image is stored multi-modally, i.e., visuo-spatial and sensori-motor. The observer recognizes the motion image, which the gesturer presents, based on her/his own repertoire of multi-modally stored mental images. To recognize the form, the observer has to follow the gesturer's hand movements and to memorize the path of the movements. This may imply that the observer mentally tunes into the gesturer's creative movement and that (s)he uses his/her own sensori-motor experience to comprehend the motion image. The mental recording of the movement path (as if the path were materialized) results in the motion image.

The NEUROGES definitions of the three *presentation* values imply a **hierarchy** between them: *motion quality presentation > spatial relation presentation > form presentation.* A *motion quality presentation* gesture may include information about a form and a spatial relation (how what moves where). A *spatial relation presentation* may include information about a form (what is where). A *form presentation* is the most basic *presentation* value as it only includes information about the form.

Form presentation: The *form presentation* gesture presents (only) a form.
"Form refers to the shape, visual appearance, and configuration of an object."[19].
"The shape and structure of anything, as distinguished from the material of which it is composed."[17].

There are different ways how information about form is transformed into a gesture. The gesturer shapes her/his hand(s) according to an actually present or a mental image of the form. With the hand(s), (s)he establishes a static form. Or, the gesturer creates a motion image of a form by tracing or by palpating along the mental image of the form that is projected into the gesture/action space. The cognitive perspective that the gesturer takes may be egocentric or mento-heliocentric.

The *form presentation* gesture includes **neither** information where the form is situated nor how the form moves/is moved.

Spatial relation presentation: *Spatial relation presentation* gestures present a spatial relation from a mento-heliocentric perspective.

Space is defined as "Extension, considered independently of anything which it may contain", "the unlimited expanse in which everything is located"[17];

"Space is the boundless, three-dimensional extent in which objects and events (motions) occur and have relative position and direction."[18]. "... space was a collection of relations between objects, given by their distance and direction from one another..."[18]. The latter definitions underline the importance of spatial relations to define space. Accordingly, if a gesturer processes or provides spatial information, (s)he needs to establish in gesture a spatial relation. A location in space can only be defined relative to another. Thus, to present spatial information in gesture, at least two points have to be presented.

Spatial relation presentation gestures are based on a mento-heliocentric perspective. The gesturer mentally takes the perspective of the sun and looks down on the imaginary spatial scenery: "In the presented environment, it would be over there." The mental image on the environment that is generated from a mento-heliocentric perspective is projected into the gesture/action space, typically onto the horizontal or frontal plane. On this imaginary map, the gesturer may show a position or a route. The mento-heliocentric perspective is reflected in the movement by the hand orientation. If the imaginary map is projected to the horizontal plane, the hand axis is in line with the vertical axis. If the imaginary map is projected to the frontal plane (in an experimental setting in which animations are presented on a screen the gesturer may choose the frontal plane), the hand axis is in line with a sagittal axis. In the latter case, it is more difficult to use the hand orientation as a movement criterion to determine the cognitive perspective, as it is the same for the mento-heliocentric and egocentric perspectives. Here, the gesturer's gaze helps to identify the cognitive perspective: In the mento-heliocentric perspective the visual focus is on the imaginary map, which is projected within reach onto the frontal plane. In contrast, in the egocentric perspective the visual focus is on the target (or, if it is invisible, on its assumed position) that is typically beyond the gesturer's reach.

In contrast, if the gesturer refers to her/his actual surroundings, (s)he is most likely to use her/himself as one point of spatial reference for establishing the spatial relation to the other position. In this case, (s)he applies an egocentric frame of reference and uses *egocentric deictics* and *egocentric directions*. Note, however, that an egocentric frame of reference can also be used to indicate positions and directions in imaginary surroundings (see above).

Motion quality presentation: These gestures present a manner or a dynamics of moving from a mento-heliocentric perspective.

Motion quality presentation gestures present how something/-one moves, e.g. circulating, contracting-expanding, quick, tense, strong, light, or heavy. The gesturer displays the motion quality or the action from a mento-heliocentric perspective. For the presentation the gesturer mentally adopts the perspective of the sun. In most cases, there is an indirect reference to the ground on which the motion or action takes place. This ground is typically projected to the horizontal plane. The gesturer's hand represents an object/agent that/who moves or acts (on that ground). The hands are used as if they were marionettes and **not** as if they actually were the gesturer's hands (as in *pantomime*). The gesturer's body is not involved in the presentation. The hands are quasi separated from the gesturer's body. The wrist is often flexed such that the hand axis is in line with the vertical axis and the hand is displaced on the horizontal plane, e.g. the index and middle finger represent two legs (pars pro toto for a human being) walking on a ground. Thus, only the hand embodies a certain quality of movement, e.g. the hand re-presents that and how a person walks or that and how something rolls.

In contrast, in *pantomime* gestures the gesturer adopts an egocentric perspective to show a motion quality (especially when re-presenting how humans move). Thus, the gesturer her-/himself moves as if (s)he were the person, e.g. re-presenting how a person walks or plays the drums.

The Function value *emblem / social convention* can only be assessed reliably by a rater who knows the gesturer's (sub-) culture. Raters who are not familiar with the gesturer's culture proceed by coding the gesture or action with the other Function values. By **not** assessing a gesture or action as an *emblem* or *social convention*, respectively, only the information is lost that the gesture or action is conventionalized and has a specific meaning or specific social context, respectively.

Emblem: The Function value *emblem* differs from the other Function values for gestures, as it only refers to the fact that signs are used, i.e., how the information is communicated. It provides no information about what is communicated. In contrast, the Function values *egocentric deictic, egocentric direction, pantomime, form presentation, spatial relation presentation,* and *motion quality presentation* provide information on how the information is communicated (indicated, pantomimed, or presented) and on what is communicated (a location, a direction, an action, a form, a spatial relation, or a motion quality).

In NEUROGES, at least the first three criteria have to be fulfilled to classify a gesture as an *emblem*:

(i) conventionality: The movement form and the meaning of the *emblem* gesture is familiar to most members in a specific culture or subculture. Thus, *emblems* are conventionalized body movements with a specific meaning. The movement form is invariant with regard to the gesture/action space, path during complex phase, hand orientation, and hand shape. If one criterion would be changed, the emblem could no longer be reliably recognized. The specific meaning is fully conveyed without words and it could be translated into language.

(ii) isolation / distal distinction: An *emblem* can be identified by the movement of the hand alone and eventually, by the specific orientation of the hand to another body part, e.g. in the Crazy sign the finger tips are oriented to the temple. Movements of other parts of the body are not necessary to understand the meaning of the *emblem*. Therefore, for icons of *emblems* it sufficient to depict the hand, e.g. the icon of a Peace sign only shows the hand. As complex information is conveyed by the hand alone (and its relation to another body part), the isolated body movement is distally often very distinct, e.g. the 'Keep one's fingers crossed' gesture.

(iii) explicitness: The gesturer is aware of displaying the gesture.[20]

(iv) relating to the addressee: As *emblems* are conventionalized in movement form and meaning, they are perfectly suited for interacting with the addressee. Many *emblems* are instructions for the addressee or show the gesturer's opinion about the addressee.

(v) novel meaning: *Emblems* that contain pointing, directing, pantomiming, depicting of a form or a motion have to be differentiated from *egocentric deictic, egocentric direction, pantomime, form presentation,* or *motion quality presentation* gestures that show a similar movement forms. In the respective *emblems*, the movement form is highly conventionalized and the meaning is novel, i.e., it differs from the meaning that a simple *egocentric deictic, egocentric direction, pantomime, form presentation,* or *motion quality presentation* gesture would have. Examples:

A *form presentation* gesture that presents the form of a T has to be differentiated from an *emblem* gesture that shows the form of a T in a highly conventionalized form and that means Time out. The criterion iv relating to the addressee is also fulfilled and the hand is typically moved into the direction of the addressee or in the upper space to be visible for the addressee, whereas for the mere depiction of a T-shape in gesturing the hand typically remains in the body midline gesture/action space.

A *motion quality* gesture that presents a fast opening and closing has to be differentiated from an *emblem* gesture in which the hand is formed in conventionalized movement form as if it were a mouth with the thumb being the lower jaw and the other four fingers being the upper jaw and which opens and closes to indicate that a person is a blabbermouth.

An *egocentric deictic* that points to the temple to indicate the temple has to be differentiated from an *emblem* gesture that points to the temple in a highly conventionalized repetitive manner and that means that somebody is nuts.

A *pantomime* gesture that presents the action of sweeping away dirt from the clothes has to be differentiated from an *emblem* gesture that sweeps away imaginary dirt from the shoulder (this location is part of the conventionalization) and that indicates contempt.

There are, however, few emblems in which only the form is conventionalized, e.g. the telephone-sign, but the meaning is that of the concrete action, i.e., the meaning does not differ from that of an equivalent *pantomime* gesture.

---

20 As an exception reported by Ekman & Friesen (1969), in certain mental states the gesturer may not be aware of (or at least, pretend to not be so) the display of the *emblem*. This applies typically to obscene or insulting *emblems*.

Social convention: These are actions or gestures that are displayed in a conventionalized manner quasi obligatorily in a specific social context, such as in a greeting situation.

The movement form and the social context of the *social convention* is familiar to most members in a specific culture or subculture. The movement form is invariant with regard to the gesture/action space, path during complex phase, hand orientation, and hand shape. If one criterion would be changed, the *social convention* could no longer be reliably recognized.

The gesturer is aware of displaying the *social convention*.

The Function values described above have been developed based on Efron's gesture classification system. The three Function values described below refer non-gestural body movements (not included in Efron's system).

Emotion/attitude: Any gesture can be performed with a certain emotional connotation or attitude, e.g. a *deictic* can be performed with firmness or an *emblem* with anger. Coded with the Function value *emotion/attitude*, however, are only those body movements that **only** express an emotion such as happiness, sadness, fear, anger, surprise, and disgust, or an attitude such as helplessness, openness, etc.. The observer will typically be able to name the emotion or the attitude that is reflected or expressed by the movement. The *emotion/attitude* movements constitute the motor component of an emotional process. The movement is obligatorily accompanied by a specific vegetative activation pattern, a specific facial expression (even if only recognizable in micro-analysis), and a specific whole body muscle innervation pattern. The body movement is part of the embodiment of the emotion. The patterns of motor expression are innate and universal, e.g. the arms *rise* with surprise or joy. The display of intrinsic *emotion/attitude* movements is initiated beyond the gesturer's awareness. The gesturer can, however, become aware of his/her moving hand during or immediately after the display. However, it is hard to perfectly suppress the display.

In contrast to these intrinsic *emotion/attitude* movements, learned conventionalized patterns of emotional expression are coded with the value *emblem/social convention*. The movement form of these gestures is coined by the rules of emotional expression in a certain (sub-) culture. Extrinsic *emotion/attitude* movements are most often displayed explicitly, and their display can be suppressed.

Object-oriented action: Action is defined as "an intentional (wilful) human body movement, a behaviour caused by an agent in a particular situation"[19], "something done"[17], " the exertion of power or force, as when one body acts on another "[17]. The exertion of power on something results in a change of that thing. Given this definition, in NEUROGES *phasic* and *repetitive* units are defined as actions if they act on something and change it.

The term *object-oriented* refers to all material things that are outside the gesturer's body. Typical body movements that cause changes in the external physical world are **tool-specific** manipulation of tools (praxis), e.g. winding up a watch changes the indicated time on the watch, writing results in a written text on a piece of paper, hammering results in a change of the position of a nail, taking a pen out of the pocket and putting it on the table results in a change in the position of a pen, or combing another person's hair results in a different order of the hair. Only in rare cases **tool-unspecific** manipulations, e.g. hammering with scissors, are *object-oriented actions*. Most often, tool-unspecific actions, such as chewing on a pen, are *subject-oriented actions*.

It is obvious that *object-oriented action* units often have the Focus values *on separate object, on attached object,* or *on person. Object-oriented actions* with the Focus value *in space* are an absolute rarity. In this case, the air is the physical substrate that is manipulated, e.g. fanning air with the hand or swimming in the water.

Non-material changes in the external world such as changes in social relations are **not** given the value *object-oriented action*.

Subject-oriented action: The term *subject-oriented* refers to the gesturer's psychosomatic state. A *subject-oriented action* can directly aim at (i) changing the gesturer's body state, (ii) changing her/his visual appearance, or, (iii) indirectly - via the body - changing the mental state.

(i) changing one's body state: *Subject-oriented actions* that aim at changing body states give relief from unpleasant physical states or they produce pleasant states. They are reactions to sensory perceptions. Perceiving pain, being cold, being hot, being hungry, etc. triggers actions to regulate the body state. Thus, for the observer, the action has a clear effect on the body, e.g. rubbing the skin, improving vision.

(ii) changing one's visual appearance: Coded here are actions on the own body that - in contrast to (i) - aim at changing the socially visible body. They may be specific reactions to actual deviations in the visual appearance, e.g. if the tie is not straight or if the hair is not in place. However, most often these *subject-oriented actions* are preening behaviour that reflect the gesturer's desire to look more attractive. Occasionally these actions serve to look superior, less attractive, inferior, etc. In these latter cases, the actions aim at changing the gesturer's social role, and their movement form is rather stereotypical and no deviation in the visual appearance is recognizable. As an example, to please the addressee the female gesturer repeatedly strokes the hair behind the ear (despite the fact that actually the hair is in place). In contrast, if actual deviations in the visual appearance need to be corrected, the actions are specific.

(iii) changing one's mental state: These actions serve to improve the gesturer's mental state, e.g. to calm down, to improve concentration. The most important movement feature of this subtype is that the individual displays the actions repeatedly in a stereotypical manner (see Section 2.3 on movement patterns). As compared to *irregular* movements, this subtype of *phasic* and *repetitive* movements represents a higher level of self-regulation.

In NEUROGES, the Function values referring to emotional expressions and gestures are ordered on a polar axis (Figure 7). Signs (*emblems/social conventions*) and actions (*object-oriented actions, subject-oriented actions*) are not included in the model.

One pole represents movements that are simple with regard to the above listed movement criteria and they are associated with emotional functions or with cognitive functions with an egocentric perspective (Figure 7 on the left). The other pole represents movements that are motorically complex and they are associated with cognitive functions with a mento-heliocentric perspective (Figure 7 on the right).

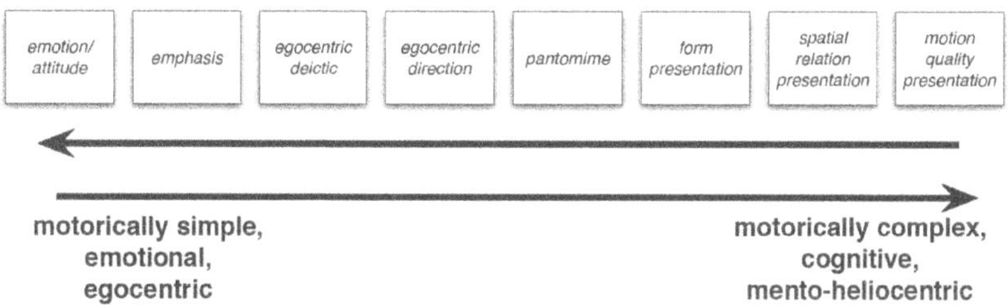

Figure 7 Function values referring to emotional expressions and gestures

Emotion/attitude movements are the visible embodiment of emotions. They are motorically simple movements with a *phasic* Structure. The complex phase is characterized by one-dimensional trajectory and they often lack either the transport phase or the retraction phase.

Emphasis gestures share some features with *emotion/attitude* movements. They often have an emotional connotation, and regarding the movement form the complex phase is one-dimensional. However, they may be *repetitive* and they are bound to speech.

Egocentric deictics are motorically simple but the hand often adopts a shape. They refer to targets from an egocentric perspective, and they do not present something.

Egocentric directions are still motorically simple. The gesturer adopts an egocentric perspective and shows the direction of an agent. There is relation with *pantomime* as *egocentric directions* may be transitive. *Pantomime* gestures are motorically complex and the movement form is variant depending on the action that is pantomimed. The gesturer adopts an egocentric perspective and presents something by acting "as if".

Form presentation gestures are motorically complex and the movement form is variant depending on the form that is represented. The gesturer adopts an egocentric or a mento-heliocentric perspective.

Spatial relation presentations are motorically highly complex, as they depict spatial relations and potentially forms, often requiring asymmetrical bimanual gestures. The movement form is variant depending on the spatial relation and the form that are represented. The gesturer adopts a mento-heliocentric perspective.

Motion quality presentations are motorically highly complex, as they depict qualities of motions and potentially spatial relations and forms. The movement form is variant depending on the movement quality, the spatial relation, and the form that are represented. The gesturer adopts a mento-heliocentric perspective.

Table 7 shows that the same concept can be displayed with an egocentric or a mento-heliocentric perspective resulting in different Function values.

Table 7 Analogous Function values for the same concept in the egocentric and the mento-heliocentric perspectives

Concept	Egocentric perspective	Mento-heliocentric perspective
a position in space	*egocentric deictic*	*spatial relation presentation* (Type *position*)
a direction in space	*egocentric direction*	*spatial relation presentation* (Type *route*)
a quality of motion or an action	*pantomime*	*motion presentation*

5.1.4.2 The Type category

The Type category offers a further assessment of hand/arm movements, since these are the most complex body movements. Some of the values can theoretically also be used for foot/leg movements as well as for head movements.

The Type category differs from the previous NEUROGES categories as it directly depends on the previous Function category. In other words, the Function value of a unit determines the range of Type values that can be coded. With the exception of the Function values *emblem, subject-oriented action,* and *object-oriented action*, each Function value is specified by several Type values.

The Function values register groups of expressive motions, gestures, and actions that share essential visually perceivable movement features and that have the same main function. As the Type values are subtypes of these Function values, they describe smaller groups of expressive motions and gestures. Accordingly, the definitions of the movement features are more specific and less general than those of the Function values. Therefore, the Type category coding can be used as a control for the Function coding. For some movements, it might be even easier to identify the Type value in the first line, e.g. a *baton* or a *shrug*, and then to note the Function value. Therefore, some raters might be tempted to skip the Function category and to directly code the Type category. Note, however, that occasionally a Function unit can contain several Type units, e.g. a *spatial relation presentation* unit may contain a *position* unit and a *route* unit. However, as compared to the previous steps, this subunit generation occurs relatively infrequently. Most often, the Type units match the Function units. Furthermore, since for statistical analyses the number of subjects needs to be substantially higher than the number of values, for most empirical investigations the Function category will be more useful than the Type category.

The Type category registers different types of Function values. The typification depends on the Function value. For *emotion/attitude* movements, the Type values refer to the direction of the movement as an embodiment of emotion and attitude. For *emphasis* gestures, the Type values refer to the movement form used to create emphasis. For *egocentric deictic* gestures, they specify the target. For *egocentric direction* gestures, the Type values specify the agent who takes the direction. For *pantomime* gestures, they register transitivity. For *form presentation*, *spatial relation presentation*, and *motion quality presentation*, the Type values classify the geometric aspects and the quality, respectively, that is presented in gesture. For *emblems*, instead of specific Type values a list of different *emblem* gestures is provided. Table 8 provides an overview on the short definitions of the Type values. For the same reason as for the Function values, only the short definitions of the specific functions are given.

Table 8 Short definitions of the Type values

Type value	Short definition
emotion/attitude - rise	dynamic fast raising up of the arm
emotion/attitude - fall	letting the arm fall down heavily
emotion/attitude - clap/beat	clapping, beating, or punching resulting in contact
emotion/attitude - shrug	shrug with falling of the shoulders
emotion/attitude - palming	presenting the palms to the interactive partner
emotion/attitude - fist clenching	clenching the fists
emotion/attitude - opening	abduction and outward rotation of the arms
emotion/attitude - closing	adduction and inward rotation of the arms
emphasis - baton	up-down movements of lower arm or hand with downward accent

emphasis - super-imposed	up-down or back-forth movements with downward or forward accent that directly follow the static complex phase of another gesture type
emphasis - back-toss	small up-down movements with an upward accent with back of hand leading
emphasis - palm-out	small supination-pronation movements with outward accent
deictic - external target	indicating a target in the external space by using an egocentric frame of reference
deictic - You	referring to the addressee as a person (2nd person) or to a part of her/his body
deictic - self	referring to oneself as a person (1rst person)
deictic - body	referring to parts of the own body
direction - neutral	indicating a direction without specifying an agent/object
direction - imperative	indicating to the addressee to move (something) in a specific direction
direction - self-related	showing the direction of oneself's (body or mental) movement
pantomime - transitive	acting as if with an imaginary object or counterpart
pantomime - intransitive / passive	acting as if without an imaginary object or counterpart or with a separate object or agent / acting as if a separate object or agent acts on oneself
form - shape	presenting a shape
form - size	presenting a length
space - route	indicating or marking a route or indicating a direction by using a mento-heliocentric frame of reference (from where to where, where along, towards where on an imaginary map)
space - position	indicating or marking a position relative to another one in a mento-heliocentric frame of reference (where on an imaginary map)
motion - manner	presenting a specific manner of movement
motion - dynamics	presenting a specific dynamics of movement

5.2 Psychometric properties

5.2.1 Objectivity

All NEUROGES categories and their values are precisely defined by movement criteria that refer to the visually perceivable aspects of movement. The objectivity of these criteria and of the values is demonstrated by the fact that some of them have successfully been used for kinematographic examinations and for developing algorithms for automatic recognition.

The detailed definitions are provided in 230 pages comprising coding manual (forthcoming as a separate book). An example for a NEUROGES value definition is given in see Subsection 4.5.3).

5.2.2 Reliability

Interrater reliability

It is a specific feature of the NEUROGES coding procedure that it comprises segmentation and coding. Therefore, the assessment of the interrater agreement has to register not only the raters' agreement concerning the values but also concerning the segmentation, i.e., if two raters agree on if there is a unit (or none, or more than one) and on when the unit begins and ends. While at first glance, this decision seems to be trivial, it turns out in the assessment of behaviour to be the most difficult one to achieve interrater agreement for.

Since among the existing statistical procedures no algorithm was available to calculate the interrater agreement for the segmentation of behaviour, as part of the NEUROGES project such a procedure has been developed by Holle & Rein. The detailed description of their algorithm, the modified Cohen's Kappa, is given in Chapter 15. As the modified Cohen's Kappa procedure can only not be applied to binary classifications but only to categories with more than two values, a further procedure for the segmentation and coding of binary categories is described in Chapter 14. It applies to the Activation category that includes only the two values *movement* versus *no movement.* To examine the interrater agreement for the NEUROGES values a meta-analysis was conducted on seven studies with different experimental designs, in which altogether 13 rater dyads coded 222 individuals (Chapter 16). The comparison of the modified Cohen's Kappa scores with the classical Cohen's Kappa scores evidenced that with a few exceptions, for all NEUROGES values the interrater agreement is moderate to substantial. Given the overall importance of interrater agreement in evaluation of behaviour, part V of this book is entirely dedicated to the achievement and the control of interrater reliability. In addition to the calculation and assessment of interrater agreement for segmentation and coding (Chapters 14 - 16), Chapters 12 and 13 describe how to train raters and how to set up the rating procedure.

Intra-rater reliability

To examine intra-rater reliability for Module I, the same rater coded the same videos after a time interval of 2 years. The agreement for the concatenated StructureFocus values - as the end product of Module I - was measured with the modified Cohen's Kappa. Particularly given the fact that not only the agreement for the values but also for the segmentation of the behaviour was considered, the intra-rater agreement was substantial: *irregular on body* 1.00, *irregular on attached object* 1.00, *phasic in space* 0.96, *phasic on body* 0.94, *phasic on at-*

tached object 1.00, *phasic on separate object* 1.00, *repetitive in space* 0.95, *repetitive on body* 0.79, *shift* 1.00.

Parallel-forms reliability

As the operationalization of the Module I Structure values essentially relies on kinematic criteria, these value definitions can be used for behavioural coding by human raters as well as for a kinematographic analysis of movement behaviour. Therefore, for the Structure category, kinematography could be used to establish parallel-forms reliability. Movement units that had been previously assessed by human raters with the Structure category were analysed with kinematography. The five Structure values *phasic, repetitive, shift, aborted,* and *irregular* were identified based on the kinematographic investigation. These kinematographic identification of the five Structure values perfectly matched the raters' classifications (Chapter 6).

5.2.3 Validity

The validity of the NEUROGES categories and values is subject of ongoing empirical investigation. Several granted research projects focussing on different aspects of movement behaviour apply the NEUROGES system and they - directly or indirectly - contribute its validation. These projects deal with the neurobiological correlates of different NEUROGES values (Deutsche Forschungsgemeinschaft DFG LA 1249/1-1, LA 1249/1-2; VolkswagenStiftung II/82175), the association between hand movements and cognitive processes (DFG LA 1249/1-3; grants by the Max Planck Society, Studienstiftung des Deutschen Volkes, and Berlin School of Mind and Brain), the association between hand movements and emotional processes in adults and children (Excellence Cluster Languages of Emotions 307-1 and 307-2; Sinergia-Förderung), the relation between prosody, semantics, and hand movements in the segmentation of events in different cultures (Bundesministerium für Bildung und Forschung BMBF 01UG1240D), hand movement behaviour in binge eating disorder in childhood (Schweizerische Nationalfonds SNF 26041079: SUN-Studie), interactive hand movement behaviour in psychotherapy (VolkswagenStiftung II/82175), and the development of algorithms for an automatic registration of the NEUROGES values (Bundesministerium für Bildung und Forschung BMBF 01UG1240D; Foundation for Polish Science INTER). These projects and further non-granted projects have investigated the relation between NEUROGES values and personality, level of intelligence, state of mental health, quality of interaction, effectiveness of psychotherapy, cognitive perspectives, brain anatomy, and hemispheric specialization (e.g. Lausberg et al. 2007; Dvoretska 2009; Wartenburger et al. 2010; Kryger 2010; Skomroch et al. 2010; Sassenberg et al. 2010; Masneri et al., 2010; Sassenberg et al. 2011; Hogrefe et al. submitted; Lausberg et al. 2010; Wartenburger et al. 2010; Helmich et al.

2011; Rein forthcoming, Bryjovà et al., 2013, Lausberg, 2013; Dvoretska et al., 2013; Dvoretska and Lausberg, 2013; Helmich et al., 2011; Helmich and Lausberg, 2012, 2013; Skomroch et al., 2013, Skomroch and Lausberg, 2013, Postma et al., 2013). While many studies are currently in progress, some results are already available. In the paragraphs below, the relevance of the various findings for the validity of the theoretical models of the NEUROGES categories can only be touched (for the detailed discussion, see the respective publications of the studies).

5.2.3.1 The Activation category

Alexithymia is a personality trait characterized by the inability to verbally express emotions. A study on alexithymic individuals and matched non-alexithymic ones evidenced that alexithymic individuals spent a significantly smaller proportion of time with *movement* units than non-alexithymic ones (Sassenberg et al. 2010; Helmich et al., 2011; Lausberg et al., in prep.). On this general level, the results indicate a reduced level of motor activation. The finding is well compatible with the concept of alexithymia. The analyses of the subsequent categories, however, allow a more differentiated view on this finding, as they reveal gender-specific and context-specific differences (see below).

5.2.3.2 The Structure category

As proposed in 5.1.1.2, *irregular, repetitive,* and *phasic* units rely on processes with different levels of cognitive complexity ranging from non-conceptual via automatic conceptual to novel conceptual. While *repetitive* and *phasic* units reflect and potentially support conceptual processes, *irregular* movements serve to regulate arousal. A high frequency of *shifts,* which are transitions between two *rest positions / postures,* may indicate physical (and mental) restlessness.
Aborted units comprise different forms of disruptions in the execution of conceptual movements and *shifts*.

Evidence for these propositions is provided by the comparison of different experimental settings, which challenge the participants differently. A meta-analysis including studies using intelligence tests (HAWIE), psychological interviews (LEAS), narration of cartoons (Sylvester & Tweety), and descriptions of drawings of everyday activities with (Motion Scenes VG) and without words (Motion Scenes VG) examined the effect of experimental design on hand movement behaviour. The patterns of the Structure values differed significantly between the experiments. Experimental settings that induced a pressure to perform (prototyp: intelligence test) were associated with a high frequency of *irregular* and *shift*s units. In contrast, experiments that animated the participants (prototyp: narration of animated cartoons) showed a high frequency of *phasic*, *repetitive*, and *aborted* units (Table 8).

In the above presented study by Dvoretska & Lausberg (2013), the evaluation of the Focus category specified the role of gestures among the conceptual hand movements: The positive correlation between Performance Intelligence Quotient (PIQ) applied to all left hand *in space* movements. The value *in space* quasi only contains hand movements that are functionally classified as gestures. The finding is in line with the propositions that gesture production represents an alternative visuo-spatial-motor way of thinking (see 2.1.1). The left hand preference further suggests that in individuals with a high PIQ these *in space* hand movements are generated in the right hemisphere. In fact, the right hemisphere is specialized for visuo-constructive processes. In line with the findings on the LBD patients, the result suggests that the generation of *in space* movements can be associated with right hemispheric visuo-constructive cognitive processes.

Dvoretska (2009) examined the relation between StructureFocus values and the personality inventory NEO-FFI in dyadic interactions. Neuroticism correlated negatively with the frequency of (*phasic* and *repetitive) in space* gestures. Furthermore, there was a negative correlation between the amount of agreeableness and the frequency of *on body* movements. The findings are compatible with the NEUROGES Focus model on pre-motor spatial attention. Neurotic and less agreeable individuals show a stronger focus of pre-motor attention on the own body. *In space* movements are externalizations of cognitive and emotional processes. As such, they are indirectly or directly accompanied by a shift of pre-motor attention to the body-external space. In the given experimental setting of dyadic interaction, the body-external space is characterized by the presence of an interactive partner.

In the Alexithymia study, the investigation of the Focus category revealed that alexithymic females displayed significantly less *in space* hand movements than the non-alexithymic females. Thus, in the interview situations, alexithymic females show a reduced externalization of thoughts and emotions and a reduced attention to the body-external space (notably the interviewer).

Kryger (2010) examined hand movement behaviour in the course of two successful psychotherapies in patients with eating disorders. The decrease of *irregular on body* movements correlated with clinical improvement. The finding supports the proposition that *irregular on body* movements serve to regulate hyper- or hypoarousal. As the patient's state improved, there was less need of self-regulation.

The above mentioned meta-analysis comparing different experimental settings showed for the Focus category a clear grouping of *in space* - dominant and *on body* - dominant experiments. Experiments providing visual stimuli (movies) were accompanied by a high frequency of *in space* units. Assuming that the renarration of these scenes elicits visual imagery, the finding supports the proposition that *in space* movements reflect conceptual visuo-constructive processes. In contrast, stress-inducing experiments were characterized by a high frequency of *on body* units. The pre-motor focus of attention is on the gesturer's body and the movement effectively serves the regulation of the mental state.

In the Gesture Only (GO) experiment as compared to the Verbal (VG) experiment, there were more *phasic in space* and more *repetitive in space* movements and less *irregular within body* and *irregular on body / on attached object* movements. Since in the GO condition, the gestural demonstration was the only means to communicate information, *in space* movements, which externalize, among others, visual concepts, are suitable to communicate information about the events. In contrast, in the VG condition is a **relative** shift of the focus of hand movements to more body-internal processes.

5.3.2.4 The Contact and Formal Relation categories

The Contact and Formal Relation categories are suitable for research questions on hemispheric interaction and hemispheric dominance. Furthermore, the two categories supplement the analyses concerning the level of cognitive complexity and the focus of pre-motor attention.

Skomroch et al. (2013) reported significant gender differences for the Contact category. Men performed significantly more *act on each other* movements than women, while women performed non-significantly more *act apart* units than men. Currently, for further clarification the Structure and Focus values of the *act on each other* and *act apart* units are analyzed statistically. Tentatively, it can be speculated that men, who show a stronger hemispheric asymmetry than women, employ *act on each other* units to stabilize the inter-hemispheric cooperation.

In the GO/VG experiment, the analysis of the Contact category showed that in the Gestures Only condition (GO) as compared to the Verbal condition (VG), there were more *act apart* units. Since among the bilateral movements, the *act apart* units allow for the most freedom of expression, this value is strongly preferred to demonstrate in gesture the everyday actions in the stimuli.

In the Alexithymia study, in the interview about emotional scenarios but not in the intelligence test, alexithymic females displayed significantly less *act apart* units than non-alexithymic females. The confrontation with the emotional scenarios led to reduction of those bilateral hand movements that are - in terms of neurological control - most instable but that, on the other hand, give the most expressive options. Furthermore, both alexithymic men and women showed a significant reduction in the duration of *act apart* units in the interview about emotional scenarios but not in the intelligence test.

The study on Performance IQ and Verbal IQ showed for the Formal Relation category that both IQ types correlated positively with the frequency and the proportion of time spent with *symmetrical* bimanual movements. The display of *symmetrical* movements may be interpreted as an indicator of an effective motor (and hypothetically also cognitive-emotional) organization.

Furthermore, the frequency and the proportion of time spent with *left hand dominance* and *asymmetrical* movements correlated positively with the PIQ. As a high PIQ indicates a high competence for visuo-constructive cognition, which is lateralized to the right hemisphere, the finding of *left hand dominance* units is highly plausible. Furthermore, *asymmetrical* movements rely on highly complex movement concepts, which typically require visuo-constructive abilities.

In the GO/VG experiment, the analysis of the Formal Relation category revealed more *asymmetrical* and *symmetrical* units in the Gestures Only condition (GO) as compared to the Verbal condition (VG). These two Formal Relation values are characterized by equal dominance of the two hands. This constellation enables to exploit the full expressive potential of each hand. Therefore, in the Gesture Only condition many bimanual movements with equal dominance of the two hands were displayed.

5.3.2.5 The Function and Type categories

The empirical studies on the Function and Type values often focused on specific values. Accordingly, below the empirical findings are described for the single Function values.

Emphasis

The verbal IQ but not the Performance IQ correlated positively with the proportion of time spent with *emphasis* gestures, specifically with Type values bimanual *batons*, bimanual *superimposed*, and right hand *back-toss* movements. Since these gestures accompany speech it is highly plausible that they correlate positively with the Verbal IQ. Individuals with a high Verbal IQ show a high competence in verbal functions and language skills and accordingly, they use those gesture Function values that support speech.

The results for this Function value as well as for the Function values described below, evidences that the different Function values are associated with different forms of intelligence.

Egocentric deictic

An *egocentric deictic* indicates where something is located by using an egocentric frame of reference. The gesturer is the point of reference. *Egocentric deictics* can often be observed in psychotherapy sessions when patients refer subjectively to other persons or to symptomatic parts of their body.

In a psychotherapy patient with eating disorders, the use of *egocentric deictics* in the course of the psychotherapy was explored as an indicator of changes in the relationship to the significant other (Lausberg and Kryger 2011). Psychodynamically, at the beginning of the therapy, the patient hardly differentiated between herself and her mother. When referring to her mother in gesture, she localized the mother in the gesture space close to the body center by using *egocentric deictics.* At the end of therapy she projected her mother distant from her body by pointing to the left gesture space. This change in the localization of the mother in the gesture space as evidenced by the *egocentric deictics* concurred with the psychodynamic development. At the end of the therapy the patient experienced herself and her mother as separate persons.

Another patient referred to her symptom (lump in her throat) reliably by performing *egocentric body-deictics* (Lausberg, 2011). She almost induced the symptom by pressing the index in the throat. The therapist implicitly adopted her gesture and reliably displayed the *egocentric body-deictic* when referring to the patient's symptom. However, in the course of the therapy he gradually transformed the concrete *body-deictic* into a *form presentation* gesture that represented the symptom in an abstract manner. Thus, according to the NEUROGES Function model there was a gradual development on the Function axis from left to right. The *egocentric body-deictic* that referred to a concrete part of the body was transformed into a *form presentation* gesture that symbolically represented the symptom. The independently conducted discourse analysis of the doctor - patient interaction (Koerfer, 2011) revealed that psychodynamically the patient understood by and by that she had no problem with the throat but that she was afraid of school.

Egocentric direction

In the intelligence experiment, the verbal IQ but not the Performance IQ correlated positively with the proportion of time spent with bimanual *egocentric direction* gestures. *Egocentric direction* gestures do not present something but they often show a direction complementary to the verbal utterance. As proposed above (see *emphasis*) individuals with a high Verbal IQ, who have a high competence to express themselves verbally, use those gesture Function values that support the verbal statement.

Pantomime gestures

In split-brain patients, Lausberg et al. (2003) demonstrated that *pantomime* gestures with tool in hand can be generated in both hemispheres while only the left hemisphere is competent to execute them without tools. The authors suggested that the generation of *pantomime* gestures with an imaginary tool in hand relies on the specifically left hemispheric competence to link the movement concept for tool use with the mental representation of the tool. They proposed a hierarchy of *object-oriented action* with tool > *pantomime* with tool > *panomime* with *hand-as-object (*the hand itself represents the tool) > *pantomime* with imaginary object (*pantomime - enclosure*, i.e., holding the imaginary object in hand when demonstrating tool use).

Subsequent neuroimaging studies with functional Magnetic Resonance Imaging (fMRI) and with Near Infra-Red Spectroscopy (NIRS) supported the proposition that the different subtypes of *pantomime* gestures are associated with different cognitive processes (Lausberg et al. 2010; Helmich et al. 2011). *Pantomime* with tool in hand was associated with bi-hemispheric activation. In contrast, *pantomime - enclosure* gestures were accompanied by left hemispheric activation and *pantomime - hand-as-object* by right hemisphere activation. The findings support the propsed hierarchy of different subtypes of *pantomimes*. *Pantomimes* with tool in hand, which are most akin to *object-oriented* actions, seem to be cognitively the simplest ones. Both hemispheres are able to execute them. *Pantomimes* in which the hand itself represents the tool can be generated in the right hemisphere. They do not require abstract cognitive operations, i.e., linking a mental representation of the tool to the movement concept. Finally, *pantomimes* which require that the hand acts with an imaginary object in hand are cognitively the most complex ones. In fact, their production crucially depends on a specific left hemispheric competence.

In the GO/VG experiment, in the Gestures Only condition (GO) as compared to the Verbal condition (VG), there were more *pantomime* units. Since the stimuli depicted individuals during everyday actions, it was likely that the participants adopted the egocentric perspective and thus, that they chose *pantomime* gestures to depict the action. In contrast, in the VG condition, the action per se was described verbally and relatively more non-presentative Function values were displayed. The hands were used significantly more often for *emotion/attitude* movements and for *subject-oriented* actions.

Presentation gestures

Wartenburger et al. (2010) related cortical thickness as measured with structural Magnetic Resonance Imaging (MRI) to hand movement behaviour during a geometric analogy task. They found a larger cortical thickness in the left Broca's area and transverse temporal cortex in those participants who produced *presen-*

tation gestures as compared to those who did not. In particular, the first group displayed more *motion quality presentation* gestures. The findings support the NEUROGES Function model proposing that *presentation* and particularly *motion quality presentation* gestures rely on complex cognitive processes. The adoption of mento-heliocentric cognitive perspective relies on the competence for abstract thinking.

This proposition is further supported in a study by Sassenberg et al. (2011). Individuals scoring high in fluid intelligence showed a higher accuracy in a geometric analogy task and they produced more gestures - as identified by the Function category - when relating to the most relevant aspect of the task. More specifically, their gestural behaviour was characterized by a high freqeuncy of *motion quality presentation* gestures. The correlation of this Function value with a high fluid intelligence strongly suggests the proposition that it relies on complex cognitive operations.

In the intelligence experiment, the Verbal IQ but not the Performance IQ correlated negatively with the proportion of time spent with left hand and right hand *spatial relation presentation* gestures. *Spatial relation* gestures are assumed to be associated specifically with visuo-constructive competence. As suggested above, individuals with a high VIQ display rather those gesture Function values that support speech and than gesture Function values that present concepts.

5.2.4 Future perspectives

As the Module I value definitions are objective and precise referring to the visual appearance of movement, the value definitions not only provide a basis to define kinematographic types but - in line with the aims of the NEUROGES system - they also suit as a basis to develop for automatized approaches for recognition of the NEUROGES values. This aim is pursued in a current research project granted by the Bundesministerium für Bildung und Forschung (BMBF 01UG1240D).

Another aim of the NEUROGES project is to gain normative data on the NEUROGES values. Since the frequency of the values is strongly influenced by the study design (see Part IV), the normative data compilation concentrates on the durations of the value units, e.g. how long a *phasic* unit typically lasts. Pilot-studies have demonstrated that the duration of a specific value unit shows little inter-individual variation and that it is reliable across different experimental settings. These normative data are intended to provide a frame of reference for assessing the individual movement behaviour. As an example, a depressive person may display longer lasting *irregular* units than the healthy reference sample.

Acknowledgments

The development of the NEUROGES coding system was supported by the German Research Association (DFG) grants LA 1249/1 - 3.

References

Akelaitis, A.J. (1945). Studies on the corpus callosum. IV. Diagonistic dyspraxia in epileptics following partial and complete section of the corpus callosum. *American Journal of Psychiatry, 101*, 594-9.

Berridge, C.W., Mitton, E., Clark, W., & Roth, R.H. (1999). Engagement in a Non-Escape (Displacement) Behaviour Elicits a Selective and Lateralized Suppression of Frontal Cortical Dopaminergic Utilization in Stress. *Synapse*, 32, 187-197.

Blonder, L.X., Burns, A.F., Bowers, D., Moores, R.W., & Heilman, K.M. (1995). Spontaneous gestures following right hemisphere infarct. *Neuropsychologia, 33*(2), 203-213.

Bogen, J.E. (1993). The callosal syndromes. In: K. M. Heilman and Edward Valenstein (Eds.), *Clinical Neuropsychology*, 337-408. New York, Oxford: Oxford University Press.

Bryjova, J., Munsch, S., Puder, J., & Hoffmann, J. (2013). *Die Reaktivität auf einen akuten Stressor und Emotionsregulationsmechanismen bei Kindern im Vorschulalter*. Paper presented at the 8. Workshop Kongress für Klinische Psychologie und Psychotherapie, 9.-11. Mai, Universität Trier.

Burton, C.L., Chatterjee, D., Chatterjee-Chakraborty, M., Lovic, V., Grella, S.L., Steiner, M., & Fleming, A.S. (2007). Prenatal restraint stress and motherless rearing disrupts expression of plasticity markers and stress-induced orticosterone release in adult female Sprague-Dawley rats. *Brain Research, 1158*, 28-38.

Chatterjee, D., Chatterjee-Chakraborty, M., Rees, S., Cauchi, J., de Medeiros, C.B., & Fleming, A.S. (2007). Maternal isolation alters the expression of neural proteins during development: "stroking" stimulation reverses these effects. *Brain Research, 1158*, 11-27

Chelazzi, L., Biscaldi, M., Corbetta, M., Peru, A., Tassinari, G., & Berlucchi, G. (1996). Oculomotor activity and visual spatial attention. . *Behavioural Brain Research, 71, 81-88.*

Condon, W.S., & Brosin, H.W. (1969). *Micro Linguistic-Kinesic Events in Schizophrenic Behaviour*. In G. Bateson, Birdwhistell, R., Brosin, H.W., Hockett, C., & McQuown, N.A. The Natural History of an Interview. Grune & Stratton, pp. 812-837.

Davis M. (1978). Movement characteristics of hospitalized psychiatric patients. In: M Costonis (ed.). *Therapy in Motion.* Urbana: University of Illinois 89-112.

Dvoretska, D., Joraschky, P., & Lausberg, H. . (2013). *Kinesische Interaktion als Prädiktor für Therapieerfolg.* Paper presented at the Deutscher Kongress für Psychosomatische Medizin und Psychotherapie, München.

Dvoretska, D., Denissen, J., & Lausberg, H. (2013). *Kinesic Turn Taking and Mutual Understanding in Interactive Dyads.* Paper presented at the TiGeR, Tilburg.

Dvoretska, D., & Lausberg, H. (2013). *Verbal and Nonverbal Intelligence Show Different Patterns of Hand Movement.* Paper presented at the 55th Conference of Experimental Psychologist, Vienna.

Efron, D. (1941, 2nd ed. 1972). *Gesture and culture*. The Hague: Mouton.

Ekman, P., & Friesen, W.V. (1969). The Repertoire of Nonverbal Behaviour: Categories, Origins, Usage and Coding. *Semiotica, 1*, 49-99.

Freedman, N., & Bucci, W. (1981). On kinetic filtering in associative monologue. *Semiotica*, 34(3/4), 225-249.

Helmich, I., Lausberg, H., & Sassenberg, U. (2011). *Bewegungsverhalten als Indikator impliziter emotionaler Prozesse alexithymer und nicht-alexithymer Probanden (Poster).* Paper presented at the 62. Jahrestagung des Deutschen Kollegiums für Psychosomatische Medizin (DKPM) und 19. Jahrestagung der Deutschen Gesellschaft für Psychosomatische Medizin und ärztliche Psychotherapie (DGPM). Deutscher Kongress für Psychosomatische Medizin und Psychotherapie, 23.-26.03.2011, Essen.

Helmich, I., & Lausberg, H. (2012). *Hand movement behavior with or without speech differs in its kinetic structure of nonverbal communication*. Paper presented at the Measuring Behavior, Utrecht, The Netherlands

Helmich, I., & Lausberg, H. (2013). *Hand movement behavior with or without speech.* Paper presented at the Tilburg Gesture Research Meeting, Tilburg, The Netherlands.

Helmich, I., & Lausberg, H. (2013 in prep.). Hand movements that accompany verbal descriptions differ from those during gestural demonstrations. *Brain and Language, in prep.*

Huys, R., Studenka, B.E., Rheaume, N.L., Zelaznik, H.N., & Jirsa, V.K. (2008). Distinct Timing Mechanisms Produce Discrete and Continuous Movements. *PLoS computational Biology, 4*(4), 1-8.

Kendon, A. (1972). *Some relationships between body motion and speech.* In A. Siegman and B. Pope (eds). Studies in dyadic communication, 177-210, Pergamon Press, New York.

Laban, R. (1988). *The Mastery of Movement.* Worcester: Northcote House.

Lausberg, H. (2013). NEUROGES – A coding system for the empirical analysis of hand movement behaviour as a reflection of cognitive, emotional, and interactive processes. In C. Müller, Fricke, Ladewig, McNeill, Teßendorf (Ed.), *Body - Language - Communication* (pp. 1018-1033): de Gruyter.

Lausberg, H., Davis, M., & Rothenhäusler, A. (2000). Hemispheric specialization in spontaneous gesticulation in a patient with callosal disonnection. *Neuropsychologia, 38*, 1654-1663.

Lausberg, H., Kita, S., Zaidel, E., & Ptito, A. (2003). Split-brain patients neglect left personal space during right-handed gestures. *Neuropsychologia, 1595*, 1-13.

Lausberg, H., Cruz, R.F., Kita, S., Zaidel, E., & Ptito, A. (2003b). Pantomime to visual presentation of objects: Left hand dyspraxia in patients with complete callosotomy. *Brain, 126*, 343-360.

Lausberg, H., Zaidel, E., Cruz, R.F., & Ptito, A. (2007). Speech-independent production of communicative gestures: Evidence from patients with complete callosal disconnection. *Neuropsychologia, 45*, 3092-3104.

Masneri, S., Schreer, O., Schneider, D., Tschöpel, S., Bardeli, R., Bordag, S., Auer, E., Sloetjes, H., & Wittenburg, P. (2010). *Towards Semi-Automatic Annotations for Video and Audio Corpora.* Paper presented at the 4th Workshop on Representation and Processing of Sign Languages: Corpora and Sign Language Technologies in conjunction with 7th Int. Conf. on Language Resources and Evaluation (LREC), June 22, 2010.

McNeill, D. (1992). *Hand and Mind: What gestures reveal about thought.* Chicago: The University of Chicago Press.

Mechsner, F., Kerzel, D., Knoblich, G., & Prinz, W. (2001). Perceptual basis of bimanual coordination. *Nature, 414*(6859), 69-73.

Mourik van, A. M., & Beek, P. J. (2004). Discrete and cyclical movements: unified dynamics or separate control? *Acta Psychologica, 117*, 121-138.

Postma-Nilsenová, M., Postma, E., Balsters, M., Krahmer, E., Schaafsma, J., Swerts, M., Vingerhoets, A., & Mol, L. (2013). *Automatic Detection of Hand/Upper Body Movement and Facial Expressions as Cues to Feelings of Exclusion*. Paper presented at the Tilburg Gesture Research Meeting, Tilburg, The Netherlands

Preilowsky, B.F.B. (1975). Bilateral motor interaction: Perceptual-motor performance of partial and complete "split-brain" patients. In K. J. Zülch,

Creutzfeldt, O., Galbraith, G.C. (Ed.), *Cerebral Localization* (pp. 115-132). Berlin, Heidelberg, New York: Springer-Verlag.

Rizzolatti, G., Riggio, L., & Sheliga, B.M. (1994). Space and selective attention. In: C. Umilità & M. Moscovitch (Eds.). *Attention & Performance XV. Conscious and nonconscious information processing* (pp. 231-265). Cambridge, MA: MIT Press.

Rothwell, J. (1994). *Control of Human Voluntary Movement (2nd edition)*. London: Chapman & Hall.

Skomroch, H., Petermann, K., Helmich, I., Dvoretska, D., Rein, R., Kim, Z. H., Sassenberg, U., & Lausberg, H. (2013). *Gender differences in Hand Movement Behavior*. Paper presented at the Tilburg Gesture Research Meeting (TiGeR), Tilburg, The Netherlands.

Skomroch, H., Rein, R., Hogrefe, K., Goldenberg, G, & Lausberg, H. (2013). *Gesture production in the right and left hemispheres during narration of short movies.* Paper presented at the Tilburg Gesture Research Meeting (TiGeR) Tilburg, The Netherlands.

Skomroch, H., & Lausberg, H. (2013). *AUVIS - Audiovisuelles Data-Mining am Beispiel der Ereignis-Segmentierung in multimodalen Sprachdaten.* Poster presented at the Kick-Off Workshop der eHumanities-Verbundprojekte Leipzig, 8./9. April 2013.

Seyfeddinipur, M. (2006). *Disfluency: Interrupting speech and gesture.* Njimegen: Max Planck Institute of Psycholinguistics.

Schaal, S., Sternad, D., Osu, R., & Kawato, M. (2004). Rhythmic arm movement is not discrete. *Nature Neuroscience, 7*(10).

Schanberg, S.M., & Field, T.M. (1987). Sensory deprivation stress and supplemental stimulation in the rat pup and preterm human neonate. *Child Development,* 58, 1431-1447.

Schneider, W.X., & Deubel, H. (1996). Visual attention and saccadic eye movements: Evidence for obligatory and selective spatial coupling. In: J.M. Findlay et al. (Eds.). Eye movement research: Mechanisms, processes and applications (pp. 317-324). Amsterdam Elsevier.

Shepherd, M., Findlay, J.M., & Hockey, R.J. (1986). The relationship between eye movements and spatial attention. *Quarterly Journal of Experimental Psychology, 38A*, 475-491.

Spencer, R.M.C., Zelaznik, H.N., Diedrichse, J., & Ivry, R.B. (2003). Disrupted Timing of Discontinuous But Not Continuous Movements by Cerebellar Lesions. *Science, 300*, 3.

Tanaka, Y., Yoshida, A., Kawahata, N. Hashimoto, R., & Obayashi, T. (1996) Diagnostic dyspraxia - Clinical characteristics, responsible lesion and possible underlying mechanism. *Brain, 119*, 859-873.

Vignolo, L.A. (1999). Disorders of Conceptual Thinking in Aphasia. In: G. Denes, & L. Pizzamiglio (Ed.), *Handbook of Clinical and Experimental Neuropsychology* (pp. 273-288). Hove, East Sussex, U.K.: Psychology Press.

Westenberg, Y., Smits-Engelsman, B.C., & Duysens, J. (2004). Development of unimanual versus bimanual task performance in an isometric task. *Hum Mov Sci, 23*(3-4), 461-474.

Zaidel, D., & Sperry, R.W. (1977). Some Long-term Motor Effects of Cerebral Commissurotomy in Man. *Neuropsychologia, 15*, 193-204.

Zülch, K.J., & Müller, N. (1969, 1980). Associated movements in man. In G. W. B. P.J. Vinken (Ed.), *Disturbances of Nervous Function*. Amsterdam: North-Holland Publishing Company.

Zijdewind, I., & Kernell, D. (2001). Bilateral interactions during contractions of intrinsic hand muscles. *Journal of Neurophysiology 85*, 1907-1913.

6. Using 3 D Kinematics for the Analysis of Hand Movement Behaviour: A Pilot Study and some further Suggestions

Robert Rein

6.1 Introduction

As gestures are inherently visual, traditional research on communicative gestures is based on video recordings using consumer cameras where participants are recorded whilst gesturing (compare for example Kita, van Gijn, & van der Hulst, 1998; McNeill, 1992, p.81). The recorded video clips are subsequently annotated using specialized tools like the NEUROGES system (Lausberg & Sloetjes, 2009) to extract more specific information about the gestures performed by the actor. This recording set-up allows for the most natural data recording context as the hand movements made by participants are not obstructed by any markers or cables common to recording procedures used in more biomechanics oriented research (see for example Cappozzo, Croce, Leradini, & Chiari, 2005; Winter, 2005). A particular advantage of this set-up is that the participants are not necessarily aware of the fact that their hand movements are investigated. Thus, one obtains an almost natural reaction and behavioural bias with a minimal recording set-up. Consequently, this approach presents a cost-effective and simple experimental methodology.

This freedom comes at a cost however as video based approaches using of the shell equipment provide only low temporal and spatial resolution. Temporal resolution refers to the number of frames collected per second, whereas spatial resolution describes the smallest object, which can be made visible. For example, DV-cameras use a resolution of 720x576 (PAL) or 720x480 (NTSC) points and record pictures with a frequency of 50Hz for half-pictures (PAL) resulting in an effective recording frequency of 25Hz (30Hz NTSC). This becomes problematic when analyzing fast hand movements. Therefore, specialized motion capturing systems have nowadays much increased resolutions of more than 1600x1280 pixels at 500Hz allowing much greater precision when analyzing bodily movements. Therefore, as the analysis of the behaviour of hand movements relies on the identification of offsets and onsets, standard video analysis provides only limited accuracy and especially with regard to exact movements of single digit, the resolution is not sufficient.

To overcome these limitations when analyzing hand gestures researchers typically resort to rules-of-thumb like the first "blurred" picture (Kita, et al., 1998) to identify on- and offsets of hand gestures. Naturally such informal criteria increase the difficulty to reliably identify gesture events across raters and prevent the application of automatic routines. In addition, hand movements are typically three dimensional in nature but video recordings using a single video camera provide only a projection of the movement onto a two dimensional plane. This further increases the difficulty to apply automatic routines to segment the stream of data into different parts and phases (see Chen, Fu, & Huang, 2003 for an example). Thus, to further the knowledge about what characteristics are subject to different hand movement behaviours, additional approaches seem warranted. First however, a scheme is needed which makes the reliable identification of gestures events possible. In the following, whenever to the kinematic properties of a movement is referred to, the term kinematics is applied in a strict physical sense, meaning referring either to position, velocity, or acceleration only.

6.2 Analysis of movement phases

When analyzing general hand movement behaviours and in particular gestures in a communicative context, the hand movements can be divided into distinct phases based on their kinematic characteristics (Kendon, 1972; Kita, et al., 1998; McNeill, 1992). A simple scheme for the analysis of hand movement behaviour can be established using three main phases only: preparation, stroke, and retraction (Kita, et al., 1998; compare also McNeill, 1992, p. 83ff; and Seyfeddinipur, 2006, p. 83ff). The different phases are defined in the following way (adapted from McNeill, 1992, p.83).

- Preparation: limb moves away from its rest position to a position in the gesture space where the stroke begins.
- Stroke: peak effort of the gesture.
- Retraction: return of the hand to a rest position.

Thereby, no fixed sequence of phases can be expected as several gestures can be stringed together which entails that different units can be grouped in arbitrary ways. The only exception is the stroke which marks the core unit as the "*content-bearing part of the gesture*" and therefore is always present (Kita, et al., 1998, p.27). Although the stroke marks the main part of the gestures, the other optional phases are important with regard to the timing of the gesture during the discourse. Gestures phases belonging together can be collected into a single behavioural unit, the so-called gesture unit. The identification of the gesture unit is important in order to not lose the semantic content of the behaviour.

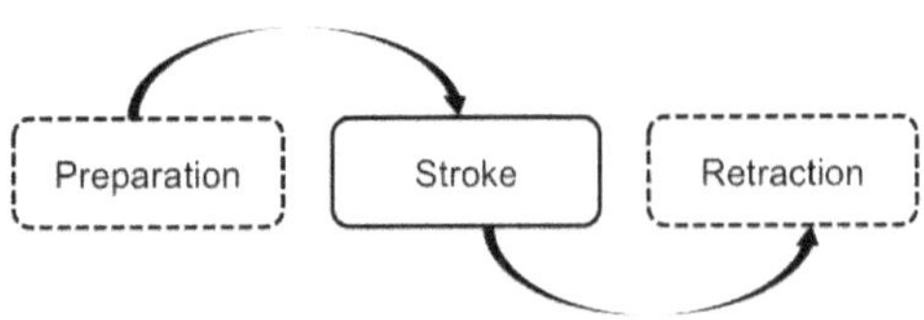

Figure 1 Sequence of gesture phases within a gesture unit (dashed phases are optional)

In Figure 1 the sequence of gesture phases are depicted. Again, the figure highlights that the core part of the gesture is marked by the stroke and the additional phases are optional. This scheme allows segmentation of the gesture stream using movement features only.

In Chapter 1, the different hand movement behaviour categories and values of the NEUROGES system have been introduced and it has been hypothesized that the different categories, which are related to different cognitive states, also exhibit distinctly different kinematic features. Thus, it seems plausible that the different values also exhibit distinct differences at the finer kinematic level with regard to gesture phases. For example, one would expect that those gestures, which have a clear communicative feature like *phasic* and *repetitive* gestures, should exhibit a preparation and a retraction phase although the latter can be omitted when one gesture is directly followed by another (McNeil, 1992, p.83). Accordingly, an *aborted* gesture, which is characterized by the lack of a stroke, should only display features of a preparation and retraction phase. Similarly, aborted gestures just like *shifts*, which do not possess an inherent semantic content on their own, should lack a clear stroke as well (compare Chapter 2). In contrast, *irregular* movements, which mostly serve auto regulative purposes, should start without neither a dedicated preparation nor a retraction phase. However, to identify this finer kinematic level, a measurement approach is necessary, which allows for better identification of the kinematics beyond what is possible with standard video recordings.

In summary, adopting techniques developed for biomechanical movement analysis and apply them to gesture research, might provide some new insights into the structure of gestures, which go beyond a pure linguistic or cognitive interpretation. In addition, analyzing the hand behaviour movements at a finer level might provide additional support for specific categories of hand behaviours, which are currently to some extent based on the inventiveness of the researcher. Thus, finding some clear quantitative characteristics for certain categories might strengthen their justification and help annotators when tagging gestures.

6.3 Electromagnetic Motion Capturing

Here, we present an approach based on an electromagnetic motion capture system. The Polhemus Liberty© (Colchester, VT) records the position and orientation of cable based markers with a recording frequency of 240Hz. As the system is cable based, it is probably less suited for the analysis of implicit gestures, as the markers obstruct to some extent arm movements and also makes it to some extent obvious to the participants that the experimenter is interested in hand movements, which might affect individual behaviour. However, as no large camera set-up is necessary, it is possible to use some sort of a cover-up story for the participants, which distracts her from the fact that her movements are recorded and analyzed.

Electromagnetic marker systems have been used in various movement settings. For example, hammering (Bril, Rein, Nonaka, Wenban-Smith, & Dietrich, 2010), grasping (Prokopenko, Frolov, Biryukova, & Roby-Brami, 2001; Weigelt & Bock, 2007), baseball (Tsai, Wu, & Wu, 2007), tennis (Konda, Yanai, & Sakurai, 2010), throwing (Hore, Watts, & Tweed, 1994) and gestures (Fröhlich & Wachsmuth, 1997; Unzueta & Goenetxea, 2010).

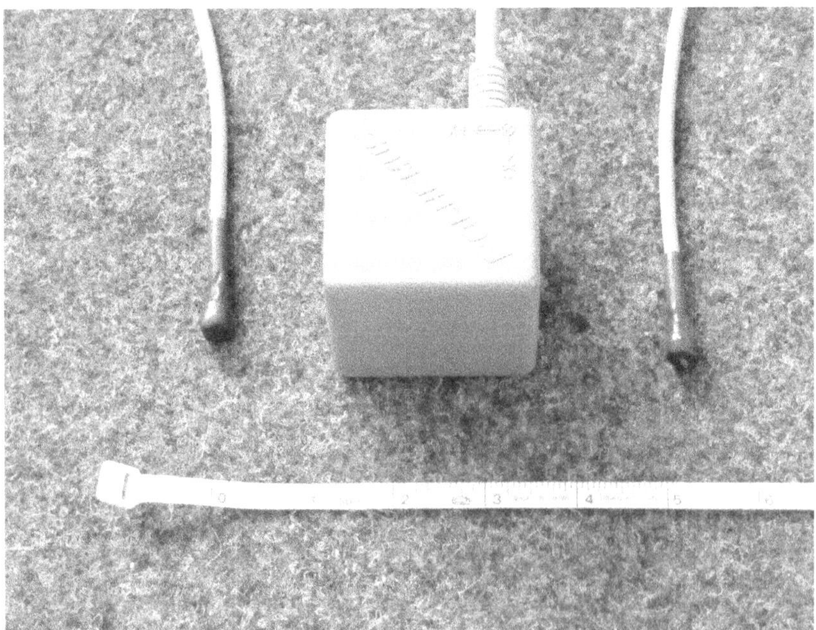

Figure 2 Polhemus Liberty© (Colchester, VT) source and markers. Scale at the bottom in centimeters.

In Figure 2, the so-called source and two markers are shown. As can be seen, the markers are relatively small and therefore, they can be placed on any body segment desired, with only limited interference to movements, especially when participants are seated. The source in the middle is also relatively small and can be placed discretely behind the participant, to mask the intentions of the experimenter. The source generates a time-varying electromagnetic dipole field and the markers measure changes in the field strength. This information is used to calculate the position and orientation of the sensors with respect to the source (Kuipers, 1999; Raab, Blood, Steiner, & Jones, 1979). The position and orientation of the markers is recorded with a maximum frequency of 240Hz, providing excellent time resolution. Typical precision is under 1mm, with angle deviations <2° (Day, Dumas, & Murdoch, 1998), thus, also providing excellent spatial resolution. As one obtains not only position data but also orientation, it is possible to calculate the position and orientation of body segments with only one marker per body segment.
When markers are applied to each arm segment (hand, forearm, humerus, and the shoulder) the calculation of a 7 degrees of freedom biomechanical arm is possible (Biryukova, Roby-Brami, Frolov, & Mokhtari, 2000). Thus, more specific statements about hand movements become possible, for example regarding the position of the hand with regard to the body or in general gesture space (see McNeill, 1992, p. 89, for an explanation of gesture space). One advantage of electromagnetic systems is their cost effectiveness as the price is only a fracture of optical motion capture systems. In addition, the system is operational within minutes without the need for any calibration or other elaborate preparation procedures. Their great disadvantage, apart from the cables, is that there must not be any large metal implements close to the measuring volume as this would distort the electromagnetic field and increase measurement errors. In the following the results form a single subject pilot study using an electromagnetic motion capture system will be presented.

6.4 Method and data analysis

The present study has only pilot character and we plan to follow up this initial work with further studies to provide stronger support for the results. Implicit hand movements of one participant were recorded using the Polhemus Liberty motion capture system. A single teardrop-shaped marker was attached to the index finger of the dominant hand using medical tape. As the orientation of the marker was not important only position data were used for further processing. The origin of the recording space was located behind the participant with the positive x-axis pointing in anterior position, positive y-axis pointing in the left direction, and the positive z-axis pointing in the upward direction.
The participant performed *phasic*, *repetitive*, *shift*, *aborted*, and *irregular* hand movements at her own pace with 30 seconds of rest between hand movements

whilst seated. In total, 10 *phasic*, 13 *repetitive*, 11 *shifts*, 5 *aborted* and 2 *irregular* hand movements were recorded. Real-time data was streamed to a standard PC and stored on the hard disk for further analysis. All calculations were performed using custom routines written in MathWorks MATLAB© R2009a (Natick, MA) and R 2.12.0 (R Development Core Team, 2008). The data was filtered using a 2nd-order, zero-lag Butterworth filter with a cut-off frequency of 8Hz after visual inspection of the frequency-spectra (Gordon, Robertson, & Dowling, 2003). This was necessary as typically raw data is always contaminated with measurement noise. Position measures of the marker were normalized to the rest position before gesturing, yielding values around zero before gesturing for the position data.

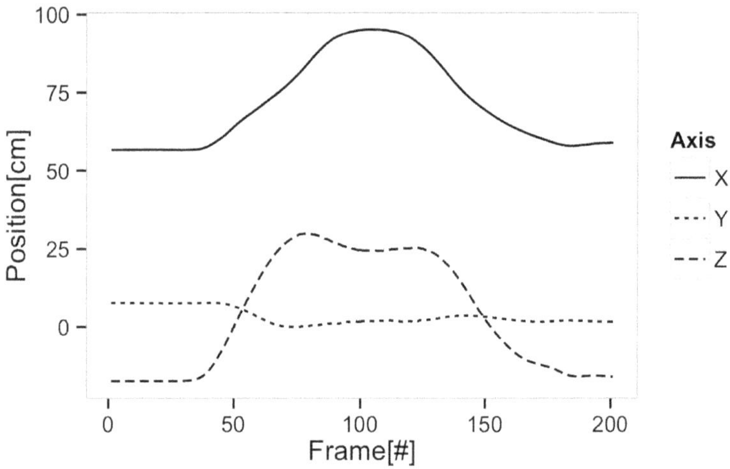

Figure 3 Position data of the finger marker during a hand movement.

In Figure 3 an example of the data obtained from the motion capture is depicted without normalization of the initial position. There are three time series, one for each axis (x, y, z), indicating the position of the marker with respect to the source. As can be seen from the plot, the curves are smooth and there are clearly visible differences between static and dynamic movement phases. In this particular case, the finger followed a backwards-forward direction mainly along the x-axis and was raised first and subsequently lowered.

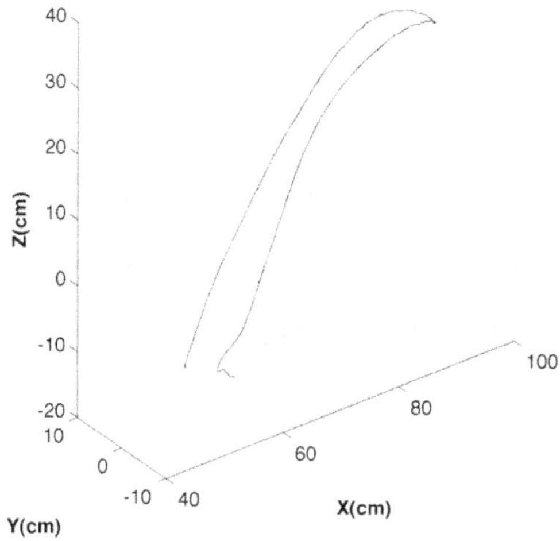

Figure 4 3D trajectory of the hand movement

In Figure 4 the actual trajectory in 3D space is shown. From this plot, the movement of the finger is easier to visualize. Thus, the finger moved from the initial position to the front of the person and returned back afterwards finishing close to the initial position resulting in a small final displacement (6.6cm).
By projecting the 3D coordinates onto the Y-Z plane (coronal plane), one obtains the view of the kinematics typically obtained by video cinematography.

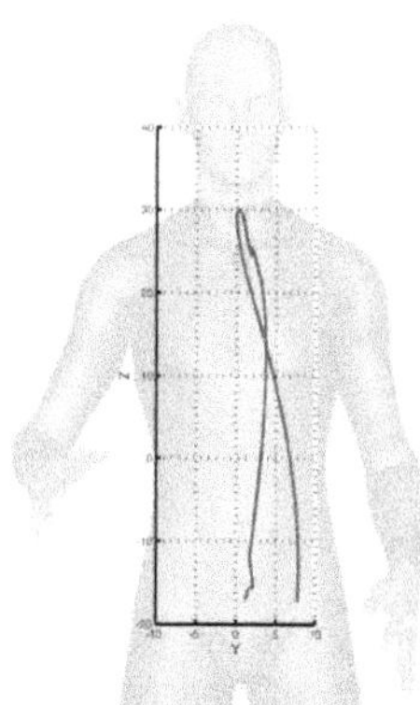

Figure 5 Projection of the kinematics onto the coronal plane

From the position data the velocity of the marker can be obtained through a three-point difference algorithm. Hereby, the difference between three successive points is calculated and divided by the time difference between the first and the third frame.

$$v(t) = \frac{x(t+1) - x(t-1)}{2\Delta t}$$

In this way, an estimate of the velocity at frame t is obtained as opposed to the velocity in-between frames, when only two points are subtracted from each other. A disadvantage of this procedure is that one frame at the beginning and one frame at the end are lost, which usually is not a problem if some additional time at the beginning and the end of the recording is allowed. As the velocity is calculated for each individual axis, a resultant velocity can be obtained by calculating the Euclidean norm across the three dimensions for each time frame.

$$|v(t)| = \sqrt{v_x(t)^2 + v_y(t)^2 + v_z(t)^2}$$

The resultant velocity is a scalar value and is always greater zero. The velocity provides further information about the movement. For example the resultant velocity can be used to differentiating between static and dynamic movement phases.

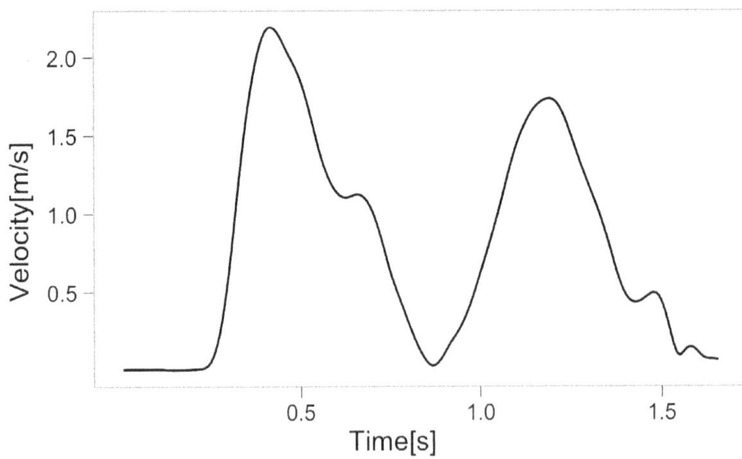

Figure 6 Resultant velocity of a hand movement

In Figure 6, the resultant velocity for the position data is shown. The velocity indicates clearly different movement phases with static and dynamic components. Again, supporting the impression obtained from the position data shown

in Figure 3 and 4. Thus, it can be concluded that these features of the movement clearly help in characterizing the hand movement and make it much easier to determine different phases of the hand movement behaviour correctly.
In the following, the detailed results from several explicit hand movements will be discussed and analyzed with regard to differences between different structure categories.

6.5 Results

Group Data

First, the average statistics for the kinematics of representative hand movements made by the participant will be shown. This section is followed by a more detailed analysis of representative individual hand movements. One has to bear in mind that the analysis is only descriptive as the present study has only pilot character.

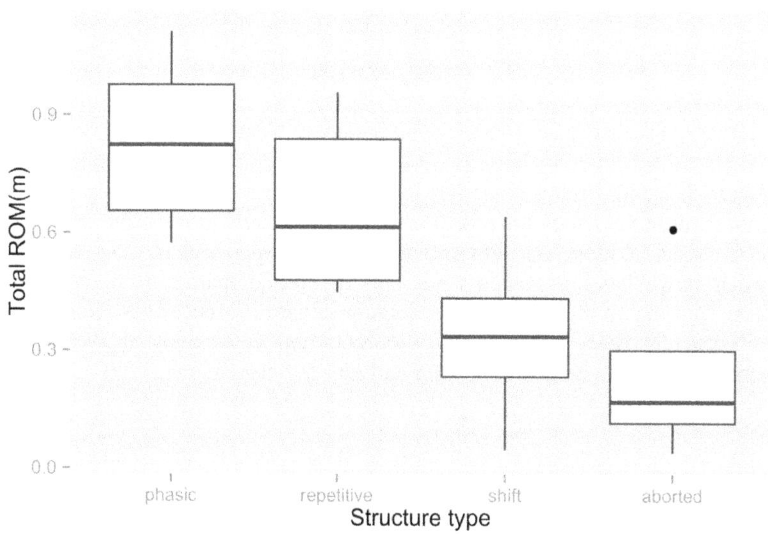

Figure 7 Absolute displacement magnitudes of the finger marker for each hand movement.

In Figure 7, the absolute magnitude of the ranges of motion (ROM) of the marker in x-, y-, and z-directions are shown. Although no statistical testing was performed, the figure suggests that there seems to be an ordering between the different structure categories, with *phasic* hand movements showing a tendency to exhibit to largest movements, followed by *repetitive* and *shift* hand movements with *aborted* hand movements exhibiting the smallest motions. *Irregular* hand movements were not included because of the small sample size.

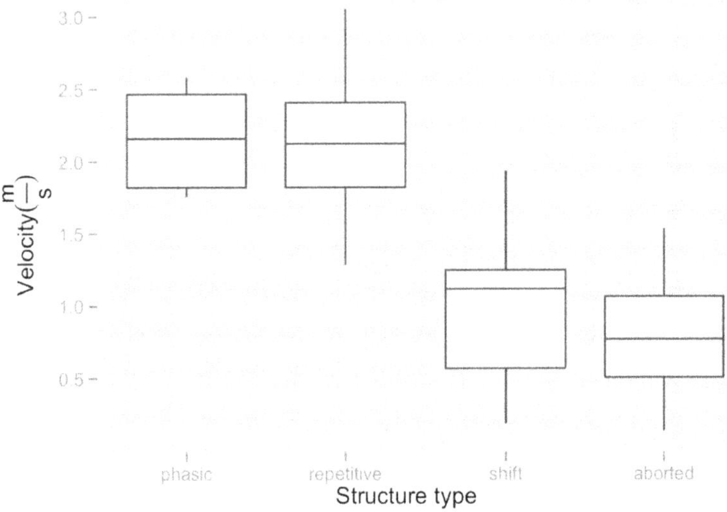

Figure 8 Maximum velocities of the finger marker for each hand movement value.

In Figure 8, the maximum velocities for each structure type are shown. The median maximum velocities for *phasic* and *repetitive* hand movements are almost twice as great as those for *shift* and *aborted* hand movements. The variability between *phasic* hand movements was also smaller compared to the other three values. Thus, again the plot suggests some peculiar differences between the different structure types: *Phasic* and *repetitive* hand movements display greater maximum velocities compared to *shift* and *aborted* movements.

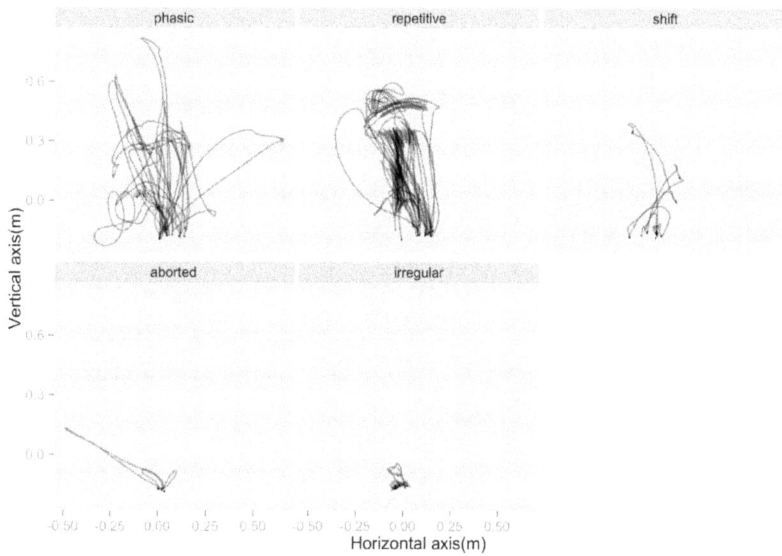

Figure 9 Finger trajectories projected onto Y-Z plane.

In Figure 9, the projections of the trajectories onto the coronal plane are shown. Speaking only qualitatively, there are some large differences between the different structure types. Both, *phasic* and *repetitive* hand movements show the largest movement and cover a greater area of the gesture space. This supports the interpretation of the ROM data in Figure 7. The two *irregular* hand movements are confined to only a small part of the gesture space whereas *aborted* and *shift* hand movements are somewhat in between the auto-regulative and the communicative gesture.

In summary, although no statistical testing was performed, the plots indicate that there are some specific differences between the different structure types and that a more detailed analysis of the hand movement behaviour kinematics can add important information to classify gestures.

In the following, some representative hand movements will be analyzed in more detail, especially with regard to their concrete characteristics sequence of gesture phases.

Example of a complex *phasic* hand movement

Movement data was downsampled to 120Hz to reduce file sizes.

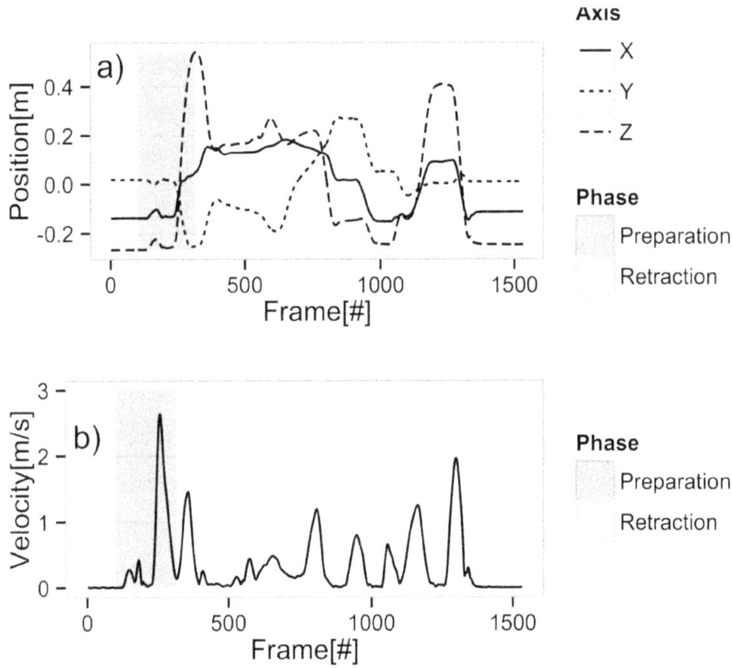

Figure 10 *Phasic* movement. (a) Position data, (b) Resulting velocity.

In Figure 10, the kinematics for a complex *phasic* hand movement are shown. The top plot (a) shows the position data for the three axes (x, y, and z), whereas the lower plot (b) shows the resulting velocity. Preparation and retraction phases are emphasized by gray rectangles. The movement lasted for approximately just over 11 seconds as the participant performed a complex concept. The position plots indicate a small movement occurring just prior to the execution of the main hand movement, which is framed by two peaks in the resultant velocity plot, characterizing the preparation and retraction phases. In between these phases, the stroke of the hand movement is quite complex and changes the direction several times throughout the stroke. Thus, a three dimensional trajectory had been used by the participant. Each part of the trajectory is traced only once in forward and backwards direction underscoring the categorization as a *phasic* hand movement. The resultant velocity plots further suggest that several brief holding phases occurred as indicated through periods of zero velocity. The initial peak of the resultant velocity plot is around 2.5m/s.

Examples of *repetitive* hand movements

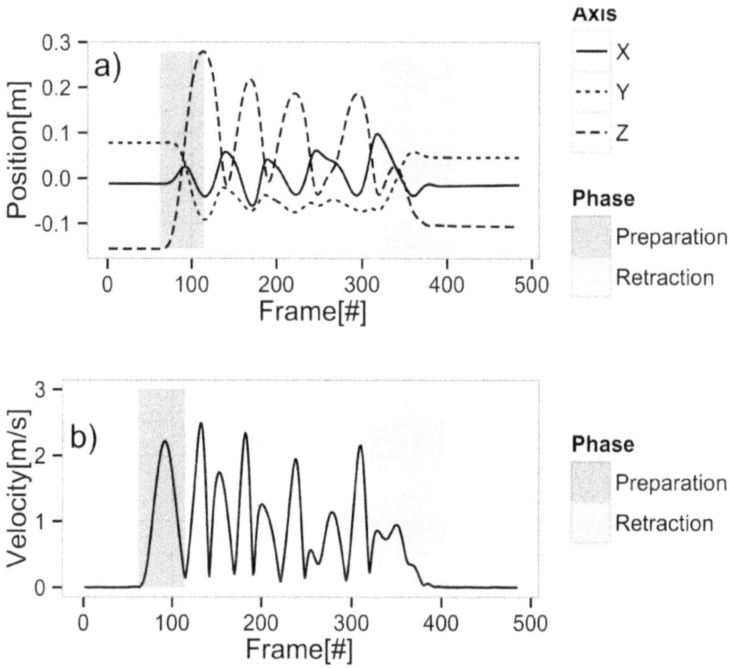

Figure 11 *Repetitive* movement. (a) Position data, (b) Resulting velocity.

In Figure 11, an example for a *repetitive* hand movement is shown. When investigating the movements, especially along the z-axis, a clear repetitive pattern is visible (Figure 11.a). The position plots further indicate that the path is based on movements in all three dimensions. The resultant velocity plot suggests several peaks, which are quite uniformly distributed. There appears to be also a sub-patterning, where a large peak is followed by a smaller curve (compare Figure 11.b). The velocity never quite reaches zero between the peaks. At the end of the hand movement there is a much smaller peak compared to the remaining peaks indicative of a retraction phase. Overall, maximum velocity peaks are around 2m/s similar to the *phasic* hand movement described above.

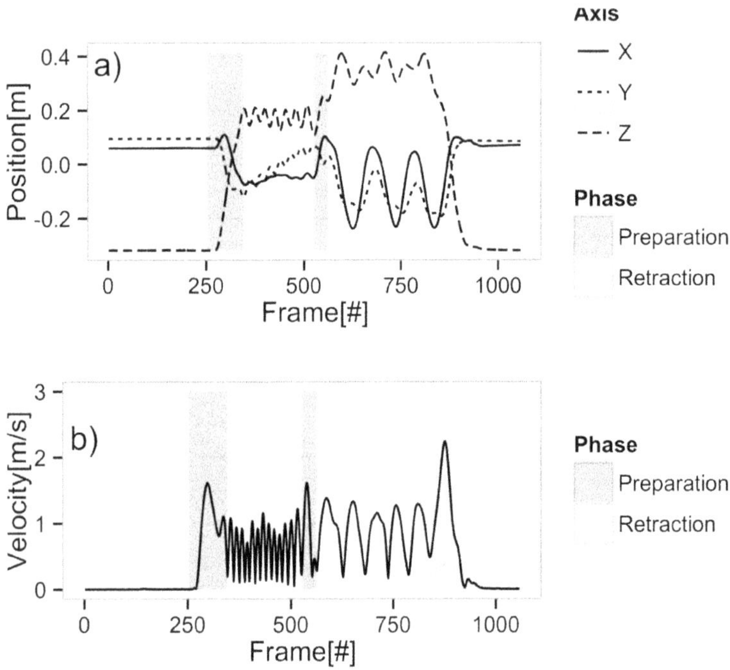

Figure 12 *Repetitive* movement. (a) Position data, (b) Resulting velocity.

In Figure 12, another representative example for a *repetitive* movement is shown. In this case, the figures suggest that instead of a single *repetitive* movement the participant concatenated two *repetitive* movements. At the beginning, the velocity plot shows a clear peak, which is much larger compared to the following peaks. Here, the hand is lifted to the starting position, thus indicating a clear preparation phase. This phase if followed by the first stroke which is characterized by a vertical zig-zag movement (compare z-axis in Figure 12a). The peaks in the velocity plots are relatively uniformly distributed following a sinusoidal pattern. Investigation of the position graphs further suggests increasing values for the y-axis, thus the finger is drifting to the left during the stroke. Position values on the x-axis are almost constant, thus the participant performs a movement in the frontal plane. At the end of the first stroke, a clear change in the patterning is visible, which is also demarked by a greater velocity peak around frame 550. Here, the hand is transported to different location in the gesture space using a second preparation phase. Subsequently, another repetitive movement is performed, this time describing a horizontal, circle-like movement, which is indicated by the almost sinusoidal plots for the x- and y-axis and much smaller movements on the z-axis. Thus, again a two dimensional movement on a plane is performed where the plane is tilted horizontally in comparison to the first stroke. Finally, a much larger peak is shown in the resultant velocity plot which marks the retraction phase of the hand movement where the hand moves back to the previous res-position. In Figure 13 the actual 3D trajectory of the finger is shown.

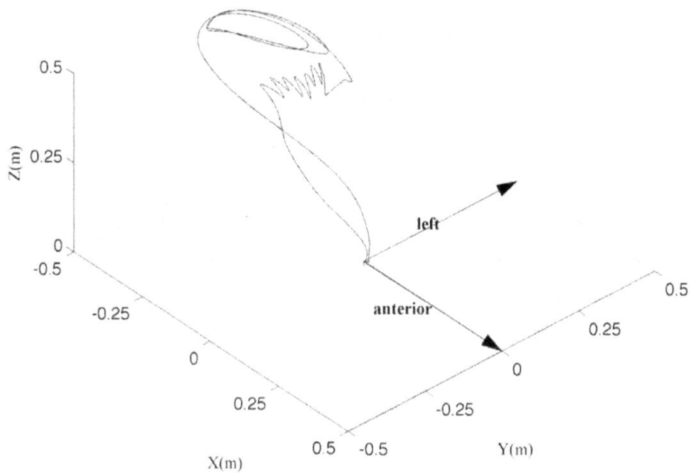

Figure 13 3D trajectory of *repetitive* movement

The plot clearly supports the interpretation above with two distinct repetitive phases, which are each preceded by a preparation phase.

Example of a *shift* hand movement

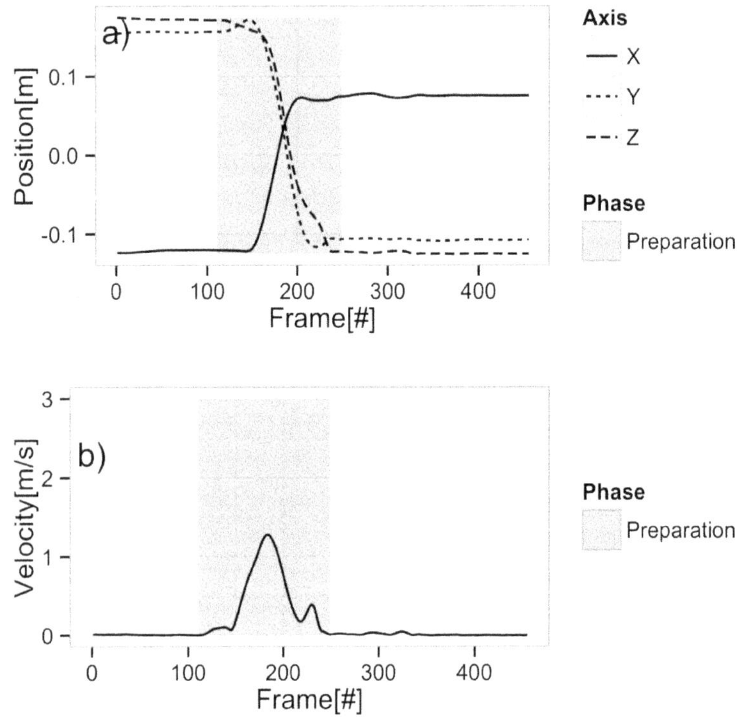

Figure 14 *Shift* movement. (a) Position data, (b) Resulting velocity.

In Figure 14, a representative *shift* hand movement is depicted. The resultant velocity plot shows mainly a single peak. Thus, only a preparation phase can be identified from the plots. The position data indicates that the participant moved the hand upwards and to the left, towards a new resting-position using a relatively straight path. The maximum velocity is much smaller compared to the *phasic* and *repetitive* movements displaying maximum velocity of around 1.2m/s. Overall, the movement can be characterized by two static phases which delimit a single short movement bout.

Example of an *aborted* hand movement

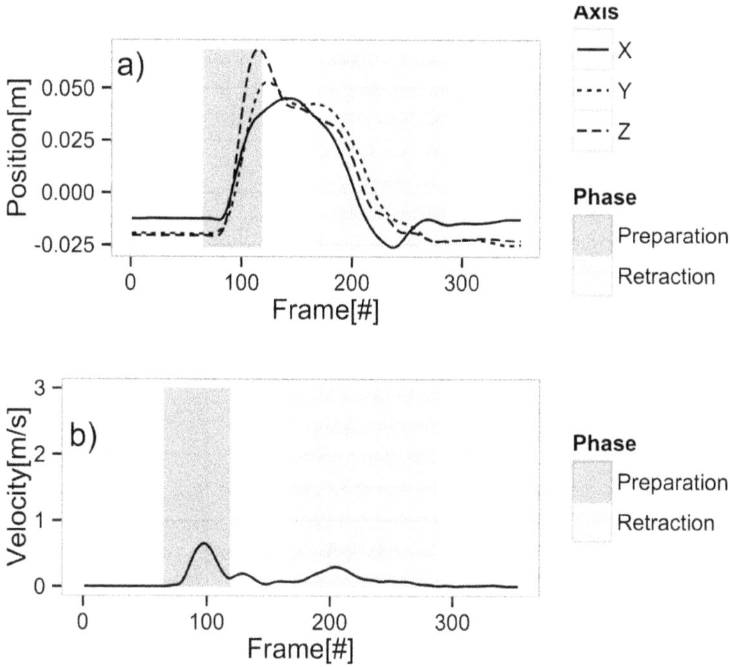

Figure 15 Aborted movement. (a) Position data, (b) Resulting velocity.

In Figure 15, an example for an *aborted* hand movement is shown. Investigating the ROM of the position data (Figure 15a) shows that the movement is relatively constrained. The resultant velocity plot shows a peak at the beginning followed by a holding phase, which is maintained for almost a whole second where the hand is held against gravity. Subsequently, the hand drifts slowly back into the base-position suggesting a retraction phase. Thus, a preparation phase is initiated but the stroke is never followed by a retraction phase. Maximum gesture velocities are much smaller compared to the *phasic* and *repetitive* movements.

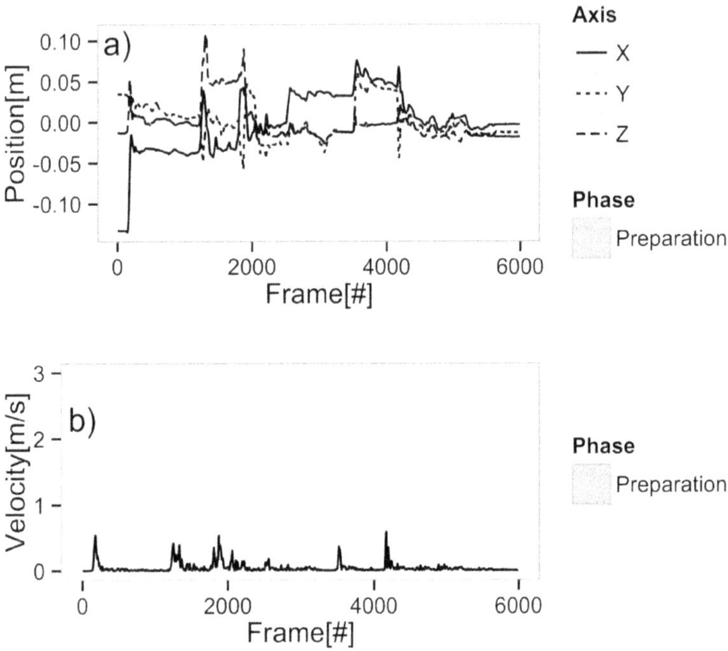

Figure 16 Irregular movement. (a) Position data, (b) Resulting velocity.

Finally, in Figure 16, an example of the kinematics for an *irregular* hand movement is given. The data clear shows that the movement follows a somewhat erratic pattern with only small displacements of the hand in various directions. Thus, the hand remains within a relatively confined area. The resultant velocity plot is interspersed with small peaks followed by short resting phases. Peak velocities never exceed 1m/s and on average are quite low. Although, at the beginning the velocity plot depicts an initial peak, the movement is much smaller, thus, the participant did not displayed a preparation phase. Similarly, the movement fades at the end thus, no retraction is visible. Regarding the length of the movement, the *irregular* hand movement persists much longer compared to the other hand movements.

6.6 Discussion

In the present pilot study, we investigated the kinematics of the five hand movement behaviour values introduced by the NEUROGES system as performed explicitly by a single participant. The kinematics of the hand movements were recorded using an electromagnetic motion capture system with great precision and time resolution. Investigation of the kinematics gave clear indications about the detailed movements underlying the gestures and further suggested clear differences with regard to the different structure categories used by the NEUROGES coding system. This provides further support for the validity of the values as they are not only linked to specific mental functions but are also clearly distinguishable based on their respective kinematics and overall form. However, as this study has only pilot character, further research is necessary before more conclusive statements can be made.

Knowledge of the kinematics provided clear indication about the structure of the movement and considerably eases the task of identifying hand movement behaviours, as typically changes in gesturing are depicted by clear changes in the kinematics. Thus, when faced with the time consuming challenge of annotating hand movement behaviours from video recording, having these additional information should provide clear hints, especially when segmenting video data. This should increase interrater reliability (compare also Holle and Rein, this book) and easing comparisons across studies. As ELAN already provides the possibility to include time-series there should be in principle no problem to augment the classical video based approach with motion capture data.

One interesting aspect pertains to the shape of the velocity curves of the preparation and retraction phases. There seemed to be a recurrent scheme where the velocity plots of the preparation phases followed more closely a bell-shaped profile which is well known from pointing and prehension movement in studies of motor control (Morasso, 1981, 1983). Potentially, this difference is related to differences in intention with regard to the two gesture phases. Under this view the preparation phase can be seen as an intentional motor act, where the hand is transported to a specific location in gesture space in order to allow the execution of the desired gesture. In contrast, the retraction phase might not be under direct intentional control of the actor anymore, thus relying more on automatic processes. Clearly however, more research is needed.

Finally, with regard to the scheme of preparation, stroke, and retraction phases introduced earlier, the present work showed that this simple scheme might already be sufficient to allow for precise segmentation of the hand movement behaviours further allowing the identification of different hand movement categories.

6.7 Outlook

The identification of kinematic differences between different hand movement behaviour values might also help to implement numerical routines, which could assist gesture researchers in identifying gestures and decrease the time necessary to analyse gestures. In

Figure 17, the number of articles indexed by PubMed and ISI Web of Knowledge in October 2010, which contain the phrase "gesture recognition", are shown.

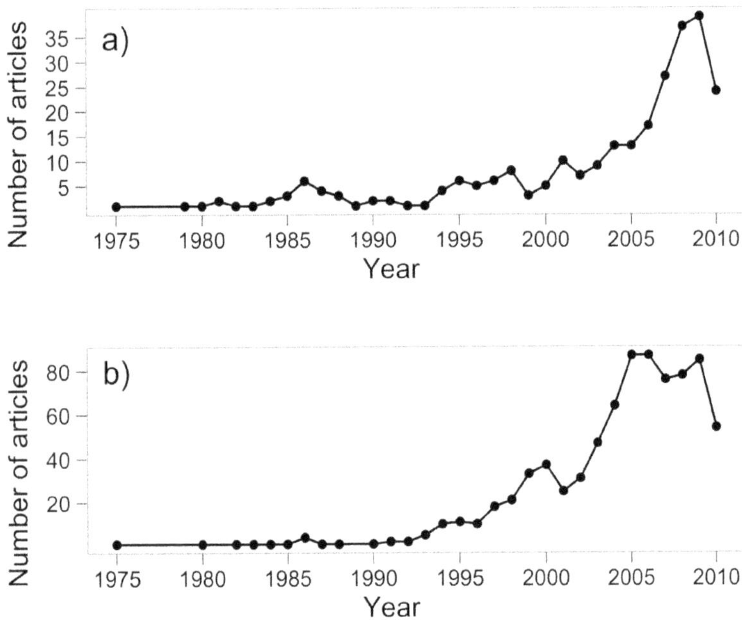

Figure 17 Number of articles per year resulting from "gesture recognition" search query at PubMed (a) and ISI Web of Knowledge (b).

As can be clearly seen, there is growing interest on the topic of gesture recognition, both, in the life sciences as indicated by PubMed as well as in general science as indicated by ISI Web of Knowledge.

One of the hot topics in computer science deals with novel ways for human machine interaction, and there is a large body of literature on routines to automatically recognize gestures in order to simplify and automate this interaction (Kraemer & Ratamess, 2004; Pavlovic, Sharma, & Huang, 1997; Wu & Huang, 1999). As computer scientists have worked on this problem for quite some time, there are some impressive algorithms already available. For example, Unzueta & Goenetxea (2010) implemented an algorithm which automatically identifies cyclical and non-cyclical gestures. Another example by Fröhlich & Wachsmuth (1997) translates speech and gestures into semiotic symbols based on an upper body model of the actor. However, many of these algorithms are based on learning schemes and code books, which are probably only of limited value for natural communicative contexts and leave much to be desired from a humanities perspective. Nevertheless, it seems quite surprising, that there is very little interaction between researchers from computer science and researchers from the humanities, although the problems are quite similar if not the same. One suggestion for the future should be to enhance the information flow between these two domains, maybe with the inclusion of researchers from the domain of motor control.

With regard to the future of motion capture, two new streams are emerging which might be particular relevant for gesture research. These are the invention of range imaging cameras and multiple view scenarios. The former allows the collection of 2.5 dimensional data, where in addition to normal visual image a second depth image is collected. As this depth data is only from a single perspective the data is not truly three-dimensional but delivers some depth data and therefore is called 2.5 dimensional. This approach has already been successfully adopted for video game control (Microsoft, 2010) and first attempts have already be done with regard to the automatic recognition of hand movement behaviours (Westfeld, 2007). The second approach is based on a multiple camera view approach. By processing the information gained from several synchronous viewpoints it is possible to calculate 3D data of objects and actors and there are already attempts to use this for gesture recognition as well (Canton-Ferrer, Casas, & Montse, 2006). Both approaches have the advantage that no markers are necessary.

In summary, including more quantitative measures like the one presented here, supports gesture researchers during data analysis and should help to establish gesture values based on some "hard" criteria. Much more empirical work is needed however. It should be clear that automatic classification of hand movement behaviour with 100% accuracy will probably not be achievable within the nearer future, as abstract entities like meaning and intent of the actor are very unlikely to be completely coded at the kinematic level. Thus, annotators will always rely to some extent on some contextual information beyond the pure hand kinematics. A possible approach could be to apply automatic routines to identify simple gestures only. This would already shorten the time necessary to analyze complex hand movement behaviour data considerably (Wittenburg, 2010).

Acknowledgements

The present work has been funded by the Volkswagenstiftung through the project "Towards a grammar of gestures: Evolution, Brain, and Linguistic Structures" (Project-code. II/82175).

References

Biryukova, E.V., Roby-Brami, A., Frolov, A.A., & Mokhtari, M. (2000). Kinematics of human arm reconstructed from spatial tracking system recording. *Journal of Biomechanics, 33*, 985-995.

Bril, B., Rein, R., Nonaka, T., Wenban-Smith, F., & Dietrich, G. (2010). The role of expertise in tool use: Skill differences in functional action adaptations to task constraints. *Journal of Experimental Psychology: Human Perception and Performance, 36*(4), 825-839.

Canton-Ferrer, C., Casas, J.R., & Montse, P. (2006). *Human model and motion based 3D action recognition in multiple view scenarios*. Paper presented at the 14th European Signal Processing Conference (EUSIPCO 2006), Florence, Italy.
Cappozzo, A., Croce, U. D., Leradini, A., & Chiari, L. (2005). Human movement analysis using stereophotogrammetry Part 1: theoretical background. *Gait and Posture, 21*(2), 186-196.

Cappozzo, A., Croce, U.D., Leradini, A., & Chiari, L. (2005). Human movement analysis using stereophotogrammetry Part 1: theoretical background. *Gait and Posture, 21*(2), 186-196.

Chen, F.-S., Fu, C.-M., & Huang, C.-L. (2003). Hand gestures recognition using a real-time tracking method and hidden Markov models. *Image and Vision Computing, 21*, 745-758.

Day, J.S., Dumas, G.A., & Murdoch, D.J. (1998). Evaluation of a long-range transmitter for use with a magnetic tracking device in motion analysis. *Journal of Biomechanics, 31*(10), 957-961.

Fröhlich, M., & Wachsmuth, I. (1997). *Gesture recognition of the upper limbs - From signal to symbol*. Paper presented at the Gesture and sign language in humancomputer interaction, gesture workshop.

Gordon, D., Robertson, E., & Dowling, J.J. (2003). Design and responses of butterworth and critically damped digital filters. *Journal of Electromyography and Kinesiology, 13*, 569-573.

Hore, J., Watts, S., & Tweed, D. (1994). Arm position contraints when throwing in three dimensions. *Journal of Neurophsiology, 72*(3), 1171-1180.

Kendon, A. (1972). Some relationships between body motion and speech. In A. W. Siegman & B. Pope (Eds.), *Studies in dyadic communication*. New York: Pergamon Press.

Kita, S., van Gijn, I., & van der Hulst, H. (1998). Movement phases in signs and co-speech gestures, and their transcription by human coders *Gesture and Sign Language in Human-Computer Interaction* (Vol. 1371/1998, pp. 23-35). Berlin/Heidelberg: Springer.

Konda, S., Yanai, T., & Sakurai, S. (2010). Scapular rotation to attain the peak shoulder external rotation in tennis serve. *Medicine and Science in Sports and Exercise, 42*(9), 1745-1753.

Kraemer, W.J., & Ratamess, N.A. (2004). Fundamentals of resistance training; Progression and exercise prescription. *Medicine and Science in Sports and Exercise, 36*(4), 674-688.

Kuipers, J.B. (1999). *Quaternions and rotation sequences: A primer with applications to orbits, aerospace, and virtual reality*. Princeton, New Jersey: Princeton University Press.

Lausberg, H., & Sloetjes, H. (2009). Coding gestural behavior with the NEUROGES-ELAN system. *Behavioral Research Methods, 41*(3), 841-849.

McNeill, D. (1992). *Hand and Mind: What gestures reveal about thought*. Chicago: The University of Chicago Press.

Microsoft (Producer). (2010). XBox Kinect. Retrieved from http://www.xbox.com/de-de/kinect

Morasso, P. (1981). Spatial control of arm movements. *Experimental Brain Research, 42*(2), 223-227.

Morasso, P. (1983). Three dimensional arm trajectories. *Biological Cybernetics, 48*(3), 187-194.

Pavlovic, V.I., Sharma, R., & Huang, T.S. (1997). Visual interpretation of hand gestures for human-computer interaction: A review. *IEEE Transactions on Pattern Analysis and Machine Intelligence, 19*(7), 677-695.

Prokopenko, R.A., Frolov, A.A., Biryukova, E.V., & Roby-Brami, A. (2001). Assessment of the accuracy of a human arm model with seven degrees of freedom. *Journal of Biomechanics, 34*, 177-185.

R Development Core Team. (2008). R: A language and environment for statistical computing. Vienna, Austria: R Foundation for Statistical Computing. Retrieved from http://www.R-project.org

Raab, F.H., Blood, E.B., Steiner, T.O., & Jones, H.R. (1979). Magnetic position and orientation tracking system. *IEEE Transactions on Aerospace and Electronic Systems, 15*(5), 709-718.

Seyfeddinipur, M. (2006). *Disfluency: Interrupting speech and gesture*. Njimegen: Max Planck Institute of Psycholinguistics.

Tsai, Y.S., Wu, P.L., & Wu, T.Y. (2007). Throwing kinematics in youth baseball players with and without elbow injury. *Journal of Biomechanics, 40*(S2), S292.

Unzueta, L., & Goenetxea. (2010). Cyclic and non-cyclic gesture spotting and classification in real-time applications. In F. J. Perales & R. B. Fisher (Eds.), *Articulated motion and deformable objects* (pp. 172-181): Springer.

Weigelt, C., & Bock, O. (2007). Adaptation of grasping responses to distorted object size and orientation. *Experimental Brain Research, 181*(1), 139-146.

Westfeld, P. (2007). *Development of approaches for 3-D human motion behaviour analysis based on range imaging data*. Paper presented at the Optical 3-D Measurment Techniques VIII, Zürich.

Winter, D.A. (2005). *Biomechanics and motor control of human movement* (3rd ed.). Hoboken, N.J.: John Wiley & Sons.

Wittenburg, P. (2010). [AVATecH Expert Workshop].

Wu, Y., & Huang, T.S. (1999). *Vision-based gesture recognition: A review*. Paper presented at the International Gesture Workshop on Gesture-Based Communication in Human-Computer Interaction.

III. Coding Movement Behaviour with the NEUROGES-ELAN System

7. The ELAN Annotation Tool

7.1 An introduction to the ELAN system

Han Slöetjes

7.1.1 Beginnings of ELAN

The development of ELAN was initiated by the Technical Group of the Max Planck Institute for Psycholinguistics (MPI-PL) at the end of the twentieth century. ELAN was one of the annotation tools that were developed with the maturation of digital media. It was designed to support the annotation of audio as well as video recordings and to accommodate different fields of research. Some tools specialized to accommodate a specific field of research, e.g. field linguistics, or a specific type of tasks, e.g. speech analysis but ELAN have always been a multipurpose, multimodal annotation tool (Brugman & Russel, 2004).

One of the predecessor tools developed at the MPI-PL was Media Tagger. This application was a MacOS-only application that stored its data in a proprietary, binary QuickTime type of file. This approach soon proved to be untenable. By the time ELAN evolved from several components in a client-server corpus system, both Java as a platform-independent programming language and XML as a format for structured textual data were on the way to become standard solutions. These technologies were adopted for most of the MPI-PL tools and ELAN is now available for Windows, MacOS X and Linux. EAF, the native file format of ELAN, is based on an XML-Schema, all annotation data is Unicode text.

7.1.2 Handling of audio and video in ELAN

The handling of media files turned out to be the disadvantage of Java as programming language. The Java Media Framework (JMF), designed to provide a multiplatform media solution, was never according to expectations. A high performance, "pure Java" media solution was still missing. Therefore, several platform specific ("native") components were developed, using different programming languages and building on various frameworks, to improve accuracy and performance of media playback and to increase the number of supported file formats. For Windows, components were developed based on Direct Show and on the Microsoft Media Foundation. For Mac OS X, a player was developed based on the QTKit Framework (as an addition to the QuickTime for Java player, which is provided by Apple). In the Linux version of ELAN, the media files are still processed by JMF.

ELAN can display up to four video files that can either be integrated in the main window or detached in a separate, resizable window. But it is possible to associate more than four video files. Each can be hidden or shown through a selection menu. A rich set of media controls is available that allow to pass through the media with different step sizes. The time-unit used by ELAN and EAF is milliseconds. Segmentation with video frame precision is sufficient for video annotation tasks without sound, the default procedure in NEUROGES.

7.1.3 Annotations and tiers, the basic building blocks

An annotation in its most elementary form is a textual label or tag associated with a segment of the media, which is defined by a begin time and an end time. Most annotation tasks start with identifying the segments and applying a value to each one. Annotations are grouped on tiers, which are a kind of layers; a tier acts as a container for annotations. Annotations on the same tier cannot overlap and typically, annotations on the same tier refer to the same kind of events (speech, gestures, posture etc.). The user can define and create as many tiers as needed and the tiers can be grouped hierarchically. When a tier is part of a hierarchy, additional constraints apply to its annotations. In general, tier dependencies are used to add annotations to annotations. Whether or not to use tier dependencies depends entirely on the focus of the research and the taste of the user. For any kind of tier, the user can fill in several attributes.

In the case of NEUROGES, the tiers are not part of hierarchies; instead, separate, independent tiers are created for all gesture categories to be coded. Two of the tier attributes are used to create tier groups; the "participant" attribute that specifies to which subject the annotations refer and the "annotator" attribute to specify who created the annotations on a certain tier, i.e. the rater.

In the naming convention of the NEUROGES tiers, these attributes re-appear, e.g. the tiers are named "A_rh_unit_R1" and "A_rh_unit_R2" etc. The prefix, i.e., "A" or "B", refers to the participant, the suffix, i.e., "R1" or "R2", to the rater. With tiers for each hand separately and for both hands combined, this can easily count up to dozens of tiers per transcription. In the visualization of the data, the tiers can be hidden and they can be sorted in several ways. This level of detail, expressed merely by the number of tiers, accommodates assessment of interrater agreement per gesture type. This is considered as an important step in validation of the system. With respect to this kind of calculations, experiences with the NEUROGES system have led to new requirements for ELAN.

7.2 Development over the years

ELAN found application in a variety of research areas being a generic multimedia annotation tool: sign language research, field linguistics, gesture studies, multimodal interaction research, behavioural studies etc. The development has largely been determined by the input and feedback of users from these communities. Long-term commitment is a must for continued use and acceptance by these communities. One of the objectives of establishing a new department at the MPI-PL in 2010, The Language Archive (tla.mpi.nl), was to ensure this long-term availability. The digital archive and most of the software tools are now maintained and further developed by this unit.

In about one decade the requirements of the users increased considerably. These requirements have grown qualitatively, i.e. growing demands on usability/ease-of-use and transcription speed and quantitatively, i.e. an increase can be observed in media file sizes, in the amount of the recordings and in the number of annotation levels created.

7.2.1 Media recording, from low resolution to high definition

The media recording equipment nowadays supports much higher resolutions (high definition) and has enormous storage capacity, leading to the production of large quantities of data. Not only in lab/studio situations, but also in the field it has become much easier to record for many hours and sometimes even with more than one camera. The original files are often too big and too unpractical to be used in ELAN directly, therefore often smaller files, of still high quality, are extracted. The .mp4/H.264 format has emerged as the standard in many projects and particularly on Windows this still presents problems. Only from Windows 7 on, support for mp4 is built-in in the Microsoft Media Foundation and a special effort has been made to build a (Java based) media player on top of that framework. MacOS mp4 has been supported for a long time, but here also efforts will be needed to further support it. A new 64-bits media framework, AVFoundation, is available and ideally ELAN will have a player build on it in the future.

7.2.2 Working modes

In addition to the media file size, the number of layers of analysis added to the primary data is increasing, resulting in transcription files containing, in some cases, several dozens of tiers.

The introduction of task oriented working modes is an attempt to improve the efficiency of common tasks. The traditional user interface, which is optimized for precision rather than speed, is now referred to as "Annotation mode". Two new modes each concentrate on one of two major steps in the common transcription process: segment and label. The Segmentation mode allows segmenting the media while it is playing. Annotations can be created on different tiers by one or two keystrokes identifying the start or end time of a segment (=annotation). The alignment of annotations can easily be adjusted by mouse-drag. The Transcription mode, on the other hand, does not allow changing the alignment of annotations but instead focuses on input of text (labelling). The annotations are presented in tabular form with the timeline going top-down. The workflow is keyboard oriented. Type in text, hit the Enter key, the next segment starts playing and the text can be entered immediately. The media synchronization mode has been available for many years already and has been updated to also visualize the waveform of audio files, making synchronization of different types of media (video, audio and time-series data) more convenient. Although it is still most suitable to clip media files beforehand so that they are in sync, this mode allows setting an offset per file in case they do not accord.

7.2.3 Multiple file functions

Although multiple documents can be opened simultaneously in ELAN, most actions perform on the one document in the active window. But a growing number of functions are added that execute on multiple files selected by the user. These functions reduce the time needed for a task so that it often would not be possible to perform it when it had to be done on a file-by-file basis. Two categories of operations can be distinguished: editing and non-editing. The latter do not change the files in the domain (e.g. export functions), while the former do change the files and can generally not be undone easily.

A first example of multiple file processing is the possibility to create multiple annotation files for a collection of media files in a single action. The user can select a folder, maybe including sub-folders, containing media files, select a template for the tier setup and generate eaf files for the recordings. Videos of multiple camera recordings can be combined in a single transcription on the basis of a different prefix or suffix in the file name.

Then, there are several “export from multiple files” options. The most important one is the export as tab-delimited text. The result is an accumulated single file export. This export has been improved by the option to create a separate column for each tier (resulting in annotations with the same time boundaries appearing in the same row).

For corpora holding transcriptions containing several dozens of tiers, it can be advantageous to be able to export a selection of the tiers of each file as new eaf files. Depending on the targeted audience, different views on the transcriptions can be represented by the choice of included tiers.

One example of a multiple file editing action is the find-and-replace in multiple files. All files can be changed by this action and therefore it is important that the user keeps save copies. A replace can usually not simply be undone by a reverse find-and-replace. Once the files have been added to the domain, it is possible to specify a selection of tiers to work on, the search query and the replace value can be entered and the type of matching (regular expressions are supported) can be chosen.

A powerful search engine for structured search in local corpora is included in the distribution as well. It allows for constructing and executing complex queries based on structural and temporal relations of annotations within and over tiers. Annotation content can be disclosed, patterns detected and hypotheses tested. The results can be exported to tab-delimited text for further processing in spreadsheet and statistical analysis applications.

A number of tier based operations can be performed on a collection of files, with the common options available when performing these operations in a single file. The rationale behind these operations is discussed in the next section. Currently available are new annotations from overlaps of annotations on different tiers, annotations by merging tiers and annotations by subtracting annotations on different tiers.

7.2.4 Tier-based operations

Creation and manipulation of annotations and tiers is a tedious, time consuming task. Therefore, functions have been added to speed up the transcription process and to reduce the number of mouse clicks and keystrokes to get to a certain result. Some of the tier oriented functions involve two tiers or more and apply a certain logic to the annotations on those tiers.

One of the tier functions allows creating annotations based on the gaps between annotations on one or more selected tiers. The gaps can represent intervals of silence, when the tier contains speech annotations, or a rest phase in the case of a gesture tier. By creating the new annotations on a different tier than the original tier, the transcription is conveniently and efficiently enriched with a silence or rest positions tier. The hierarchical nature of tier structures can be turned to advantage by the options to automatically create child annotations on depending tiers, either per parent annotation when it is created, or for all annotations of selected tiers in one go.

The triple consisting of the functions to create annotations based on the overlaps of annotations of two tiers, to merge annotations of two tiers onto a third tier and to create annotations by subtracting the annotations of one tier from those of another, together represent the logical AND, OR and XOR (exclusive or) operations applied to time segments. Although, e.g. overlaps can be found and extracted by the search facilities, there can be good reasons to use the overlap function to (permanently) create a new tier. The new tier itself can hold and represent meaningful units and it can in turn become a source tier for following tier operations.

A combination of the overlap and merge routines is applied in the non-standardized “compare annotators” feature. Implementations of more commonly accepted interrater agreement algorithms are expected to be added in the future.

8. NEUROGES in Combination with the Annotation Tool ELAN

H. Lausberg & Han Slöetjes

The combination of the NEUROGES coding system and the annotation tool ELAN results in an effective tool for empirical research on movement behaviour. It is evident that in numerous aspects ELAN provides the perfect technical basis for applying the NEUROGES coding system. Therefore, since 2006, NEUROGES has been combined with ELAN (Lausberg & Slöetjes, 2009).

Over the years, the developments of the NEUROGES coding system and the annotation tool ELAN have substantially influenced each other. The experiences with the NEUROGES system provided useful information and insights for the refinement of ELAN. Wishes of the NEUROGES researchers such as functions for assessing interrater agreement or for creating overlaps of units of different tiers have inspired the development of ELAN, resulting in new or improved tool functionality such as the determination of interrater agreement, the creation of overlaps of units of different tiers, and the fully integrated calculation of contingency tables. On the other hand, new functions in ELAN such as merging units of different tiers and concatenating values have substantially coined and further facilitated the NEUROGES coding procedure.

For the application of NEUROGES with ELAN the NEUROGES coding algorithms have been translated into a NEUROGES-ELAN template, which is basically an electronic coding sheet. Thus, NEUROGES is available as ready-to-use ELAN template file. Table 1 shows how the categories of the Modules I - III are represented as tiers in the NEUROGES-ELAN template.

Table 1 Tiers of the NEUROGES-ELAN template

Module	Step	Tier
Module I	Step 1	rh_Activation_R0 lh_Activation_R0
	Step 2	rh_Structure_R0 lh_Structure_R0
	Step 3	rh_Focus_R0 lh_Focus_R0

Module II	Step 1	bh_Contact_R0
	Step 2	bh_Formal Relation_R0
Module III	Step 1	bh_Function_R0 rh_Function_R0 lh_Function_R0
	Step 2	bh_Type_R0 rh_Type_R0 lh_Type_R0

References

Lausberg, H., & Slöetjes, H. (2009). Coding gestural behaviour with the NEUROGES - ELAN system. Behaviour Research Methods 41(3), 841-849.

9. Step by Step Instruction in NEUROGES Coding with ELAN

Han Slöetjes

9.1 Download and install ELAN

Download ELAN at http://tla.mpi.nl/tools/tla-tools/elan/download/. Select the variant that corresponds to your operating system and save the installer on your computer. Run the installer and then launch ELAN.

9.2 Create a new annotation document

In the *File* menu, select *New...*

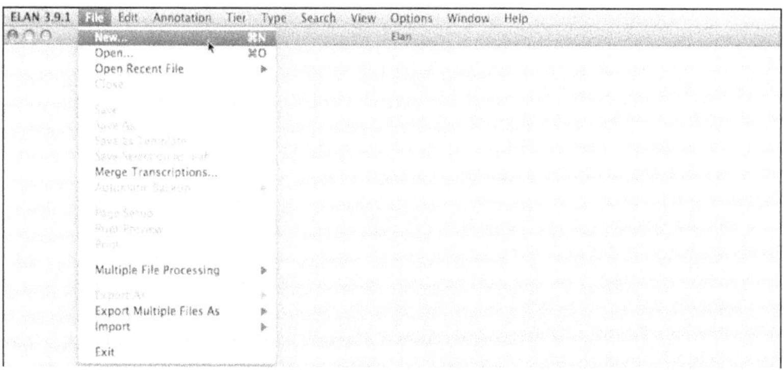

In the file browser, navigate to the folder containing the media file(s) and select one or more media files. Click the "copy to right" button (">>") or double-click the media file. The right panel lists the selected file(s) for the new document.

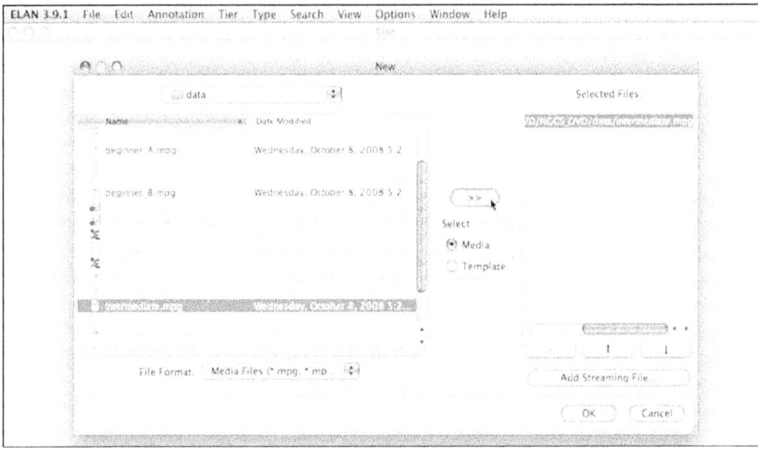

Then select the *Template* button and browse to the folder containing the NEUROGES template. Select the template and click the "copy to right" button (">>") or just double click it. With the template file and a video file in the right area of the window, confirm by clicking *OK*.

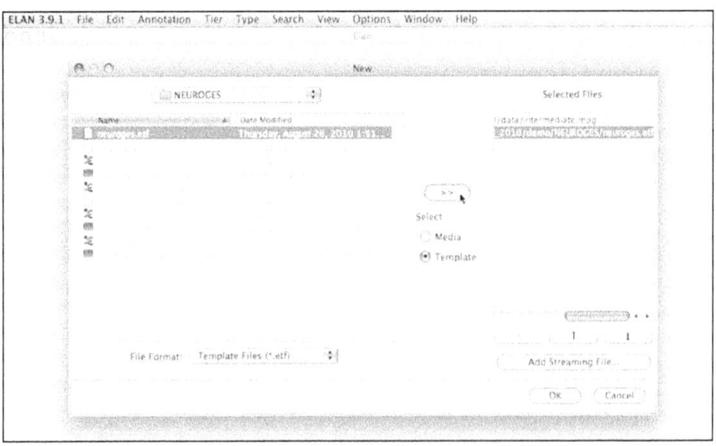

A new document is created with the media player and the tiers as defined in the template*.

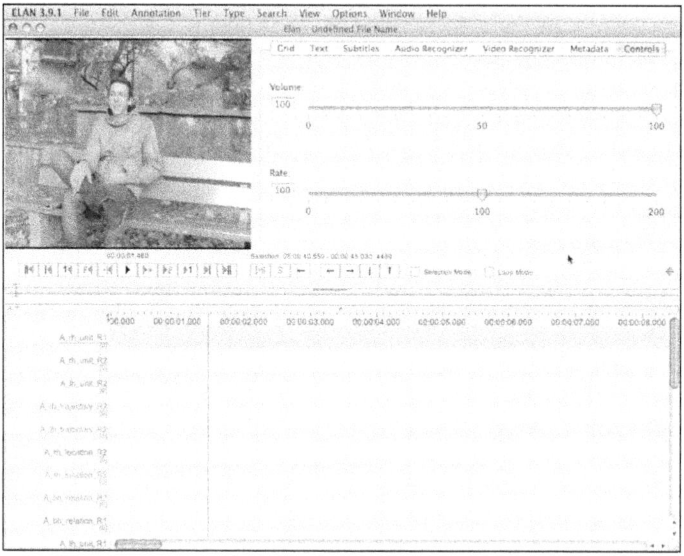

In the *File* menu select *Save...* or *Save As...* and save the new document as an ELAN Annotation File (.eaf).

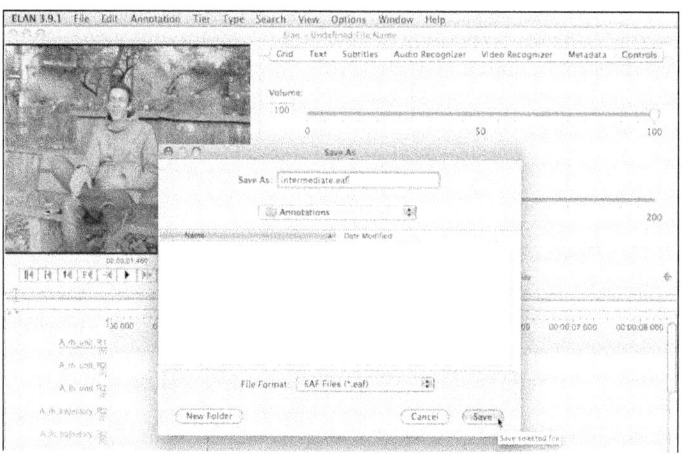

9.3 Organize the tiers

Click the right mouse button in the area of the tier labels and select the option *Show/Hide More...* in the context menu. In the window that appears click the *Hide All* button and then check the tiers that you want to be visible. If you are the first annotator hide all the tiers ending with "_R2". Confirm by clicking *OK*. Alternatively in the *Visible Tiers* menu select the *Show Annotator(s)* submenu and select "R1", hiding all tiers not belonging to R1.

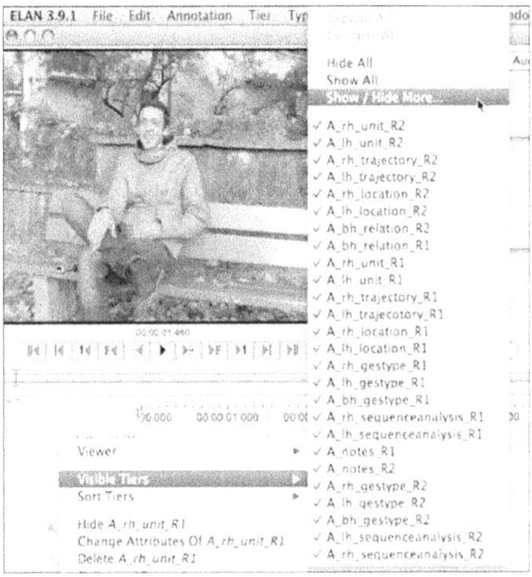

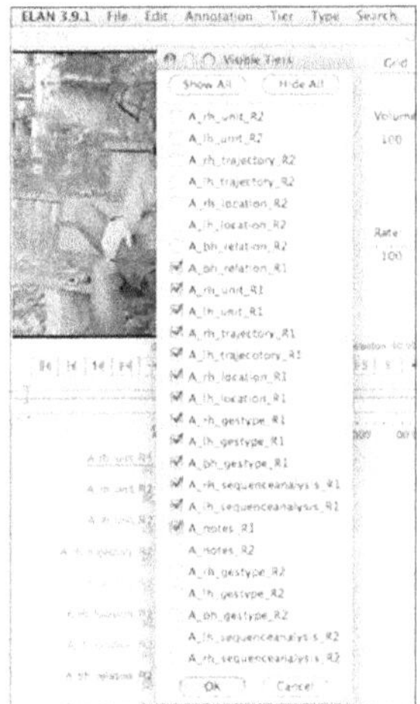

Change the order of the tiers using drag-and-drop on the tier name labels. The "active" tier has a red, underlined label and a light red background color. A tier can be made the "active" tier by double-clicking the name label.

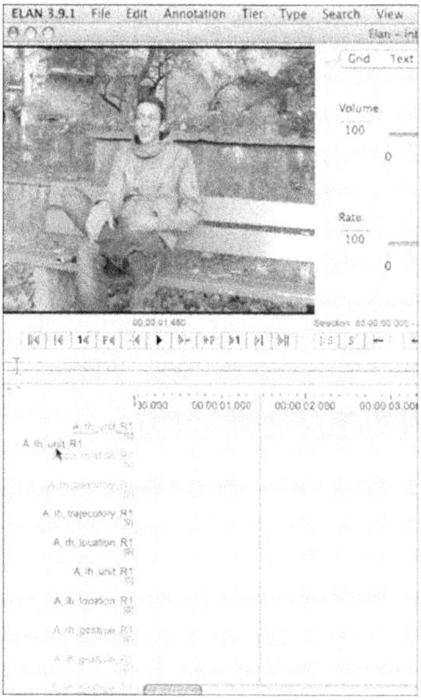

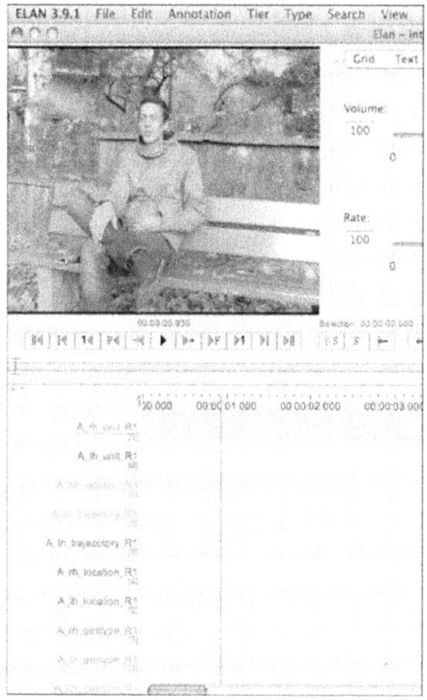

9.4 Create annotations

Start with "A_rh_unit" as the active tier. The play/pause and forward/backward buttons of the video player can be used to inspect the video and identify *movement* units, in this case of the right hand.

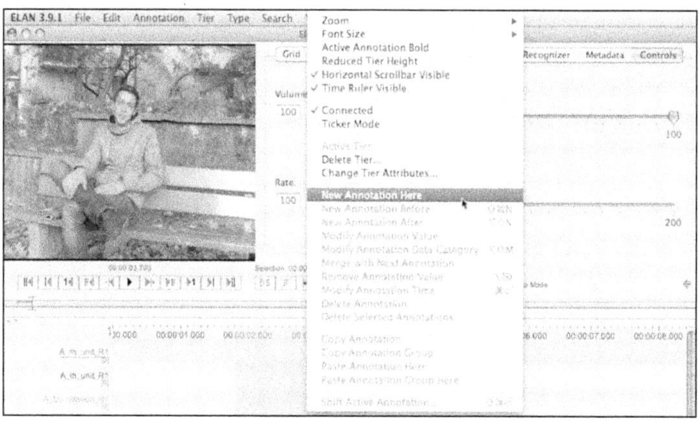

By dragging the mouse with the left button down a segment of the video can be selected (marked light blue). Dragging can be performed left-to-right or right-to-left, the video image is updated while dragging.

A selection can also be made by activating the Selection Mode and using the player's forward and backward buttons (or just the play/pause button) to select a segment of the video. This method is especially useful for long segments, segments longer than the width of the view.

An annotation can now be created on the active tier by a keyboard shortcut (Alt+N) or by right-clicking on a tier inside the selected interval and choosing *New Annotation Here* from the context menu.

It is also possible to create an annotation by double-clicking within the intersection of the selection and a tier.

Alternatively, an annotation can be created by first moving the crosshair to the begin time, marking it with the key combination Shift+Enter and then moving the crosshair to the end and marking that again with Shift+Enter.

When a new annotation is created on this tier a list of values pops up. Select "unit" as the annotation value.

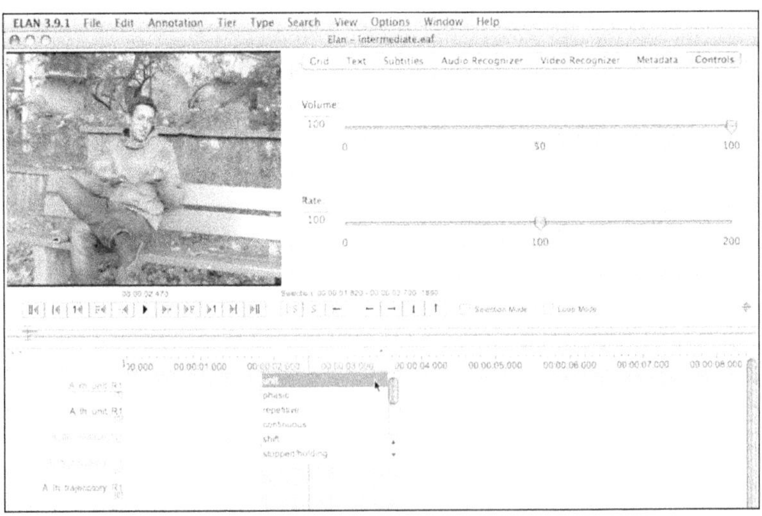

9.5 Change annotations

It may be necessary at some point to change the alignment and/or duration of an existing annotation. There are several ways to achieve this.
Activate the annotation (annotation in dark blue).

With the Alt key down drag the annotation to the left or to the right (annotation in green)-

To only change the begin or end time of the annotation, click close to the boundary while holding down the Alt key and drag the boundary to a new location.

It is also possible to change the alignment by activating the annotation, changing the selection (e.g. by holding down the Shift key and clicking at the new begin or end boundary) and then updating the annotation with Control+Enter.

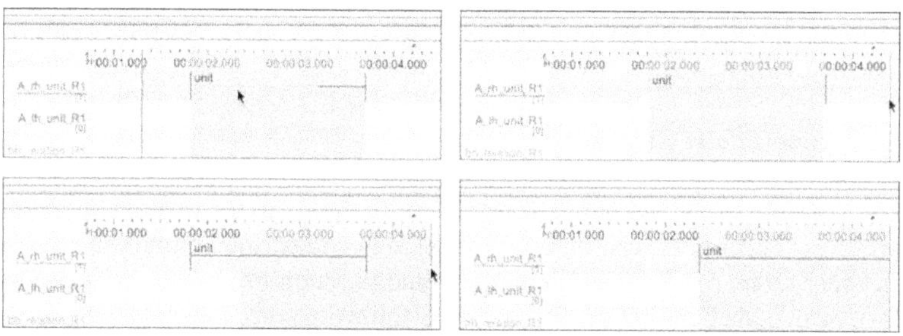

The contents or value of an annotation can be changed by double clicking it and selecting a new value from the drop down list or by entering the new value in the text edit box.

An annotation can be deleted by activating it and selecting the option *Delete Annotation* from the right mouse button context menu.

An annotation can be copied to the clipboard and pasted on the same or on an other tier. Once activated select *Copy Annotation* from the *Annotation* menu or from the context menu. Activate any other tier and select *Paste Annotation* to paste the annotation to the other tier while retaining the time information. It is possible to paste the annotation somewhere else by selecting *Paste Annotation Here* from the context menu after right-clicking a tier at the desired location.

An annotation can be duplicated onto another tier by making that other tier active and selecting *Duplicate Annotation* from the *Annotation* menu.

9.6 Tier-based operations

9.6.1 Copy a tier

While creating annotations on the different tiers according to the modules of the NEUROGES coding system, a few tier-based actions can be helpful. First of all, there is the option to create a copy of an entire tier, including the annotations. If you have several tiers with mostly the same segmentation, you can create a copy of the first tier and change the annotation values on the copy of the tier. To copy a tier, do as follows:

1. In the *Tier* menu select *Copy Tier...*
2. In the first screen of the window select the tier, in the second screen select *No Parent* and in the third screen the type as required for the copy, the destination tier. Click *Finish* to create the copy.
3. Change the name of the new tier (which has the name of the original and the suffix "-cp") via *Change Tier Attributes...* in the *Tier* menu. Select the copied tier in the table, enter a new tier name and click *Change*

The function *Remove Annotation or Annotation Value* from the *Tier* menu can be used to remove those annotation values that do not conform to the coding scheme of the new tier.

9.6.2 Annotations from overlaps

It is possible to create annotations based on the overlaps of the annotations of two tiers. This option can be used as a step in comparing annotations created by different raters or to detect the amount and duration of co-occurring events that have been coded on different tiers. Do as follows:

1. in the *Tier* menu select *Create Annotations from Overlaps...*
2. in the first step of the window select two tiers, in the second step enter a name for the new tier, select a type and customize some options concerning the contents of the annotations. Click *Finish*
3. the new tier with the overlapping segments is created

In case this function is applied to two equivalent tiers of which one is coding the left hand and the other the right hand, concatenating the values of the two overlapping annotations automatically codes the bimanual units.

9.6.3 Merge tiers

This is the counterpart of the *Annotations from Overlaps* function. Based on the total extent of overlapping annotations of two tiers, annotations are created on a new tier. *Merge Tiers...* is accessible via the *Tier* menu. The same options are available as for *Annotations from Overlap*, like concatenating the values of the annotations.

9.6.4 Compare annotators

Algorithms to calculate kappa values for interrater agreement, as described in other chapters, have not been implemented in ELAN yet. But there is a function to compare the annotations of two annotators expressed as the quotient of the overlap of two annotations and the total time span of these annotations. The value is a number between 0 and 1; closer to 1 is better. This is a non standard way of assessing agreement. *Compare Annotators* is accessible in the *Tier* menu.

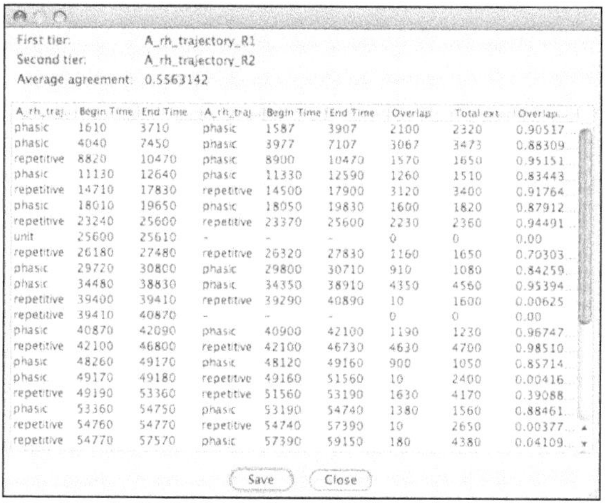

First tier: A_rh_trajectory_R1
Second tier: A_rh_trajectory_R2
Average agreement: 0.5563142

A_rh_traj...	Begin Time	End Time	A_rh_traj...	Begin Time	End Time	Overlap	Total ext...	Overlap...
phasic	1610	3710	phasic	1587	3907	2100	2320	0.90517...
phasic	4040	7450	phasic	3977	7107	3067	3473	0.88309...
repetitive	8820	10470	phasic	8900	10470	1570	1650	0.95151...
phasic	11130	12640	phasic	11330	12590	1260	1510	0.83443...
repetitive	14710	17830	repetitive	14500	17900	3120	3400	0.91764...
phasic	18010	19650	phasic	18050	19830	1600	1820	0.87912...
repetitive	23240	25600	repetitive	23370	25600	2230	2360	0.94491...
unit	25600	25610	-	-	-	0	0	0.00
repetitive	26180	27480	repetitive	26320	27830	1160	1650	0.70303...
phasic	29720	30800	phasic	29800	30710	910	1080	0.84259...
phasic	34480	38830	phasic	34350	38910	4350	4560	0.95394...
repetitive	39400	39410	repetitive	39290	40890	10	1600	0.00625
repetitive	39410	40870	-	-	-	0	0	0.00
phasic	40870	42090	phasic	40900	42100	1190	1230	0.96747...
repetitive	42100	46800	repetitive	42100	46730	4630	4700	0.98510...
phasic	48260	49170	phasic	48120	49160	900	1050	0.85714...
phasic	49170	49180	repetitive	49160	51560	10	2400	0.00416...
repetitive	49190	53360	repetitive	51560	53190	1630	4170	0.39088...
phasic	53360	54750	phasic	53190	54740	1380	1560	0.88461...
repetitive	54760	54770	repetitive	54740	57390	10	2650	0.00377...
repetitive	54770	57570	phasic	57390	59150	180	4380	0.04109...

Save Close

9.7 Annotation statistics

Some basic statistical information on the annotations in a file can be obtained via *Annotation Statistics* in the *View* menu. There are tabs for several categories (annotation, tier, type, participant, annotator), each one showing a table with an overview of the number of occurrences of (i) either individual annotation values (ii) or all annotations taken together and their minimal, maximal, average and median durations. Each tab can be saved as tab-delimited text.

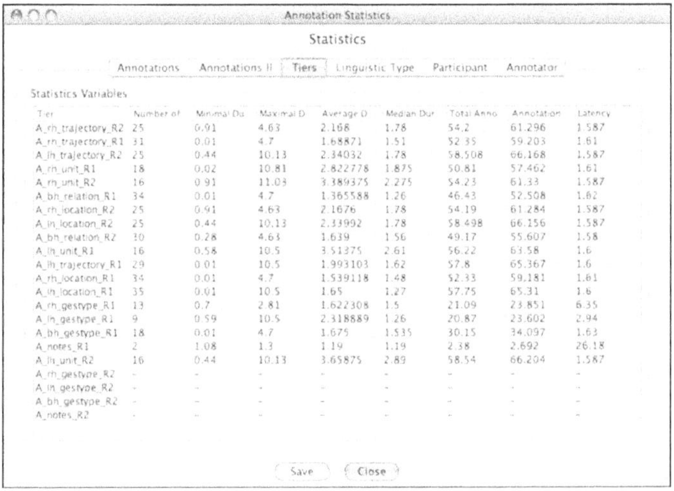

Tier	Number of	Minimal Du	Maximal D	Average D	Median Dur	Total Anno	Annotation	Latency
A_rh_trajectory_R2	25	0.91	4.63	2.168	1.78	54.2	61.296	1.587
A_rh_trajectory_R1	31	0.01	4.7	1.68871	1.51	52.35	59.203	1.61
A_lh_trajectory_R2	25	0.44	10.13	2.34032	1.78	58.508	66.168	1.587
A_rh_unit_R1	18	0.02	10.81	2.822778	1.875	50.81	57.462	1.61
A_rh_unit_R2	16	0.91	11.03	3.389375	2.275	54.23	61.33	1.587
A_bh_relation_R1	34	0.01	4.7	1.365588	1.26	46.43	52.508	1.62
A_rh_location_R2	25	0.91	4.63	2.1676	1.78	54.19	61.284	1.587
A_lh_location_R2	25	0.44	10.13	2.33992	1.78	58.498	66.156	1.587
A_bh_relation_R2	30	0.28	4.63	1.639	1.56	49.17	55.607	1.58
A_lh_unit_R1	16	0.58	10.5	3.51375	2.61	56.22	63.58	1.6
A_lh_trajectory_R1	29	0.01	10.5	1.993103	1.62	57.8	65.367	1.6
A_rh_location_R1	34	0.01	4.7	1.539118	1.48	52.33	59.181	1.61
A_lh_location_R1	35	0.01	10.5	1.65	1.27	57.75	65.31	1.6
A_rh_gestype_R1	13	0.7	2.81	1.622308	1.5	21.09	23.851	6.35
A_lh_gestype_R1	9	0.59	10.5	2.318889	1.26	20.87	23.602	2.94
A_bh_gestype_R1	18	0.01	4.7	1.675	1.535	30.15	34.097	1.63
A_notes_R1	2	1.08	1.3	1.19	1.19	2.38	2.692	26.18
A_lh_unit_R2	16	0.44	10.13	3.65875	2.89	58.54	66.204	1.587
A_rh_gestype_R2	-	-	-	-	-	-	-	-
A_lh_gestype_R2	-	-	-	-	-	-	-	-
A_bh_gestype_R2	-	-	-	-	-	-	-	-
A_notes_R2	-	-	-	-	-	-	-	-

9.8 Merge transcriptions

If two raters (R1 and R2) have been annotating in separate files, these files can be merged into one file by selecting *Merge Transcriptions* in the *File* menu. The window allows the user to select two transcription files (.eaf) and to specify a third file, which will contain the result of the merge operation. Additionally it is possible to select which tiers from the second source should be added to those in the first file (by default all will be added). With the tiers of both raters now in one file it is easier to compare the results.

9.9 Export annotations

Annotations can be exported to tab delimited text files (amongst other types of files). This type of data can be opened or imported in spreadsheet applications (like Excel). In the *Export As...* submenu of the *File* menu one of the options is *Tab-delimited Text.* The configuration window allows selection of the tiers to export and customizing of the way the contents of the annotations is stored in the text file.

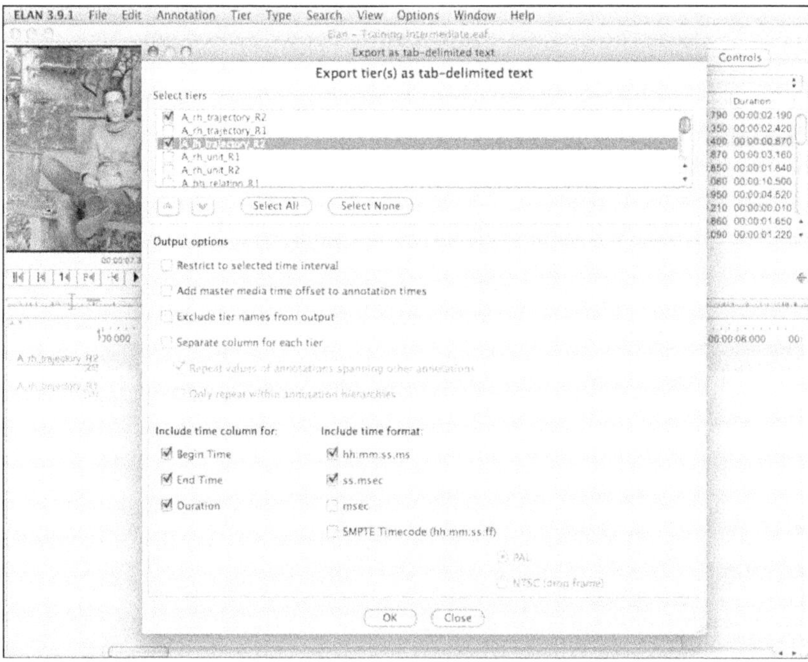

* The screenshots are based on a previous version of the NEUROGES coding system; some of the codes are no longer in use.

IV. Obtaining Data on Movement Behaviour

10. Study Designs in Movement Behaviour Research

H. Lausberg

10.1 Different types of study designs across scientific disciplines

Across scientific disciplines, different study designs are applied to obtain data on movement behaviour. In this section, three main approaches are presented and their advantages and disadvantages are discussed.

10.1.1 Movement behaviour that is spontaneously displayed in natural settings

This type of study design takes advantage of the fact that human beings tend to move spontaneously when they think, feel, act, or interact. The context is natural, e.g. dinner with friends, doctor - patient interaction, university lecture, etc. Neither directives to move nor to perform particular types of body movements are given.

The person whose movement behaviour is studied is not informed about the fact that her/his movement behaviour is subject of investigation. Of course, the person has to be informed about the video registration and (s)he has to give her/his consent. However, the information about research goals should be kept general. It should not be emphasized that the person's movement behaviour is investigated, since this information typically resuls in an inhibition of the spontaneous flow of body movements. In that case, the person might start to control his/her movement behaviour and thus, change from an implicit spontaneous display of movements to an explicit controlled one.

This methodological approach is often taken in anthropology, nonverbal communication, dance movement therapy, parent-child interaction, doctor-patient interaction, etc.

In this approach, the individual movement repertoire, as it naturally occurs, is observed. Thus, the strength of in this approach is that individual patterns can be investigated particularly well. Furthermore, the implicit movement behaviour, which is displayed beyond the mover's awarenss, is registered. As discussed in Subsection 2.2, implicit movement behaviour is of specific research interest as it enables to examine implicit cognitive, emotional, and interactive processes.

A further advantage of this design type is that no directives to perform particular movement values are needed. Therefore, the design can be applied with small children and with patients whose ability to concentrate may be limited. In general, for all groups of participants, the effectiveness of this design type does not depend on the individual's motivation, a factor that is, however, crucial in the other two designs types described below.

In addition, the assessment of movement behaviour in natural settings exactly has direct pratical implications, since the setting of investigation matches the setting of later application of the achieved knowledge. As an example, the findings on movement behaviour of those teachers who are highly effective in the class room can be used directly to improve the teachers' competence in that situation. Or, the results on the movement behaviour of an effective doctor-patient interaction can be applied to improve the interaction in less effective doctor-patient dyads.

A disadvantage of this approach is that it is difficult to examine research questions that focus on specific movement values such as exploring in which context *emphasis* gestures are displayed. As individuals vary in their movement repertoire often a large sample has to be investigated to gain enough data on a certain movement value to answer the research question. In the given example of a study on *emphasis* gestures it would need to be considered that some individuals hardly display *emphasis* gestures.

In general, care should be taken that even in a natural context the settings should be as optimal and as stable as possible to make it possible to conduct inter-individual and group comparisons. As an example, in psychotherapy sessions the patients should always sit in the same distance and orientation to the therapist. However, such a modification of the setting should not interfer with the naturality of the setting, particularly in therapy settings. For instance, it is well-known that some patients wish to sit closer or in a more frontal orientation to the therapist than other patients. Here, for ethical reasons, the therapy has priority to the research study.

10.1.2 Indirect elicitation of movement behaviour by using stimuli other than movement instructions

This design type uses stimuli to elicit movement behaviour. The term stimulus is used here in the broadest sense. Stimuli can be pictures, movies, questions, topics, improvisation tasks, music, objects, etc. The exception is any kind of instruction that demands a certain movement form (see 10.1.3). Thus, no directives to perform particular types of body movements are given. For the same reason as outlined above, the participant is not informed about the fact that her/his movement behaviour is subject of investigation, or at least, (s)he is not informed about what aspects of her/his movement behaviour are of interest.

The stimuli are administered in a semi-standardized setting with regard to the investigator and the space. Depending on the stimuli, the investigator may be more or less actively involved in the experiment. The participant may be asked to narrate the stimulus - quasi as a monologue - or there may be a semi-structured interaction between the investigator and the participant.

This design type is used in dance movement therapy, psycholinguistics, deception studies, psychology, psychosomatic and psychiatric research, etc.

The strength of this design type is that on one hand the situation is experimental and on the other hand, the observed movement behaviour is relatively natural. Thus, the setting can be designed according to the research question, e.g. to compare different groups or to examine specific movement values. Furthermore, confounding variables can be controlled. At the same time this design type enables to investigate spontaneous implicit behaviour and to observe individual variations. Obviously, with decreasing levels of task structuring inter-individual and group comparisons becomes more difficult and individual patterns manifest more clearly, and vice versa for increasing level of task structuring.

A limitation of this design type is that the participant's behaviour depends on her/his motiviation. This is relevant, for example, for the examination of patients with mental illness, who may differ in their verbal and nonverbal engagement in a narration task from the healthy participants only because of motivation deficits, caused by the illness itself, the hospitalization, etc.

Finally, it has to be considered that the participants' movement behaviour is clearly influenced by the stimulus. This aspect shall be discussed in more detail below, since often, when applying this study design type, researchers have neglected the influence of the stimulus on the movement behaviour and consequently, they have claimed that their findings are generally valid.

Gesture studies using different stimuli and different settings have reported hand preferences for co-speech gestures. A right-hand preference for co-speech gestures was found when gestures were examined during narrations of stories or during monologues on non-personal topics (Kimura, 1973 a, b; Stephens, 1983; Lavergne & Kimura, 1987). In contrast, an equally frequent use of the right and left hands was reported when co-speech gestures were investigated during free or semi-structured interviews on personal topics conducted by trained interviewers (Blonder et al., 1995; Ulrich, 1980; Lausberg et al., 2007). Few studies have directly investigated the influence of the stimulus on the hand preferences in the same individuals. In a study by Souza-Poza et al. (1979) participants used the right and left hands equally frequent during interviews with person-oriented topics, but they showed a significant right hand preference during nonperson-oriented topics. Likewise, the split-brain patient N.G. showed a right hand preference when co-speech gestures were investigated during narrations of the animated stimuli 'Tweedy and Sylvester' (McNeill, 1992; McNeill & Pedelty, 1995), while she displayed a reliable left-hand preference during the interviews (Lausberg et al., 2007). However, with the exception of the study by Souza-Poza et al. (1979), in the above mentionned studies the influences of the setting (monologue versus dialogue) versus the topic (personal versus unpersonal) cannot be disentangled, since monologues were always combined with unpersonal topics and dyadic interactions always with personal topics.

These findings of topic- and setting-related changes in hand preferences for co-speech gestures are likely to reflect that the different topics/settings elicit different gesture types. As demonstrated in Subsection 2.5, there are different hand preferences for different gesture types. A significant right hand preference has been reported for *physiographics / iconics*. Since, narrations are primarily accompanied by *iconic* gestures (Stephens, 1983), accordingly, studies examining narrations and monologues with unpersonal topics report a right hand preference for gestures (McNeill, 1992; McNeill & Pedelty, 1995; Lausberg, Davis, & Rothenhäusler, 2000; Stephens, 1983; Souza-Poza et al., 1979; Blonder et al., 1995). It follows that if, atypically, narrations are not accompanied by many *physiographics / iconics*, no right hand preference should be found. This was indeed reported for the split-brain patient L.B. whose predominant gesture type during narrations was *beats*. In split-brain patients *beats / batons* are only performed with the left hand and accordingly, this patient showed a left hand preference for co-speech gestures during the narration of Tweety & Sylvester (McNeill, 1992). Furthermore, the left hand preference for co-speech gestures during personal interviews might be secondary to the more frequent use of *batons* and *emotion/attitude* movements, which are accompanied by a facial emotional expression. Infact, for these types there is a left-hand preference (McNeill, 1992; McNeill & Pedelty, 1995; Lausberg et al., 2000; Stephens, 1983; Souza-Poza et al., 1979; Moscovitch & Olds, 1982; Blonder et al., 1995).

The example illustrates that a researcher should be cautious making general inferences based on results from experiments with specific settings and stimuli. The researcher's neglect of the context dependency of her/his findings may even lead to (falsely) controverse discussion with other reseachers. Because of the relevance of this topic, Chapters 11 and 17 further address the issue of the influence of the experimental setting and the stimulus on the choice of movement values.

10.1.3 Movement tasks - direct instructions to perform specific body movements

This design type uses directives to induce the performance of specific body movements. The instruction can be given verbally, by movement demonstration, or by tools. As examples, the investigator asks the participant to raise the right arm, (s)he shows a movement and the participant imitates it, or (s)he presents a tool and the participants demonstrates how to use it.

As the participant executes body movements on demand, most of his/her movements are displayed explicitly. Only during transition phases, e.g. in pauses between two tasks, implicit movement behaviour can be observed. Obviously, the participant is aware of that her/his body movements are subject to investigation.

This design type is often applied in clinical settings, such as in neurology, dance movement therapy, body-oriented therapies, psychomotor research, etc.

In neurology, - apart from the standard neurological examination that shall not be discussed here - specific movement tasks are administered to screen for apraxia (see 3.5.2). The tests typically examine transitive and intransitive gestures and actions. They often combine the executions on verbal command, on imitation, on visual presentation of tools, and with tool in hand (e.g. Goldenberg, 1993; Dovern et al., 2011).

In dance movement therapy, Espenak (1985), Schoop (1981), and Lausberg (1994) have developed comprehensive tests for movement behaviour diagnosics. These tests include movement tasks such as stamping, turning, falling to the ground, spinning, that are characterized by the fact that individuals and diagnostic groups perform them distinctly differently. The diagnostic specificity of these tasks is related to the fact that they elicit certain emotional states. As examples, stamping is often associated with experience of aggression. The experience of this feeling can be avoided by holding back strength during stamping. The contraction/expansion task (Schoop, 1974; Laban, 1988; Bernstein, 1991) reveals whether a person prefers to contract or expand. These movements are typically associated with the experience of opening and closing also on a psychological level. Spinning can lead to an ecstatic state (Akstein, 1981). If the individual allows this to happen, then their spinning movement is accelerated initially, the orientation space, e.g. by fixating a point, is given up, and the movement flow is free. In all these tasks, psychosomatic patients differ significantly from healthy controls (Lausberg et al., 1996). In most body-orientated therapies with or without psychotherapeutic approach, movement tasks are used for a precise body and movement behaviour diagnosis.

Psychomotor tests are used for a highly objective registration of movement behaviour. Standardized motor tests are administered to test specific psychomotor competences. This experimental psychological approach has a long-standing tradition. As early as 1931, the Russian neurologist Oseretzky developed a motor test battery with various tasks to examine static and dynamic coordination, motor activity, motor reaction, and motor adaptation. Later, further tests were developed, such as the Luria-Nebraska Neuropsychological Battery (Golden et al., 1978) or the modified Lincoln-Oseretzky-Development Scale (Günther, 1980). Normative performance scores are provided for these tests. Based on this normative data, the development of children can be assessed as well as alterations of movement behaviour associated with mental illness and brain damage.

The strength of this study design type is that the movement tasks enable to directly evaluate certain movement abilities. The participant's performance can be assessed according to a more or less documented performance standard. This can be based on the therapist's experience or on normative data such as provided for psychomotor tests.

A limitation of this approach is that the observable movement behaviour is reduced to those body movements that are asked for in the task. The individual's movement repertoire cannot be observed. Especially in psychomotor tests, movement behaviour is assessed primarily by quantitative parameters in terms of deficient versus non deficient.

Furthermore, the repeated testing with the same movement tasks, especially with psychomotor tasks, entails learning processes. The effect of learning has to be considered, for example, in pre- and post-therapy assessments. The "true" improvement in movement behaviour, e.g. as a reflection of an improvement of the patient's depressive state, may be confounded by learning effects.

Finally, the participant's performance crucially depends on his /her motivation.

10.2 Recommendations for study designs

In the first line, the research question determines what kind of study design is chosen. However, since the different types of study designs - as outlined above - all have their advantages and disadvantages, it is useful to combine different approaches. A broad methodological spectrum is particularly useful in basic research on movement behaviour that aims to explore specific movement values. The combination of different approaches enables, for example, to examine and compare the explicit versus implicit production of a movement value. While movement instruction results in the explicit generation of body movements, a great proportion of the spontaneous movement behaviour is displayed implicitly (see Subsection 2.2). With regard to neuropsychological research questions, tasks with defined movements instructions mainly challenge left hemispheric competences, whereas the examination of spontaneous movement behaviour is an important methodological approach to gain insight into motor competences of the right hemisphere. The advantage of combining methods shall be further illustrated by two examples from our own research.

To examine the research question if *pantomime* gestures with an imaginary tool in hand are primarily generated in the right or the left hemispheres, two main methods were combined in a study on split-brain patients (Lausberg et al., 2003a; Lausberg et al., 2007): (i) the spontaneous display of *pantomime* gestures during interviews, and (ii) the demonstration of *pantomime* gestures on command. In the first condition, it was striking that the split-brain patients spontaneously only used the right hand for *pantomimes*. However, the interpretation regarding hemispheric specialization was ambiguous since it could not be ruled out that in the given situations the patients had actually only referred to actions that they would actually use their right hand for, such as tooth brushing. The second condition, however, revealed that the split-brain patients had a selective left hand apraxia for *pantomime* with an imaginary tool in hand. It turned out that they were really unable to execute this subtype of *pantomime* with the left hand. Thus, the structured experiment with movement instructions helped to interpret the findings of the experiment on spontaneous behaviour.

On the other hand, in spontaneous movement behaviour, phenomena can be observed that may be not manifested in structured experiments with instructions on how to move. In a study on gesture and spatial cognition in split-brain patients (Lausberg et al., 2003b), the pattern of the spontaneous use of gesture space during gestural demonstration of animations with moving objects revealed a spatial neglect in the split-brain patients' right hand gestures. The neglect, however, did not manifest in standard neuropsychological tasks for spatial attenttion such as choosing options in the left space of Raven's Progressive Matrices by motor response (Zaidel et al., 1981), or touching the left hemibody with the right hand. In these neuropsychological examinations the manifestation of the implicit neglect of the left hemi-space was overridden by the explicit demand to pay attention to the left hemi-space in the motor response (Plourde & Sperry, 1984; Zaidel, 1979; Zaidel et al., 1981).

To summarize, if the research question aims at exploring the validity of specific movement values it is recommended to combine different methods as such as combination clearly broadens the insight. It is the premise to make more general statements about a movement value that are independent from the experimental setting.

Regarding the study sample, the following criteria, which all influence movement behaviour, should be considered for the inclusion of participants:

(i) handedness: If the laterality of limb movements is subject to investigation (see Subsection 2.5), the handedness of a participants has to be registered. Handedness influences the spontaneous laterality preferences (e.g. Kimura, 1973 a, b). Appropriate handedness measurements are, for example, the Oldfield Inventory (Oldfield, 1971), and the Montreal Handedness Questionnaire (Crovitz & Zener, 1962).

(ii) gender / sex: The gender and sex, respectively, have an impact on movement behaviour (Frances, 1979; Saucier & Elias, 2001). In the Alexithymia study (Subsection 5.2.3), alexithymic males and females even displayed opposite tendencies in some movement values. While alexithymic males increased the frequency of *phasic in space* units during the LEAS interview as compared to the HAWIE interview, females showed a clear decrease of this movement value.

(iii) mental illness, brain disease, or brain damage: Mental illness, brain disease, and brain damage all result in specific alterations of movement behaviour (see Chapters 2 and 3).

(iv) physical illness: For physical illness it has to be checked in each individual case if it has an impact on the patient's movement behaviour.

(v) medication: For medication it has to be checked if the given preparation has side effects on the movement behaviour (see 3.5.1).

Furthermore, there is some evidence that the investigator influences the participant's movement behaviour. Cold interviewers as compared to warm, empathetic ones lead to an increase of the participant's *continuous direct body-focused* activity (Freedman et al., 1972). Furthermore, the sex of the interviewer effects the participant's nonverbal behaviour (LaFrance et al., 2003). Since, thus far, there is only little empirical knowledge on the specific effects of different investigator variables on movement behaviour, it is recommended to reduce as much as possible the number of investigators in a study. This applies in particular to all experimental settings that imply an intensive interaction of the investigator and the participant. Future research should aim at clarifying the effect that the gender, personality, etc. of the investigator have on the participant's movement behaviour.

Regarding the spatial setting and the video registration, the following arrangements are recommended:

(i) standardized distance and orientation of investigator's and test subject's chairs; an angle of 120 ° is reported by most participants to be the most comfortable orientation vis-à-vis the investigator.

(ii) firm chair with armrests, i.e., no swivel chairs with wheels; if a table is necessary, this should not impair the vision on the participant and on the investigator.

(iii) optimal and standardized lighting; before the beginning of the study and of each video registration the light conditions for the video should be checked.

(iv) standardized background, optimally in monochrome high-contrast colors such as blue.

(v) high camera resolution, which is a prerequisite to detect fine body movements in the video data.

(vi) video recording of the participant's full body size in frontal view; it is recommended to additionally register the investigator, even if the investigator's behaviour is not primarily subject of investigation (see Figure 4 in Chapter 17). This enables to later clarify if certain movements of the participant are mere reactions to the investigator's movements. Furthermore, it opens the chance to later investigate the interaction of the investigator and the participant.

(vii) for studies on interaction, three cameras are recommended: one symmetrically on the dyad with each interactive partner in full body size, and the other two each on one partner registrating her/him in full body size in frontal view. Occasionally, split-screens have been used for playing the video registrations of dyads. However, the split-screen renders it difficult to unequivocally assess the direction of movements vis-à-vis the partner, e.g. it is difficult to judge if partner A directly points at partner B or more aside. Thus, the quality of the intra-dyadic relation may be hard to assess in split-screen play.

References

Akstein, D. (1981). Bewegungstrance. In H. Petzhold (Hrsg.), *Psychotherapie & Körperdynamik*, pp. 195-202. Paderborn: Junfermann.

Bernstein, P.L. (1991). Objektbeziehungen, Selbstpsychologie und Tanztherapie. In E. Willke, G. Hölter, and H. Petzhold (Ed.), *Tanztherapie, Theorie und Praxis,* pp. 217-44. Paderborn: Junfermann.

Blonder, L.X., Burns, A.F., Bowers, D., Moore, R.W., & Heilman, K.M. (1995). Spontaneous Gestures Following Right Hemisphere Infarct. *Neuropsychologia, 33*(2), 203-213.

Crovitz, H.F., & Zener, K. (1962). A group-test for assessing hand and eye-dominance. *American Journal of Psychology*, 75:271-6.

Dovern, A., Fink, G.R., & Weiss, P.H. (2011). Diagnostik und Therapie der Gliedmaßenapraxie. *Fortschritte der Neurologie-Psychiatrie, 79*, 345-357.

Espenak, L. (1985). *Tanztherapie - durch kreativen Ausdruck zur Persönlichkeitsentwicklung*. Dortmund: Sanduhr.

Frances, S. (1979). Sex Differences in Nonverbal Behavior. Sex Roles (5). 519-535.

Freedman, N., O'Hanlon, J., Oltman, P., & Witkin, H.A. (1972). The imprint of psychological differentiation on kinetic behaviour in varying communicative contexts. *Journal of Abnormal Psychology, 79*(3), 239-258.

Golden, C.J., Hammeke, T., & Purisch, A. (1978). Diagnostic Validity of a Standardized Version of Luria's Neuropsychological Version. *Journal of Consulting and Clinical Psychology, 46*, 1258-65.

Goldenberg, G. (1993). Praxie. In D. Y. von Cramon, Mai, N., and Ziegler, W. (Ed.), *Neuropsychologische Diagnostik* (pp. 259-286). Weinheim: VCH.

Günther, W. (1980). Untersuchungen zur Wirksamkeit mentaler Trainingsverfahren bei grobmotorischen Bewegungsstörungen. Unveröff. Diss. Psychologisches Institut Tübingen.

Kimura, D. (1973a). Manual Activity during Speaking - 1. Right-Handers. *Neuropsychologia, 11*, 45-50.

Kimura, D. (1973b). Manual Activity During Speaking - 2. Left-Handers. *Neuropsychologia, 11*, 51-55.

Laban, R. (1988). *The Mastery of Movement*. Worcester: Billing & Sons Ltd.

LaFrance, M., Hecht, M.A. & Paluck, E.L. (2003) The Contingent Smile: A Meta-Analysis of Sex Differences in Smiling. *Psychological Bulletin*. (129). 305-344.

Lausberg, H. (1994). *Vergleichende Bewegungsanalyse von vier Patientengruppen mit psychosomatischen Erkrankungen und einer gesunden Kontrollgruppe*. Psychosomatik und Psychotherapie. Lübeck, Medizinische Universität zu Lübeck. Dissertation.

Lausberg, H., von Wietersheim, J., & Feiereis, H. (1996). Movement Behaviour of Patients with Eating Disorders and Inflammatory Bowel Disease: A controlled Study. *Psychotherapy and Psychosomatics* 65, 272-276.

Lausberg, H., Davis, M., & Rothenhäusler, A. (2000). Hemispheric specialization in spontaneous gesticulation in a patient with callosal disconnection. *Neuropsychologia 38*, 1654-1663.

Lausberg, H., Kita, S., Zaidel, E., & Ptito, A. (2003b). Split-brain patients neglect left personal space during right-handed gestures. *Neuropsychologia 41*, 1317-1329.

Lausberg, H., Zaidel, E., Cruz, R.F., & Ptito, A. (2007). Speech-independent production of communicative gestures: Evidence from patients with complete callosal disconnection. *Neuropsychologia 45*, 3092-3104.

Lausberg, H., Cruz, R.F., Kita, S., Zaidel, E., & Ptito, A. (2003a). Pantomime to visual presentation of objects: Left hand dyspraxia in patients with complete callosotomy. *Brain 126*, 343-360.

Lavergne, J., & Kimura, D. (1987). Hand movement asymmetry during speech: no effect of speaking topic. *Neuropsychologia 25*(4), 689-693.

McNeill, D. (1992). *Hand and mind : What gestures reveal about thought*. Chicago: University of Chicago.

McNeill, D., & Pedelty, L.L. (1995). Right brain and gesture. In K. Emmorey, Reilly, J. (Ed.), *Language, Gesture, and Space* (pp. 63-85). Hillsdale, N.J. (U.S.A.): Lawrence Erlbaum Associates.

Moscovitch, M., & Olds, J. (1982). Asymmetries in spontaneous facial expressions and their possible relation to hemispheric specialization. *Neuropsychologia, 20*(1), 71-81.

Oldfield R.C. (1971). The assessment and analysis of handedness: the Edinburgh inventory. *Neuropsychologia,* 9(1): 97-113.

Oseretzky, N. (1931). Psychomotorik. *Zeitschrift für Angewandte Psychologie, Beiheft 1*, 57.

Plourde, G., Sperry R.W. (1984). Left hemisphere involvement in left spatial neglect from right-sided lesions. *Brain, 107*, 95-106.

Saucier, D.M. & Elias, L.J. (2001). Lateral and Sex Differences in Manual Gesture During Conversation. *Laterality, (6).* 239-245.

Schoop, T. (1974, 1981). *... komm und tanz mit mir*. Zürich: Musikhaus Pan.

Souza-Posa, J.F., Rohrberg, R., & Mercure, A. (1979). Effects of type of information (abstract-concrete) and field dependence on asymmetry of hand movements during speech. *Perceptual and Motor Skills 48*, 1323-1330.

Sperry, R.W. (1968). Hemisphere deconnection and unity in conscious awareness. *American Psychologist 23*, 723-733.

Stephens, D. (1983). *Hemispheric language dominance and gesture hand preference*. Ph.D. dissertation, Department of Behavioral Sciences, University of Chicago.

Ulrich, G. (1980). Lateralization of Hand-Movements in Patients with Affective Psychoses During an Interview Situation: An Attempt at a Physiological Interpretation. *Psychological Research,* 41, 249-258.

Zaidel, E. (1979). Performance on the ITPA following cerebral commissurotomy and hemispherectomy. *Neuropsychologia*, *17*, 259-80.

Zaidel, E., Zaidel, D.W., & Sperry, R.W. (1981). Left and right intelligence: case studies of Ravens' Progressive Matrices following brain bisection and hemidecortication. *Cortex*, *17*, 167-86.

11. Speakers Adapt their Hand Movement Behavior to the Content of Visual Stimuli

Harald Skomroch, Katharina Hogrefe, Robert Rein

Setting and stimulus of an experiment influence the hand preferences for co-speech gestures (see Chapter 10). A comparison of the hand movement behavior in 20 healthy subjects during Mr. Bean and Tweety and Sylvester (T & S) narrations suggests that also the choice of gesture types (Function values) is influenced by the stimulus. Participants displayed different hand movement patterns concerning *pantomime* and *presentation* gestures and hand choice during the respective interviews. Whereas participants chose an egocentric perspective for co-speech gestures more frequently when narrating clips of Mr. Bean, they performed more non-egocentric (mento-heliocentric) gestures (*motion presentation*) when describing events of clips. Additionally, in bimanual hand movements they displayed *left hand dominance* more often during cartoon narrations. These findings highlight the impact of the stimuli selection and suggest that participants adapt their gestural behavior to content they want to communicate.

11.1 Introduction

Chapter 10 proposes that the experimental setting (structured vs. unstructured) affects the hand movement (see also Bock, 2013). Further, alterations in task design can predetermine the scientific interpretation of the data as well as the likelihood of a specific behaviors' occurrence. Chapter 17 contrasts hand movement behavior analyzed according to NEUROGES Module I in description of everyday activities and in semi-structured interviews and found different patterns in the distribution of StructureFocus values in the respective settings. This finding is in line with previous studies, where the experimental setting or content was tested.

Accordingly, hand movement behavior differs when participants are engaged in cognitive tasks compared to when asked to elaborate about hypothetical emotional states or when asked to describe everyday activities (Chapter 16). Bavelas et al. (2007) could demonstrate in an experimental setting that gestural behavior is less affected by visibility of an interactional partner than by the degree of interaction in a speaking act. Participants performed significantly less gestures when their verbal description was taped as a monologue compared to when they were talking to a present interlocutor or to a person on the phone. Still, like in Alibali et al. (2001), gestural behavior during face-to-face interactions differed in some aspects compared to interactions where conversational partners cannot see each other. Representational gestures appear to decrease to a greater extent in non-visibility conditions than in *beat* gestures emphasizing prosody.

Hand movement behavior can also be affected by the presence/absence of speech. Although the general motor arousal seems unaffected when comparing participants' hand movements during silent and speech conditions, they display more *pantomime* gestures during the silent trials (Helmich & Lausberg, 2013). Additionally, in silent narrations participants produce a higher variety of spatial and kinetic aspects in their hand movements (Hogrefe et al., 2011). Further, when participants are restricted to speak when presenting spatial content they perform more bimanual gestures (simultaneous use of left and right hand) with an observer viewpoint and more unimanual gestures when they are allowed to speak (Lausberg & Kita, 2003). Lausberg and Kita (2003) were able to demonstrate that participants are accurate in their gestural representation of an object according to its spatial appearance on the screen and chose the hand accordingly. Note that this accuracy can decrease in interactional contexts depending on the spatial position and number of addresses (Özyürek, 2000). Also, deliberately controlled linguistic stimuli may alter accompanied hand movement patterns as metaphorical stimuli elicit a weaker right hand preference compared to abstract and concrete stimuli. Concrete stimuli referring to actions performed bimanually triggered a preference for bimanual gestures (Kita et al., 2007). Chapter 10 provides a more thorough overview for hand preference according to different stimuli and topics in narrations or interactions. This overview suggests that a right hand preference for *iconic* gestures in non-personal narrations shifts to equal usage of right and left hand when personal topics are elaborated or when spatial cognition is involved in the tasks and reflect stronger right hemisphere processing.

Small changes in the stimuli of various tasks can alter hand movement behavior accompanying speech. There is evidence that not only the presence of a specific object affects gestural behavior during its description but also the specific aspects of the object (Morella & Krauss, 2004). Objects that were considered to be hard to remember, difficult to describe, or lacking a clear verbal-codability elicited a higher gesture rate during descriptions. When describing everyday activities participants' gesture rates differs between activities independent of frequency of the activities occurrence suggesting that some activities are more likely (e.g. making coffee, changing batteries) to elicit gesture production than others (e.g. going by bus, ordering pizza) (see Chapter 17).

In line with these findings, Hostetter and Alibali (2008) propose a model of gesture production, which explicitly takes into consideration that gesture production is influenced by spatial imagery next to linguistic factors. More specifically, they distinguish between visual and motor imagery. Through visual imagery a person imagines an object, action, or sequence of actions as if watching it from an outside perspective whereas in motor imagery a person imagines to be a person or an object performing a specific action. Sirigu and Duhamel (2001) were able to demonstrate that participants choose different strategies concerning motor and visual imagery when confronted with a mental rotation task in a first person or third person perspective. Their results suggest that abnormal positions of the hands during this task restrain motor imagery and simultaneously enhance visual imagery. Further, this dissociation between motor and visual imagery abilities was reflected patients with neurological lesions. The model proposed by Hostetter & Alibali (2008) predicts, that if a gesture is produced in relation to visual imagery, the perspective of this gesture should be in line with the image. A person whose gesture is based on visual imagery takes an "observer point of view" for the gesture and a person whose gesture is based on a motor imagery takes a "character point of view". Note, that the terminology is taken from McNeill's (1992) investigations of persons narrating cartoon clips of Tweety and Sylvester. "Character point of view" gestures refer to movements where a speaker gestures as if being one of the characters and "observer point of view" refers to the speaker's perspective as an observer of the clip and gestures.

These terminologies can be translated to NEUROGES-Elan Function values of Module III. Although *pantomime, egocentric deictic* and *egocentric direction* do not explicitly presuppose a "character point of view", it is essential for these values that the person takes an egocentric perspective, i.e., it is constitutional that the person performs the movement from an egocentric perspective without making assumption about whether the persons incorporates the view of an alien character. Similarly, for the *presentation* values *form presentation, spatial relation presentation*, and *motion presentation* a non-egocentric (mento-heliocentric) perspective is constitutional, which relates to an "observer point of view". The gesturer projects the objects or actions s/he refers to into an imaginary space independent from her/his own person (see 5.1.4).

A common stimulus for eliciting gestures in narration tasks is cartoon clips of Tweety and Sylvester. Sequences of this series have been used extensively by various groups in gesture research in order to elicit gestural behavior (Cocks et al., 2011; Mol et al., 2009; Casey & Emmorey, 2008; Stam, 2006; Özürek, 2000). This has the advantage that results from different studies can be compared more easily. In order to elicit a broad range of gesture types, a recent study used T & S cartoons as well as Mr. Bean clips as stimuli (Hogrefe et al., 2012). Both types of stimuli are comedy series, which depict a simple plot with unambiguous characters and do not rely on verbal information.

Nevertheless, the T & S clips and Mr. Bean clips differ in some important aspects. Humans enact the characters in Mr. Bean clips whereas T & S clips are animated. Also, the amount of spatial information of the clips differs as in T & S characters change the scenery quite often whereas the plot of Mr. Bean clips takes place at a single location. Mr. Bean does not show much locomotion in space but rather acts in a static position. Close-ups and midrange shots rather emphasize Mr. Bean's actions on a second character and the way he performs them. The other character remains passive except for close-ups of his facial expressions. The characters in T & S display manual actions in static positions as well. But additionally, they move in different manners (running, jumping etc.)

between sceneries and often they are depicted simultaneously or subsequently when moving.

These differences potentially affect whether visual or motor imageries are triggered when recalling the clip. Further, the complexity of the actions can determine whether the visual information can be explained from an egocentric perspective at one point of time. Whereas in Mr. Bean spatial information is minor for the actions, in T & S the (spatial) relationship between characters is more important as it is changing and characters are also moving to and from each other as well as between sceneries. Consequently, if we assume that these clips induce different kind of imagery (visual vs. motor) in the observer, this is reflected in their hand movement behavior when re-narrating the clips. Hence, in this study, we compare hand movement behavior that was elicited with Mr. Bean clips to hand movement behavior that was produced while renarrating T & S cartoons.

11.2 Methods

11.2.1 Participants

The hand movement behavior of 20 (ten female, ten male) participants was analyzed. Participants' mean age was M = 53 (SD = 11) and all were tested on handedness according to the modified Oldfield Inventory (Salmaso & Longoni, 1985) that revealed a mean score for handedness M = 95.6 (SD= 9.56) ranging from 66 to 100. All persons were unaware of the purpose of the study and did not know that gesture was object of analyses.

11.2.2 Stimuli

Mr. Bean and the guardsman

The sequence of Mr. Bean and the guardsmen was subdivided into four short clips. The interviews, which were analyzed for this investigation, were based on the 2nd, 3rd, and 4th clip of this sequence. The clips had a mean (M) length of 86 sec (SD = 7.8 sec.) ranging between 69 and 90 sec.

Tweety and Sylvester

Clips of two sequences were used as stimuli for this study: "park" and "boot". Both sequences were subdivided into three clips. For this investigation the three "boot" clips and the third "park" clip were used. These clips had a mean length of 54 sec (SD = 21.2 sec.) ranging from 30 to 81 sec.

11.2.3 Procedure and materials

The video clips were presented to the participants who were asked to re-narrate the content of the clip after watching each clip. Then the next clip was presented to the participants. No specific instructions regarding use of gestures were given to the participants. Thus, only spontaneous gesturing was analyzed. The interviews were videotaped and converted to MPG format. The experimenter remained passive during the interviews except for affirmative signals such as nodding or verbal expressions like "hmm".

Accordingly, seven interviews were analyzed for each participant. Mean length of the interviews following Mr. Bean clips were M = 58.3 sec (SD = 17.5 sec), M = 80.2 sec (SD = 25 sec), and M = 72.8 sec (SD = 29.7 sec). Mean duration of the interviews following T & S clips were M = 77 sec (SD = 25), M = 125.3 sec (SD = 30 sec), M = 78 sec (SD = 22.7 sec), and M = 76 sec (SD = 24.6 sec).

11.2.4 Gesture coding and interrater agreement

Videotaped interviews were coded according to NEUROGES Modules I, II, and III Step I by two independent raters. One rater coded 100% and the second rater coded 25% of the material in order to control for interrater agreement. Interrater agreement was established after both raters annotated Module I, Module II, and Module III. After calculating interrater agreement according to a modified Cohen's Kappa (see Chapter 15) raters solved non converging annotations in consensus discussion. Annotations of the first rater were used as the basis for further annotations as well as for statistical analysis.

11.2.5 Statistical analysis

Data was exported from ELAN and mean frequency and proportion of time was calculated in Excel® for each value according to participant and interview. Frequency refers to the number of value units per minute and proportion of time indicates how much time participants spent with a specific value unit per minute (see Chapter 16). Mean values for interviews on Mr. Bean and T & S were accumulated and divided by three and four, respectively. On these values we performed repeated measurement ANOVAs with StructureFocus(5), Contact (3), FormalRelation (4) and Function (9) as within subject factors. Additionally, Stimuli (2) and hand (2) were included as within subject factors. For main and interactional effects, post hoc comparisons were calculated using Bonferroni corrections for multiple comparisons. Note that initially Gender was included as a between-subjects factor in these computations initially but did not reveal any significant interactions with Stimuli. Differential statistics were conducted in SPSS® 20. Significance level was set at alpha = 0.05.

11.3 Results

For all statistical computations only those results are reported, which are significant at a level of $p < 0.05$, and refer to main effects and interactional effects concerning Stimuli, if not mentioned otherwise. Further, only post hoc comparisons of interactional effects of level of analysis x Stimuli are reported, which refer to comparisons between Stimuli.

11.3.1 Interrater agreement

Interrater agreement for the values of StructureFocus, Contact, Formal relation and Function are displayed in Table 1.

Table 1 Interrater agreement according to the modified Cohen's Kappa for values of Structure, StructureFocus, Contact, Formal Relation, and Function categories with raw agreement scores in brackets

Structure	*Phasic*	*repetitive*	*Shift*	*aborted*	*irregular*	
HS-RR	0.43 (0.77)	0.5 (0.87)	0.34 (0.91)	0.32 (0.92)	0.37 (0.83)	
StructureFocus	*phasic on body*	*phasic in space*	*repetitive on body*	*repetitive in space*	*irregular on body*	*irregular in space*
HS-RR	0.35 (0.94)	0.45 (0.79)	0.4 (0.96)	0.56 (0.9)	0.44 (0.87)	0.12 (0.95)
R1-R2	0.5 (0.9)	0.6 (0.82)	0.53 (0.96)	0.67 (0.93)	0.71 (0.94)	0 (1)
Contact	*act on each other*	*act as a unit*	*act apart*			
HS-RR	0.51 (.98)	0.80 (.94)	0.78 (.90)			
Formal Relation	*Symmetrical*	*lh dominance*	*rh dominance*	*asymmetrical*		
HS-RR	0.84 (0.95)	0.73 (0.95)	0.66 (0.98)	0.32 (0.97)		
Function	*egocentric deictic*	*egocentric direction*	*emotion/ attitude*	*emphasis*	*form presentation*	*motion presentation*
HS-RR	0.59 (0.99)	0.56 (0.99)	0.69 (0.99)	0.86 (0.95)	0.68 (0.97)	0.75 (0.93)
Function	*pantomime*	*spatial relation presentation*	*subject-oriented action*			
HSRR	0.81 (0.96)	0.58 (0.97)	0.87 (0.96)			

Note, that rater dyads did not meet after coding Activation and Structure. This can affect the interrater agreement negatively because difference on the previous coding steps permeate to subsequent annotations (see Chapter 16).

11.3.2 Frequency

To test whether participants performed StructureFocus values with different frequencies during Mr. Bean and T & S narration, we performed a 2 (Stimuli: Mr. Bean, T&S) x 2 (hand: left hand (lh), right hand (rh)) x 5 (*irregular on body, phasic in space, phasic on body, repetitive in space, repetitive on body*) ANOVA on the parameter frequency, i.e., the mean number per minute of StructureFocus units. On the level of StructureFocus no significant effect for Stimuli or interactional effects of Stimuli x StructureFocus, Stimuli x Hand, and Stimuli x StructureFocus x Hand have been found.

Also, a 2 (Stimuli: Mr. Bean, T & S) x 2 (Hand: lh, rh) x 3 (Contact: *act on each other, act as a unit, act apart*) repeated measurement ANOVA did not reveal a significant main effect for Stimuli or for any interactional effect including Stimuli.

A repeated measurement ANOVA with Stimuli 2 (Mr. Bean, T & S) x Formal Relation 4 (*symmetrical, lh dominance, rh dominance asymmetrical*) revealed a significant interactional effect for Stimuli x Formal Relation (F (2, 17) = 7.242, p = 0.002). Post hoc comparisons indicate that participants performed more *left hand dominance* units per minute during the T & S narrations compared with Mr. Bean narrations (Mean difference (MD) = 1.09, $p = 0.001$).

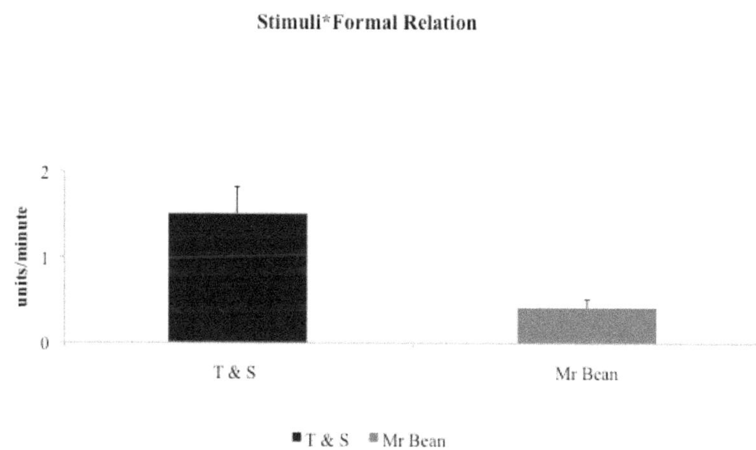

Figure 1 Means of frequency of *left hand dominance* units during T & S and Mr. Bean narrations. Error bars indicate standard error of mean (SE). Differences between mean values corresponding to the depicted bars are statistically significant with $p < 0.05$.

All Function values except for the values *emblem* and *object oriented action* were included in a repeated measurement ANOVA with Stimuli 2 (Mr. Bean, T & S) x Hand 3 (lh, rh, both hand (bh)) X Function 9 (*egocentric deictic, egocentric direction, emotion/attitude, emphasis, form presentation, motion presentation, pantomime, spatial relation presentation, subject oriented action*) as within-subject factors. Significant interactional effect for Stimuli x Hand (F (2, 18) = 8.11, p =*0.003*), and for Stimuli x Function (F (8, 12) = 3.52, p = *0.025*) were found.

A higher frequency of Function value units executed with the left hand was performed during T & S narrations compared with Mr. Bean narrations (MD = 0.17, p = *0.016*).

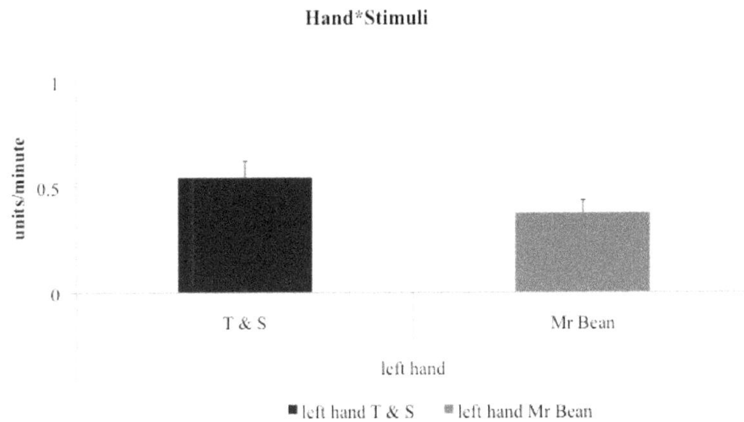

Figure 2 Means of frequency for Function units during T & S and Mr. Bean narrations. Error bars indicate SE. Differences between mean values corresponding to the depicted bars are statistically significant with $p < 0.05$.

Post hoc comparisons concerning the Stimuli x Function interaction showed that participants showed higher frequencies of *egocentric deictic* (MD = 0.162, p = *0*), *egocentric direction* units (MD = 0.11, p = *0.02*), *pantomime* units (MD = 0.226, p = *0.04*), and *form presentation* units (MD = 0.203, p = *0.009*) during Mr. Bean narrations. In contrast, participants performed *motion presentation* units at a higher frequency during narrations (MD = 0.4, p = *0.012*). As displayed in Figure 3, participants performed almost no *egocentric deictic* or *egocentric direction* gestures during narration whereas this Function value played some role during Mr. Bean narrations. Visual inspection of Figure 3 also suggests that *pantomime* gestures were predominant in Mr. Bean narrations. This pattern was different during narrations where participants' gestures were mostly *motion presentation* gestures. The frequency of all other Function values did not differ between the narrations of different stimuli. For instance, during T & S as well as Mr. Bean narration *emphasis* units (M = 1.95, M = 1.96) and *subject oriented action* units (M = 1.1, M = 1.05) were displayed most often.

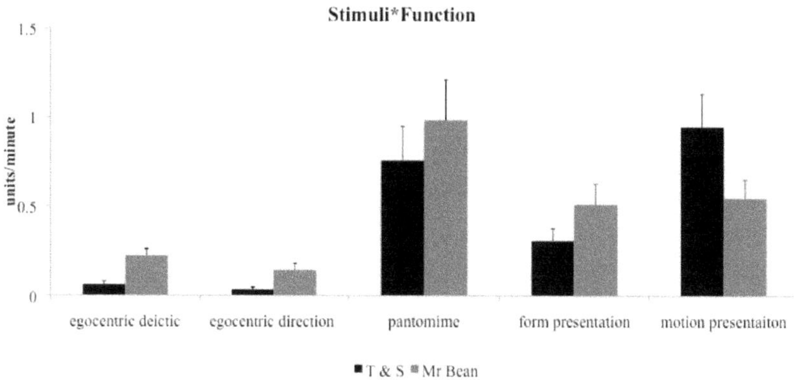

Figure 3 Means of frequency for Function value unit during T & S and Mr. Bean narrations. Error bars indicate SE. All differences between adjacent bars are all statistically significant with $p < 0.05$.

11.3.3 Proportion of time

We also included the parameter proportion of time (PoT, see Chapter 17) in the same repeated measurement ANOVAs. Only those results will be reported which differ from the Frequency analyses.

On the level of StructureFocus an additional interactional effect for Stimuli x StructureFocus was found (F (4, 16) = 7.57, $p = 0.001$).

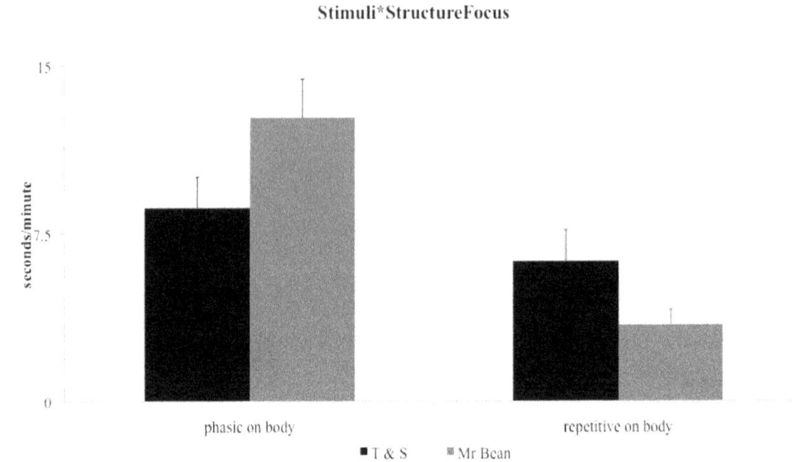

Figure 4 Means for proportion of time for StructureFocus value units during T & S and Mr. Bean narrations. Error bars indicate SE. Differences between adjacent bars are all statistically significant with $p < 0.05$.

Post-hoc comparisons revealed that whereas participants spent more time with *phasic on body* units during Mr. Bean narrations (MD = 4.04, $p = 0.001$), they spent more time with *repetitive on body* units than during T & S narrations (MD = 2.86, $p = 0.006$). As this pattern did not surface in the analysis of mean Frequencies, *phasic on body* units must have been longer during Mr. Bean narrations and *repetitive on body* units during T & S narrations.

On the level of Contact and Formal Relation analyses no structurally different patterns have been found.

On the level of Function, only the post hoc comparison between *pantomime* during T & S and Mr. Bean can be interpreted as trend (MD = 0.62, $P = 0.064$). Consequently, participants performed slightly shorter *pantomime* gestures during Mr. Bean narrations. Otherwise, the duration of the value units discussed in this chapter do not differ.

11.4 Discussion

The comparisons of the hand movement behavior during T & S and Mr. Bean narrations revealed differences in patterns on the levels of Formal Relation between right and left hand in bimanual units as well as on the level of Function. More specifically, on the level of Function the values with a higher degree of presentative function are affected. At the same time, these results highlight that idiosyncratic movement behavior patterns on the level of Structure, Contact and other Function values (*emphasis, subject-oriented action, emotion/attitude*), which rather reflect general discourse habits or emotional states, remain unaffected. Note that the frequencies of Structure, Contact, or the respective Function values are not prone to alterations of the setting at all. It rather seems that other aspects of the setting, such as the nature of the task (cognitively demanding, emotionally demanding, etc.) tend to alter these movement behaviors (see Chapters 10 and 17).

In T & S movies, characters display more locomotion in space of the characters, such as running, jumping and climbing, and between sceneries. Moreover, often two characters move simultaneously. It appears that participants reflect these motions through a higher frequency of *motion presentation* units. In contrast, the Mr. Bean clips emphasize Mr. Bean's specific actions as the guardsmen remains passive except for facial expressions. Accordingly, participants display more *pantomime*. Additionally, participants appear to reflect a higher degree of egocentric perspective through *egocentric deictics* and *directions* as well. According to the model proposed by Alibali & Hostetter (2008), this reflects a greater number of motor imageries induced by Mr. Bean clips compared to T & S clips.

Although, *motion presentation* units were performed predominantly among gestures with iconic content (*presentation/pantomime*) during T & S narrations, participants did not perform more mento-heliocentric gestures in general. It seems more likely that participants performed higher frequencies of *motion presentation* units at the expense of *spatial relation* and *form presentation* units in order to reflect the locomotion presented in the T & S video clips. Whether participants are more likely to recall motor imageries in Mr. Bean narrations because real characters are displayed or because the mode of actions is emphasized remains unclear at this stage of analysis.

Whereas participants displayed the same amount of *symmetrical, asymmetrical,* and *right hand dominance* movements, they performed more *left hand dominance* units during T & S narrations. T & S clips depict more spatial information of value than Mr. Bean clips. This might trigger a higher degree of spatial cognition during the narration and thus provoke a shift to left hand use.

11.5 Conclusion

The investigations on hand movement behavior during narrations of different kind of clips contributes to the idea that persons adapt their gestural behavior to the content of stimuli in two ways. First, it indicates that relatively specific differences in stimuli affects the choice of hand and gesture types although other aspects of the setting, such as task, interactional partner, and emotional state during the task, are stable. This emphasizes that the choice of stimuli for renarration tasks matters. Secondly, the findings presented here suggest that persons adapt their gestural behavior systematically depending on whether visual or motor imageries are triggered. However, the differentiation between T & S clips and Mr. Bean clips do not allow a clear designation of the cause for the different hand movement patterns. Further research should clarify whether the tendency for more egocentric gestures is induced by the fact that actions are presented by real persons or by the nature of the actions.

References

Alibali, M.W., Heath, D.C., & Myers, H.J. (2001). Effects of visibility between speaker and listener on gesture production: Some gestures are meant to be seen. *Journal of Memory and Language, 44,* 169-188.

Bavelas, J. Gerwing, J. Sutton, C., & Prevost, D. (2007). Gesturing on the Telephone: Independent effects of dialogue and visibility. *Journal of Memory and Language, 58,* 495-520.

Bock, O., & Züll, A. (2013). Characeristics of grasping movements in a laboratory and in an everyday-like context. *Human Movement Science, 32*, 249-256.

Casey, S., & Emmorey, K. (2008). Co-speech gesture in bimodal bilinguals. *Language and Cognitive Processes, 24(2),* 290-312.

Cocks, N. Dipper, L., Middleton, R., & Morgan, G. (2011). What can iconic gestures tell us about the language system? A case of conduction aphasia. *International Journal of Language and Communication Disorder, 46(4),* 423-436.

Helmich, I., & Lausberg, H. (2013). *Hand movement behavior with or without speech*. Paper presented at the Tilburg Gesture Research Meeting, Tilburg, The Netherlands.

Hogrefe, K., Ziegler, W., & Goldenberg, G. (2011). Hamming distance – a measure for determining the formal diversity of hand gestures. In: Stam, G. & Ishino, M. (eds.): *Intergrating gestures: the interdisciplinary nature of gesture*. Amsterdam: John Benjamins Publishing, 75-88.

Hogrefe, K., Ziegler, W., Weidinger, N., & Goldenberg, G. (2012). Nonverbal communication in severe aphasia: Influence of aphasia, apraxia, or semantic processing? *Cortex, 48*, 952-962.

Hostetter, A B., & Alibali, M.W. (2008). Visible embodiment: Gestures as simulated action. *Psychonomic Bulletin & Review, 15(3)*, 495-514.

Kita, S., de Condappa, O., & Mohr, C. (2007). Metaphor explanation attenuates the right-hand preference for depictive co-speech gestures that imitate actions. *Brain and Language, 101,* 185-197.

Lausberg, H. & Kita, S. (2003). The content of the message influences the hand choice in co-speech gestures and in gesturing without speaking. *Brain and Language, 86,* 57-69.

McNeill, D. (1992). *Hand and mind. What gestures reveal about thought.* Chicago: University press.

Mol, L., Krahmer, E., & Swerts, M. (2009) Alignment in Iconic Gestures: Does it make sense? In Theobald, B-J. & Harvey, R. W. *The eighth international conference on auditory-visual speech processing, Norwich, United Kingdom.* 3-8.

Morsella E., & Krauss R.M. (2004). The role of gestures in spatial working memory and speech. *American Journal of Psychology, 117*, 411-424.

Özyürek, A. (2000). The influence of addressee location on spatial language and representational gestures of direction. In D. McNiell (Ed.) Language and Gesture. Cambridge University Press.

Salmaso, D., & Longoni, A.M. (1985). Problems in the assessment of Hand Preference. *Cortex 21.* 533-549.

Sirigu, A., & Duhamel, J.R. (2001). Motor and Visual Imagery as Two Complementary but Neurally Dissociable Mental Processes. *Journal of Cognitive Neuroscience, 13(7),* 919-919.

Stam, G. (2006). Thinking for speaking about motion: L1 and L2 speech and gesture. In Jordens, P. & Kellerman, E. *International Review of Applied Linguistics in Language Teaching, 44(2),* 140-171.

V. Establishing Interrater Agreement

12. Rater Training and Rating Procedures

Hedda Lausberg

12.1 Naïve raters base their judgements on wrong premises

In expression psychology, a number of experiments on the interpretation of expressive behaviour have been conducted. These experiments unanimously reveal that naïve raters may agree in their judgements but that these judgements, however, do not correlate with an objective assessment or even more, that they are wrong.

Eisenberg and Reichline (1939) had naïve raters judge a person's dominance by observing the person's gait. The naïve raters agreed more among each other than with the dominance rating based upon a questionnaire (Eisenberg, 1937). Similar findings were reported by Mason (1957). 24 untrained raters were asked to judge leadership qualities of 75 candidates based on photographs. As an external criterion, the candidates' leadership qualities were assessed during a field test which required cooperation and problem solving competence by three trained raters, who applied a semi-objective checklist (interrater agreement r = .91). In addition, the candidates assessed each other after the field test. The judgements of the trained raters correlated high with those of the candidates (r = .78), i.e., the external criterion was reliable. The naïve raters, who evaluated the applicants' leadership competence based on photographs, did not agree well (r = .30), and their assessments correlated even less with those of the trained raters and of the candidates (r = .18).

In a study by Wallbott (1989), 20 naïve raters were presented without sound the videotaped movement behaviour of psychiatric patients in clinical interviews. The raters were asked to estimate, whether the videotaped behaviour was from an admission interview or from a discharge interview. It turned out that the naïve raters' admission/discharge attributions were totally invalid. Hand movements that were intensive, expansive, soft, round, not nervous, and not coarse (according to descriptive scales) and that correlated with the computer parameters large circumference, long waylength, and high velocity were systematically associated by the raters with the discharge interview. This attribution, however, was wrong.

To summarize, the results of the studies by Eisenberg and Reichline (1939), Mason (1957), and Wallbott (1989) evidence that naïve raters deviate from external objective criteria when assessing personality traits or psychopathology based on movement behaviour. In particular, Wallbott demonstrated that the naïve raters "were not 'wildly guessing' " (p. 142) but that they systematically employed specific criteria to assess whether the movement behaviour was from the admission interview or the discharge one. However, they based their judgements on wrong premises.

Three main conclusions shall be drawn from these findings: First, it is an obligatory challenge for empirical research to validate movement values in order to build a reliable corpus of scientific knowledge on movement behaviour. Popular interpretations of movement behaviour as used by naïve observers are potentially invalid.

Second, the naïve raters tended to agree more among each other than with the external measure. Untrained raters seem to ground their judgements on common (but partly invalid) premises. Accordingly, Frijda (1965) underlined that it is not only important to understand the principles of the meaning of expression but also to explore the principles of the assessment of expression. Therefore, it is worthwhile to investigate the implicit frames of reference for the interpretation of movement behaviour that determine the judgements of naïve raters.

Third, since naïve raters interpret movement behaviour partly based on wrong premises, it is evident that raters need a proper training in movement behaviour analysis. They have to acquire knowledge on movement behaviour and they have to actually learn how to analyze movement behaviour. It is noteworthy that in other diagnostic domains, as matter of course, intensive training has to be passed. As an example, neurologists who want to analyze electroencephalograms have to participate in a regular training and - according to German guidelines - they have to evaluate 1000 electroencephalograms to acquire the certificate. In Chapter 1 it has already been discussed in detail why movement behaviour research has, thus far, not developed as an academic discipline on its own. The same arguments are valid to explain why, thus far, a regular academic training in movement behaviour analysis has scarcely been established, despite the fact that empirical data clearly demonstrate the need for a professional training.

12.2 Self-perception is crucial for objective movement behaviour assessment

Further evidence for the necessity to establish a regular training in movement analysis derives from research on self-perception and social perception. There is long-standing knowledge in dance and movement therapy that therapists are better in understanding the client's movement behaviour, if they have an objective perception of their own movement behaviour. Empirical support for this practical intuition has been provided across different scientific disciplines. In expression psychology, Wolff (1943) reported that the gait of another person can only be objectively described by a rater whose self-assessment of the own gait is objective. Likewise, the performance in the identification of the own voice correlates positively with that in the identification of other persons' voices (Sackheim et al., 1978). Further insights are provided by current neuroimaging research with functional MagneticResonanceImaging (fMRI). The observation of body movements that belong to the observer's own movement repertoire is associated with a stronger cerebral activation than the observation of movements that do not belong to the own repertoire (e.g. Calvo-Merino et al., 2005; Cross et al., 2008). In contrast, the observation of movements that are only visually familiar to the observer but that do not belong to his/her own active repertoire is not associated with a stronger cerebral activation (Calvo-Merino et al., 2006). Obviously, the increase of cerebral activation during the observation of movements that belong to the own repertoire is independent of a previous visual exposition to the movement. It occurs even if these movements have not been observed in others before (Reithler et al., 2007).

Thus, there is diverse empirical evidence demonstrating that observation skills are better if the observer assesses the own movement behaviour objectively. Furthermore, neuroimaging data suggest that the observation skills will improve if the observer has performed her-/himself the movements (s)he is asked to assess. These findings demonstrate that observation skills are not only an innate gift but that they can be regularly acquired if an elaborate training is provided.

12.3 Recommendations for rater training

The above presented empirical findings have implications for rater training in the behavioural analysis of movement behaviour. The realization of these implications in rater training is illustrated by the example of the NEUROGES training.

The NEUROGES rater training consists of three components: a detailed theoretical introduction to movement behaviour research, movement exercises, and a proper coding training. Formally, the training consists of seminars, self-study, and exams.

Essential parts of the theoretical introduction are given in this book. In the movement exercise part of the training, the trainees actually learn to perform the various NEUROGES values. They are encouraged to sense the specific effects that the performances of the various body movements have on their thinking, feeling, and interacting. The own performance of the movement values clearly improves the recognition of the display of these values in other persons. To further comprehend the nature of the NEUROGES values, in self-study the trainees can use the numerous value examples in the coding manual, which describe for each value different forms of its visual appearance, as "stage directions" to exercise the body movements, and they can imitate the video-examples for each value provided on an interactive CD (Chapter 13).

For the coding training, the detailed definitions of the categories and values given in the coding manual serve as a guideline. During the seminars many video-examples are presented so that trainees learn to identify the values with their inter-individual variations. For self-study, the interactive training CD is used which also contains training videos with hideable correct solutions of the codings. During the coding training the trainees code several training videos with the NEUROGES-template. The ELAN annotated files (eaf) of all raters are compared and discussed. The Compare Annotator's function[21], which is implemented in ELAN, is used as first rough estimate to gain an impression how well the trainees code by comparing their codings with those of an expert rater. Table 1 gives an example of the agreement of a novice rater and an advanced rater with the expert rater.

Table 1 Agreement of a novice rater and an advanced rater with the expert rater

	Novice rater		Advanced rater	
	right hand: Compare Annotator's value; categorical agreement	left hand: Compare Annotator's value; categorical agreement	right hand: Compare Annotator's value; categorical agreement	left hand: Compare Annotator's value; categorical agreement
Training video 1				
Structure	0,29; 8/12	0,42; 11/13	0,81; 8/9	0,60; 9/11
Focus	0,42; 9/12	0,42; 11/13	0,39; 10/12	0,49; 10/12
Contact	0,75; 6/8		0,99; 8/8	
Formal Relation	0,75; 6/8		0,99; 8/8	
Training video 2				
Structure	0,60; 14/17	0,61; 12/13	0,97; 17/17	0,98; 13/13
Focus	0,50; 15/20	0,48; 12/15	0,84; 17/19	0,81; 13/15
Contact	0,99; 8/8		0,99; 8/8	
Formal Relation	0,99; 8/8		0,99; 8/8	
Training video 3				
Structure	0,15; 4/13	0,39; 4/8	1,0; 4/4	0,8; 8/9
Focus	0,08; 4/8	0,27; 3/8	0,74; 3/4	0,82; 7/8
Contact	0,99; 14/15		1,0; 15/15	
Formal Relation	0,99; 14/15		1,0; 15/15	
Training video 4				
Structure	0,63; 25/28	0,49; 25/30	0,85; 27/28	0,78; 27/30
Focus	0,40; 29/35	0,28; 24/35	0,60; 27/33	0,56; 26/34
Contact	0,99; 33/33		0,99; 33/33	
Formal Relation	0,85; 36/33		0,85; 37/33	

21 Note that during the coding training the Compare Annotator's function is used to estimate interrater agreement, since it can be applied immediately with the eaf files (Chapter 14). For empirical research studies, however, the modified Cohen's Kappa (Chapter 15) should be used for all NEUROGES categories with the exception of the Activation category.

The first value in each column refers to the temporal agreement only, e.g., how much both raters agree on when the unit begins and when it ends, independently of the categorical agreement concerning the Structure, Focus, Contact, or Formal Relation value.

As a technical remark it shall be noted that previous NEUROGES trainings have revealed that fine-grained temporal disagreements between the raters concerning the beginning and end of a unit may be due to different tagging techniques. If one rater tags a unit based on a frame-by-frame observation from the beginning to the end of the movement, his/her start and endpoint of the tag will differ from that of another rater who first observes the whole movement and then tags backward by moving the mouse to the left. Therefore, in order to improve the fine-grained temporal agreement, raters should use the same tagging technique in ELAN.

The second value in each column of Table 1 indicates the categorical agreement, e.g., if both raters agree on that the unit is a *phasic* unit. The above comparison of the agreements of the novice and advanced raters with the expert rater illustrates that in the course of the NEUROGES training, there is a clear improvement in the reliability of codings. In general, trainees are considered to be trained well when they achieve an agreement of > .75 with the expert's coding of the training video. To further ensure the quality of the NEUROGES training, there is an exam after each Module and the successful trainee acquires a NEUROGES certificate.

12.4 Recommendations for rating procedures in empirical studies

The rater training qualifies observers to reliably apply the NEUROGES system. Thus, given a thorough rater training, the reliability of the codings of certified raters can be assumed.

However, standards in empirical research require that the interrater agreement is re-established for every single study. To ensure the reliability of the ratings, at least two trained raters who are blind to the research hypotheses should evaluate the video data. It is sufficient to establish interrater agreement on 25% of the data of **each** subject. Thus, the first rater codes 100% and the second rater codes 25% of the data of each subject.

It is a well-known phenomenon that in the course of assessing the videos of a study sample raters slightly change their assessments due to an increasingly differentiated perception (Bergen, 1988; Owens & Johnstone, 1982). As an example, if the behaviour of 100 subjects is to be evaluated and the rater would code one subject after the other, her/his assessment will differ for subject 100 as compared to subject 1 just because of her/his increased perceptual sensitivity. This natural development is reflected in the relatively low **intra**-rater retest-reliability movement analysis studies (Bergen, 1988; Owens & Johnstone, 1982). This potential development has to be controlled especially in newly certified raters. Therefore, in empirical studies the video data of each subject should be divided into several segments and the segments of all subjects should be presented to the raters in a pseudo-random order.

Table 2 shows an example for a rating schedule for a study on 20 subjects.

Table 2 Example for a coding schedule for two raters

Scheme for Rater 1 (100%)

R1 codes 100% of data	2. →															
1. ↓ Subject (n=20)	Clip1	Clip2	Clip3	Clip4	Clip1	Clip2	Clip3	Clip4	Clip1	Clip2	Clip3	Clip4	Clip1	Clip2	Clip3	Clip4
1	x							x			x			x		
2		x			x							x			x	
3			x			x			x							x
4				x			x			x			x			
5	x							x			x			x		
6		x			x							x			x	
7			x			x			x							x
8				x			x			x			x			
9	x							x			x			x		
10		x			x							x			x	
11			x			x			x							x
12				x			x			x			x			
13	x							x			x			x		
14		x			x							x			x	
15			x			x			x							x
16				x			x			x			x			
17	x							x			x			x		
18		x			x							x			x	
19			x			x			x							x
20				x			x			x			x			

Scheme for Rater 2 (25%)

R2 codes 25% of data	2. →															
1. ↓ Subject (n=20)	Clip1	Clip2	Clip3	Clip4	Clip1	Clip2	Clip3	Clip4	Clip1	Clip2	Clip3	Clip4	Clip1	Clip2	Clip3	Clip4
1	x															
2		x														
3			x													
4				x												
5	x					x										
6		x														
7			x													
8				x												
9	x															
10		x					x									
11			x													
12				x												
13	x															
14		x														
15			x					x								
16				x												
17	x															
18		x														
19			x													
20				x	x											

The video material of each subject is divided into four segments (Clip 1 - Clip 4). On top, there is the coding schedule for rater 1 who codes 100% of the data. Below, there is coding schedule for rater 2 who codes only 25% of each subject's data. Rater 1 starts with columne 1, i.e., (s)he first codes clip 1 of subject 1, then clip 1 of subject 6, then clip 1 of subject 11, and then clip 1 of subject 16. She/he then continues with column 2, i.e., clip 2 of subject 2, clip 2 of subject 7, etc. Analogously, rater 2 starts with column 1, and then continues with column 2.

If the experiment includes more than one group or more than one condition, the groups and conditions, respectively, have to be considered as well in the pseudo-randomization of the rating schedule.

The final interrater agreement is established on the 25% of the data that both raters have coded. However, it is **strongly** recommended to check the interrater agreement repeatedly before the final agreement calculation in order to detect potential systematic disagreements between the raters that could be avoided.

Because of the above mentioned differentiation in perceptual sensitivity, furthermore in NEUROGES one category is coded after the other. First, the Activation category is coded for **all** data, following rating schedules of the sort as shown in Table 2. The interrater agreement is calculated with the ELAN Compare Annotators function (Chapter 14).

For the Structure category coding, the *movement* units of Rater 1, who has coded 100% of the data, are adopted. Thus, both raters continue with Rater 1's *movement* units. For the Structure category, they follow the same rating schedule as for the Activation category. The interrater agreement is calculated with the Modified Cohen's Kappa (Chapter 15) based on the 25% of the data, which have been coded by both raters.

For the Focus category coding, the Structure units of Rater 1 are adopted. Both raters continue with Rater 1's Structure units. Again, for the Focus category, they use the same rating schedule as for the Activation and the Structure categories. The interrater agreement is again calculated with the Modified Cohen's Kappa (Chapter 15).

The same procedure is applied for the subsequent Contact, Formal Relation, Function, and Type categories.

References

Bergen, J.A., Carter, N.B., Craig, J., MacFarlane, D., Smith, E.F., & Beumont, P.J.V. (1988). AIMS Ratings - Repeatability. *British Journal of Psychiatry, 152*, 670-673.

Calvo-Merino, B., Glaser, D.E., Grezes, J., Passingham, R.E., & Haggard, P. (2005). Action Observation and Acquired Motor Skills: An fMRI Study with Expert Dancers. *Cerebral Cortex 15*, 1243-1249.

Calvo-Merino, B., Grèzes, J., Glaser, D.E., Passingham, R.E. & Haggard, P. (2006). Seeing or Doing? Influence of Visual and Motor Familiarity in Action Observation. *Current Biology, 16*, 1905-1910.

Cross, E.S., Kraemer, D.J.M., Hamilton, C., Kelley, W.M., & Grafton, S.T. (2008). Sensitivity of the Action Observation Network to Physical and Observational Learning. *Cerebral Cortex 19*, 315-326.

Eisenberg, P. (1937). Expressive Movement related to Feelings of Dominance. *Archives of Psychology 211.*

Eisenberg, P., & Reichline, P. (1939). Judgements of Dominance Feelings from Motion Pictures of Gait. *Journal of Abnormal and Social Psychology 10.*

Frijda, N.H. (1965). Mimik und Pantomimik. In: R. Kirchhoff, Hrsg. *Handbuch der Psychologie, Band 5, Ausdruckspsychologie*. Göttingen: Hogrefe 351-422.

Mason, D.J. (1957). Judgements of Leadership based upon Physiognomonic Cues. *Journal of Abnormal and Social Psychology 54 (2),* 273-4.

Owens, D.G.C., & Johnstone, E.C. (1982). Spontaneous Involuntary Disorders of Movement. *Archives of General Psychiatry, 39.*

Reithler, J., van Mier H.I., Peters J.C., & Goebel, R. (2007). Nonvisual motor learning influences abstract action observation. *Current Biology, 17*(14), 1201-1207.

Sackheim, H.A., Packer, I.K., & Gur, R.C. (1978). Hemisphericity, Cognitive Set, and Susceptibility to Subliminal Perception. *Journal of Abnormal Psychology 86 (6), 624-30.*

Wallbott, H.G. (1989). Movement quality changes in psychopathological disorders. In: Kirkaldy, B., editor. Normalities and abnormalities in human movement. *Medicine and Sport Science 29*, 128-146.

Wolff, W. (1943). *The Expression of Personality*. New York, London: Harper & Brothers.

13. The NEUROGES Interactive Learning Tool

Jana Bryjovà

Purpose and use

The NEUROGES interactive learning tool presents an education-software that has been developed for the purpose of facilitating comprehension of the NEUROGES gesture coding system. The interactive learning tool focuses on hand/arm movements.

The main goal of developing this stand-alone flash-application was to provide a valid demonstration of the NEUROGES coding units as well as to enable coding practice. Both, teaching and learning through technology is promoted by user-friendly design as well as an easy navigation throughout the learning tool. The NEUROGES interactive learning tool imposes thus a novel extension to traditional tutoring methods.

Structure

Based on the NEUROGES coding system manual, this interactive learning tool consists of three separate Modules as well as an Exercise part. Each of the introduced Modules with their respective Steps is presented by a short description with one or several video examples, in order to promote a better understanding of the coding system obligatory criteria, such as movement dynamics or trajectory.

Modules

The structure of the NEUROGES interactive learning tool enables progressing in a step-by-step way through all three Modules and associated Steps of the NEUROGES coding system. The navigation through the learning software is equivalent to the coding procedure in NEUROGES-ELAN. In Module I, beginning with the Activation category, the *movement* and *no movement* units are explained and provided with examples. A brief demonstration of the movement Structure and Focus categories follows, respectively. In Module II, the two coding steps display the distinct kinds of relations between the both hands. Finally, in the most extensive Module III, the Function and the Type categories are specified.

Excercise

The exercise part of the NEUROGES interactive learning tool was developed in collaboration with Han Slöetjes from Max Planck Institute for Psycholinguistics (Nijmegen). A brief instruction on use of the ELAN annotation tool as well as a short video demonstration is provided in this section. The latest version of the ELAN annotation software can be launched directly from the NEUROGES interactive learning CD without the need of any additional software installation on the computer. A special NEUROGES template established for the purpose of coding with the NEUROGES coding system is also implemented in this CD, which enables custom use of the pre-set categories.

Accordingly, the exercise part enables easy rehearsal of the already acquired coding skills as well as comparison to the reference coding.

Videos

Short video examples shown in the NEUROGES interactive learning tool were recorded and cut by the author between years 2008 and 2009. The subjects appearing in those sequences were native German-speaking volunteers, who lived in distinct areas of Germany, Austria, and Switzerland at the time of recording and had been previously known and befriended by the author. A conversation on everyday topics of their own preference was established between the subjects and the author, who was seated in front of them, behind the camera during the recording.

Participants had been told in advance that the interview was video-recorded without sound, in order to establish an intimate conversation atmosphere that would enable to talk about the topics without any constraints. Subjects had not been informed about the fact that the hand movements were the subject of interest, neither were they given any specific instructions regarding their nonverbal behaviour. Thus, the hand movements that could have been observed occurred spontaneously while speaking and therefore, it can be assumed that the hand movements performed by the speakers were a part of the subjects' own natural movement repertoire.

After being informed extensively about the purposes of the video recording, all participants gave consent on publishing the videos as a part of the NEUROGES interactive learning tool. The participants were not paid any compensation money for being recorded.

After the recording was finished, the video material was analysed according to the NEUROGES coding manual by the author as well as the editor of the book (Hedda Lausberg) in order to establish reliable as well as representative video samples of the respective NEUROGES values. Subsequently, each of the previously coded units was cut and embedded into the learning tool, accompanied by an introduction text that had been adopted from the NEUROGES coding manual.

Application in use

The NEUROGES interactive learning tool has been so far used by trainers in the NEUROGES training, mostly for the purpose of demonstration of the specific values. The trainees receive the CD together with the coding manual as a part of study material. The NEUROGES interactive learning tool has proved to be a valuable lecturing support for tutors and for students.

Acknowledgements

The development of the interactive CD was supported by the DFG grant LA 1249/1-3.

14. Calculating Temporal Interrater Agreement for Binary Movement Categories

Kerstin Petermann, Harald Skomroch, Daniela Dvoretska

Interrater agreement for the Activation category cannot be specified through the modified Cohen's Kappa (see Chapter 15) as with this measure the agreement for shorter *movement* units (as compared to longer ones) would be considered disproportionally. Thus, a different strategy is necessary to calculate interrater agreement for this category. As a strategy to calculate interrater agreement for the Activation category we propose to use the ratio between total length of overlaps from both annotators and total length of movement units from both annotators. To calculate this ratio, proceed as follows:

14.1 Establish values for merged annotations

Open the ELAN file with transcriptions of both annotators merged

Merge tiers of annotations rh_activation_R1 and rh_activation_R2.
In the *Tier* menu, select *Merge Tiers...*

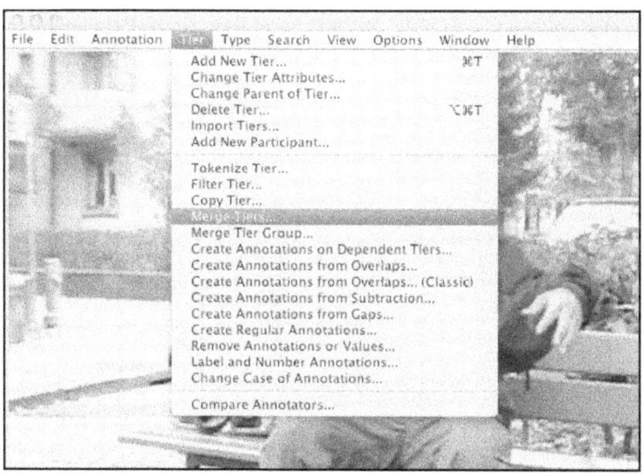

A pop-up window appears. Select the tiers you wish to merge. This will either be rh_activation for both raters or lh_activation for both raters.

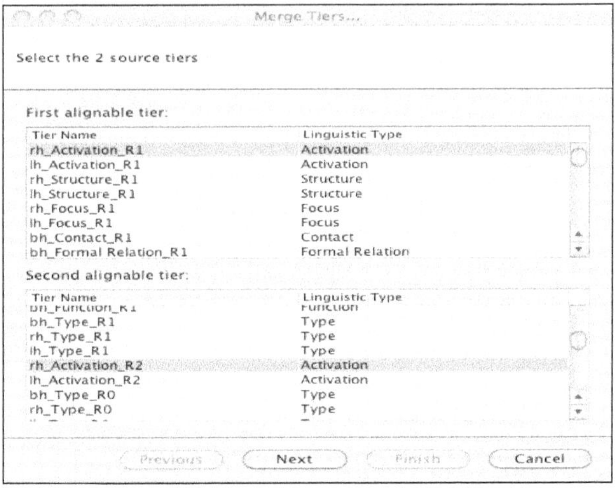

Click *Next*. You will then be asked to enter a name for the newly created tier. Assign a suitable name such as *merged_rh*. Confirm by clicking on *Finish*. A new tier with merged annotations of both raters (for rh_activation annotations) is created.

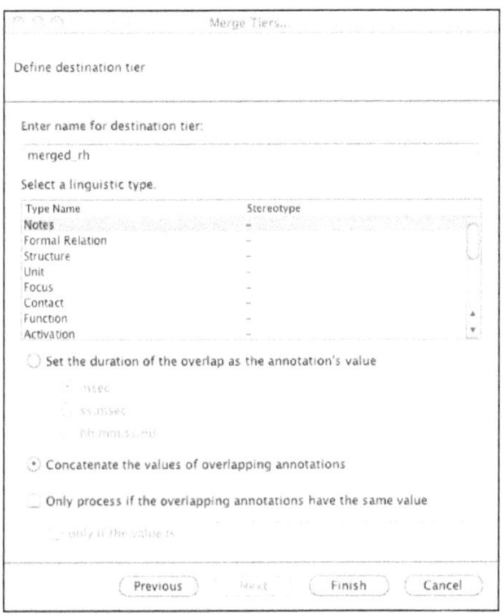

Proceed accordingly for lh_activation.

14.2 Create overlaps from annotations of both raters

In the *Tier* menu, select *Create Annotations from Overlaps... (Classic)*

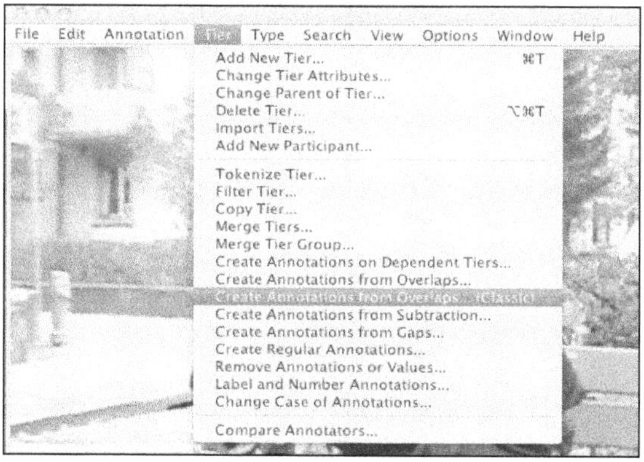

Select the tiers in the pop-up window from those overlaps you wish to create annotations from. This will either be rh_activation for both raters or lh_activation for both raters.

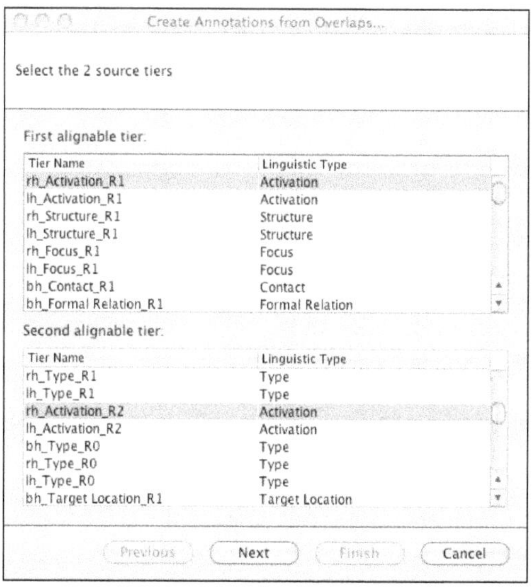

Click *Next*. You will then be asked to enter a name for the newly created tier. Assign a suitable name such as *overlaps_rh*. Confirm by clicking on *Finish*. A new tier with annotations created from overlaps of both raters (for rh_activation annotations) is created.

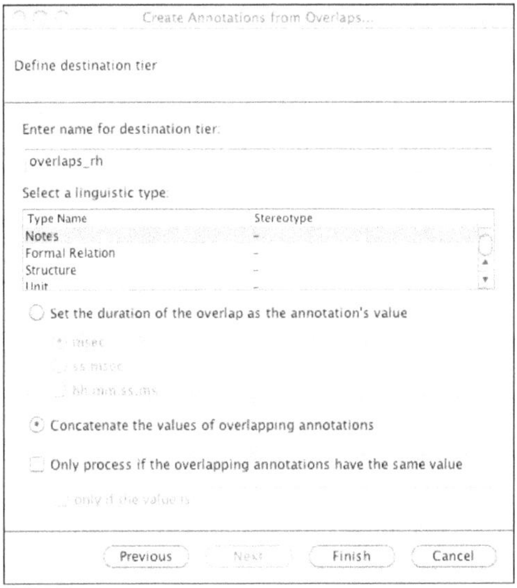

Proceed accordingly for lh_activation.

After having created new tiers with merged annotations and annotations from overlaps you should save the file.

Repeat these steps for all your data.

14.3 View statistics

The *View* > *Annotation Statistics* function in ELAN is a convenient instrument to quickly get an overview of the total length of units.

Clicking on the Menu bar item, a pop-up window will open showing the relevant data for each tier.

You have to select the *Tier* rider and then scroll down to the end where you find the tiers you have newly created.

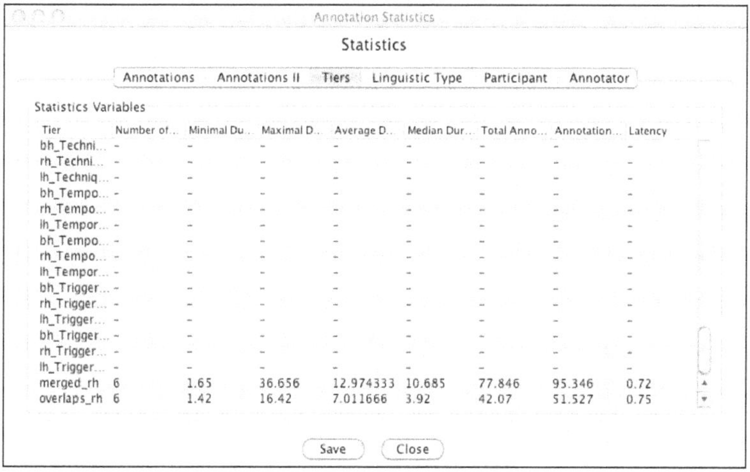

You should save the table so that you will have easy access to the data in the future. You can use these statistics to calculate the interrater agreement by entering the Average Duration of *merged_rh, merged_lh, overlaps_rh,* and *overlaps_lh* for each file manually in an Excel sheet.

It is advisable to export all your data from ELAN and compute the average duration automatically in Excel in order to avoid having to manually enter the values.

14.3.1 Export the new annotations

Proceed as follows:

Open ELAN and from the *File* menu apply the *Export Multiple Files As... Tab-delimited Text...* function.

A window pops up. Select *New Domain.* This will prompt another window to pop up in which you can select the files to export. Be sure to only select files you wish to be grouped and analyzed together.

You are then asked to assign a name to the selected domain of files. Select a suitable name specifying the group of files you wish to group and analyze together. Confirm by clicking *OK.*

Another window pops up. You can now select the tiers you wish to export. This will be the newly created tiers "merged" and "overlap" for the respective hand, i.e. either *merged_rh, overlaps_rh, merged_lh* plus *overlaps_lh.*

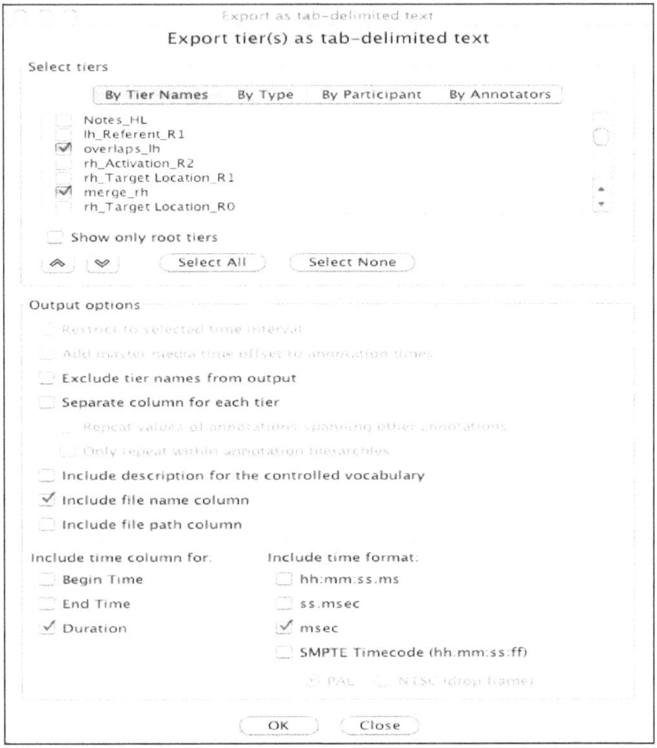

Confirm your selection by clicking *OK.* A new window will open asking you to assign a name for the export file. Having assigned a name, you can save the export text-file by clicking *Save*.

14.3.2 Enter the data into an excel file

You now have created a text file containing the Duration values of the merged annotations from Rater 1 and Rater 2 and of the overlaps respectively. The text file may now be easily imported in Excel. For doing this, click on the exported text file with the right mouse button and select *Open with > Microsoft Excel*
Name the columns: Tier, Duration, Unit, and Subject

	A	B	C	D
1	Tier	Duration	Unit	Subject
2	merged_rh	3650	movement mc	Caro
3	merged_rh	1420	movement mc	Caro
4	merged_rh	2760	movement mc	Caro
5	merged_rh	9490	movement mc	Caro
6	merged_rh	5530	movement mc	Caro
7	merged_rh	11380	movement mc	Caro
8	merged_rh	6520	movement mc	Caro

Compute the average duration in a pivot-table (*Data > PivotTable report*).Select *Subjects* for row, *Tier* for column, and *Duration* for data by dragging them from the right side.

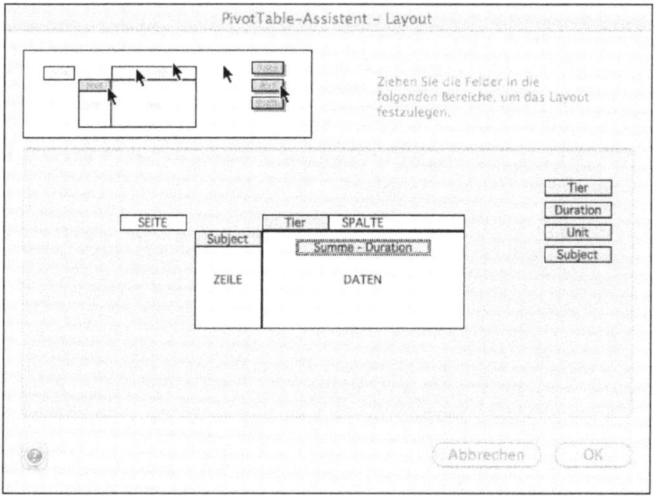

The pivot table shows the average durations for each file.

Sum - Duration	Tier				
Subject	merged_lh	merged_rh	overlaps_lh	overlaps_rh	Gesamtergebnis
Caro	86839	85395	81935	79119	333288
Nico	54959	63241	14135	21189	153524
Ann	68839	82385	51935	69123	272282
Kei	68120	77846	32200	42070	220236
Gesamtergebnis	278757	308867	180205	211501	979330

To calculate the interrater agreement, now apply the following function:

(length of annotations from overlaps) / (length of merged annotations)

Applying the above function in the sample file from the screenshots, the overall ratio is calculated. This value is the interrater agreement:

Subject	ratio_lh	ratio_rh
Caro	0,94	0,93
Nico	0,26	0,34
Ann	0,75	0,84
Kei	0,47	0,54
Average	0,61	0,66

This procedure provides a realistic estimation of the actual agreement of two independent raters without disproportionally considering disagreements on shorter *movements* units.

15. The Modified Cohen's Kappa: Calculating Interrater Agreement for Segmentation and Annotation

Henning Holle and Robert Rein

15.1 Introduction

With a new and complex manual for movement behaviour classification such as the NEUROGES-ELAN system, one naturally wants to evaluate the degree to which two (or more) raters agree in their classification decisions. Determining interrater agreement can be done with a variety of different intentions in mind, including (1) the development of reliable diagnostic rules to separate the different movement categories, (2) evaluating the effects of training on interpretation consistency and (3) determining the reliability of a classification system (cf. Crewson, 2005).

In this chapter, we will propose a new method for evaluating interrater agreement of movement classifications. The first section deals with the most basic questions of movement annotation, i.e., segmentation and annotation. Next, we introduce the properties of Cohen's kappa (Cohen, 1960), which is a widely used measure for interrater agreement. Subsequently, we describe an algorithm designed to identify those movement tags in the annotation data that fulfill certain agreement criteria. The application of this algorithm allows the calculation of kappa for the non-binary NEUROGES categories, i.e., with the exception of the binary Activation category (see Chapter 14). Finally, we present initial interrater agreement results for the NEUROGES-ELAN system, followed by a discussion of potential sources of disagreement, and suggest some possible ways of increasing interrater agreement.

15.1.1 The heart of it all: segmentation & annotation

A movement can be regarded as a dynamic signal that unfolds over time. Thus, a first question a rater has to answer is when a movement starts (onset) and when it ends (offset) in an observed video. Of course, raters will never perfectly agree in this decision. For instance, the definition of movement thresholds (e.g. what constitutes a movement and what does not?) and segmentation cues (e.g. how much time has to pass between two consecutive movements before they are considered as two separate movements rather than one single movement) may vary between raters. The question whether two raters agree in their decisions about movement onsets and offsets will be referred to as the *segmentation problem* throughout this chapter.

Once the onset and offset of a movement have been identified, a rater has to choose an appropriate label for the observed movement segment. In the Structure category of the NEUROGES system, which was used for the present analysis, a total of five different values are available (see 5.1.2.2). The question whether raters agree in their values for an observed movement segment will be called the *annotation problem* hereafter.

Within the NEUROGES-ELAN system the processes of segmentation and annotation are not implemented as independent and separate parsing steps. Instead, segmentation and annotation take turns. In a first step, raters decide for a given video segment whether a hand has moved or not (segmentation in Activation category). In the second step (Structure category), they take a closer look at the Structure of the segment (annotation). If there are different Structure values contained in the movement, the segment is demarcated into sub-units until each sub-unit contains only one Structure throughout (annotation & segmentation). Following this, in the third step (Focus category), the raters examine the Focus for all (sub)-units (annotation). If there are different Foci contained in one (sub)-unit, this unit is further demarcated into sub-units until each sub-unit contains only one focus throughout (annotation & segmentation). Thus, each tag contains the sum of all previous segmentation and annotation decisions. Accordingly, if one wants to determine whether two tags given by two raters can be considered as an *agreement*, these tags have to fulfill a number of criteria: (i) The tier type must match (e.g., both raters have placed the tag in the left hand Structure); (ii) Both tags must have the same label (e.g., *irregular*); (iii) There has to be a substantial temporal overlap between the two tags (for more information about the amount of overlap, see below).

Only if all three criteria are fulfilled, two tags can be considered as agreement between raters. Before giving a more detailed description of the algorithm used to calculate interrater agreement, we will first introduce Cohen's kappa (Cohen, 1960) which is a popular measure for interrater agreement.

15.1.2 Cohen's Kappa: calculation and properties

In order to illustrate the calculation and properties of Cohen's kappa, we will use an example unrelated to gesture. Consider two psychiatrists who frequently have to diagnose whether a patient has a depression or not. Furthermore, assume that 100 patients have been independently diagnosed by these two psychiatrists. In this example, we have a so-called binary outcome measure (depressive vs. not depressive). Because there are two raters, this results in four possible outcomes for each patient: (1) Both psychiatrists rate the patient as depressive (x x), (2) only the first psychiatrist considers the patient as depressive, the second one does not (x o), (3) only the second psychiatrists rates the patient as depressive, but not the first (o x) and (4) both psychiatrists rate the patient as non-depressive (o o). The frequency with which each of these four outcomes has occurred in the sample of 100 patients can be summarized in a 2x2 contingency table.

Table 1 A 2x2 contingency table showing the frequency of the four possible outcomes for the depression example. The right-most column and the bottom row depict the row and column sums, respectively. For more details, see text.

		Rater 1		
		X	O	Σ
Rater 2	X	13	11	n1• = 24
	O	9	67	n2• = 76
	Σ	n•1 = 22	n•2 = 78	n = 100

As can be seen from Table 1, there are two possible ways in which the raters can agree: Either they can both agree that a patient *is* depressive (positive agreement ,x x, which occurred 13 times), or they can both agree that a patient is *not* depressive (negative agreement, o o, which occurred 67 times). The combined cases of positive and negative agreement allows the calculation of a raw general agreement score which is defined as

Raw Agreement	=	number of agreeing cases / total number of cases
		(13 + 67) / 100
	=	0.8

Thus, in 80% of all patients, the two raters agreed in their diagnosis. However, the problem with such raw agreement indices is that they do not consider chance agreement. In this example, there were overall much more patients that were categorized as non-depressive than there were patients that were categorized as depressive (compare row and column sums in Table 1). Therefore, raters who would randomly rate two out of three patients as non-depressive would still be able to achieve reasonably high raw agreement scores, just because there were more non-depressive patients in the sample. One can calculate the degree of chance agreement by dividing the row and column sums by the total sum (for a more detailed description, see Crewson, 2005). In the present example, chance agreement can be determined as follows:

Chance Agreement	=	$(n_{1\cdot} / n) * (n_{\cdot 1} / n) + (n_{2\cdot} / n) * (n_{\cdot 2} / n)$
		(24 / 100) * (22 / 100) + (76 / 100) * (78 / 100)
	≈	0.65

Thus, the percentage of agreement by chance is in this case 65 %. In other words, one can expect for almost two out of three patients that the two raters would agree by chance alone. As can be seen from the formula below, the rationale of Cohen's kappa is to isolate levels of agreement that go beyond pure chance agreement:

Cohen's Kappa	=	(Raw Agreement – Chance Agreement) / (1 – Chance Agreement)
		(0.80 – 0.65) / (1 – 0.65)
	≈	0.43

Kappa represents the general agreement between two raters beyond that which would be expected by chance alone. Thus, in the example above, the agreement between the two raters was 43 % better than chance. A kappa of 1.0 would represent perfect agreement; a kappa of 0.0 would represent chance-level agreement. It is also possible that the kappa coefficient turns out to be negative. In these cases, the observed rater agreement is even worse than chance-level agreement.

There is some controversy in the literature about which values of kappa represent adequate and inadequate reliability. Landis and Koch (1977) initially proposed a classification scheme which is shown in Table 2 (left panel). Shrout (1998) discussed the labels provided by Landis and Koch and argued for a more conservative interpretation (Table 2, right panel). We will use the more conservative classification scheme provided by Shrout for the interpretation of our data.

Table 2 Classifications schemes for the interpretation of kappa. Slightly adapted from Jones (2004).

INTERPRETATION OF RELIABILITY			
Landis and Koch (1977)		Shrout (1998)	
Value of reliability	Strength of agreement	Value of reliability	Strength of agreement
<0.00	Poor		
0.00-0.20	Slight	0.00-0.10	Virtually none
0.21-0.40	Fair	0.11-0.40	Slight
0.41-0.60	Moderate	0.41-0.60	Fair
0.61-0.80	Substantial	0.61-0.80	Moderate
0.81-1.00	Almost perfect	0.81-1.00	Substantial

While the kappa value of 0.43 calculated indicates fair agreement according to Shrout (1998), it is also important to take the error margin of this estimation into account (compare also Fleiss, Cohen, & Everitt, 1969). Confidence intervals can provide important information with respect to this issue, because they inform the reader how consistent an observed agreement index is with its label [22]. For instance, the 95% confidence interval of kappa for the depression example ranges from 0.23 – 0.64. Thus, the true agreement between raters (on a population level) can be anywhere between 'slight', 'fair' and 'moderate' (see Table 1). For meaningful reliability analyses, Jones (2004) has suggested to sample enough

22 An easy and comprehensive way to obtain confidence intervals for various agreement measures of a 2x2 contingency table is through a freely available Excel®-Worksheet (Mackinnon, 2000, available online at www.mhri.edu.au/biostats/DAG_Stat)

data to be 95% confident that the value of kappa obtained from a sample will be within 0.1 of the true value of kappa (i.e., the confidence interval should be <= 0.2, as opposed to 0.41 in the present example). Jones provided tables of required sample sizes (see Table 3), given an estimate of kappa and the prevalence of the to-be-rated trait. The prevalence of depression in the example would be 23 % (Rater 1 classified 22 % of all patients as depressive, Rater 2 24 %). Taking the observed kappa of 0.43 as an estimate for the population kappa, it follows from Table 3 that a sample size of 489 subjects is in this cases required for a sufficiently precise reliability study.

Table 3 Sample size for a reliability study assuming dichotomous data, two raters, 95 % confidence interval for Kappa, and a conidence interval of <= 0.2

	Prevalence (%)				
Estimate of kappa	10	20	30	40	50
0.4	848	489	379	335	323
0.5	801	451	344	301	289
0.6	705	392	296	257	246
0.7	569	314	236	205	196
0.8	401	222	167	145	139
0.9	209	116	88	77	72
Unknown	851	505	412	387	385

15.2 Description of the algorithm

In order to transform annotation data provided by the raters into the required 2 x 2 contingency table, which subsequently allows the calculation of kappa, one essentially needs to determine which rater tags belong together and which tags do not. This decision has to be based upon (1) the tier in which the tag was placed, (2) the label of the tag and (3) the degree of temporal overlap between tags given by different raters.

In the example used to introduce kappa, the outcome measure was binary (depressive, non-depressive). However, determining a value for the NEUROGES categories system is not a binary decision. As an example, in the Structure category as each rater has to choose between 5 possible values for an observed movement, which would result in a 5 x 5 contingency table for the agreement analysis. Because it is impractical to calculate kappa for such large contingency tables (Kraemer, 1992), we perform a binary mapping of the outcome measures, as has been advocated in the literature (Wirtz & Kuschmann, 2007). More specifically, agreement is analyzed for one value at a time, which is then contrasted with the rest of all other values.

An example: Interrater agreement for *shift* units

As an example, we will explain how the algorithm classifies agreement for *shift* units. The analysis will be based on the sample data shown in Figure 1.

Two tags by two raters are considered as agreement, if and only if all of the following criteria are fulfilled:

i) both tags are placed in the same tier (e.g., lh_Structure_R0).

ii) both tags have the same Structure value (e.g., *shift*).

iii) Both tags have a temporal overlap.

The temporal overlap covers at least 60% of the length of the longer tag[23].

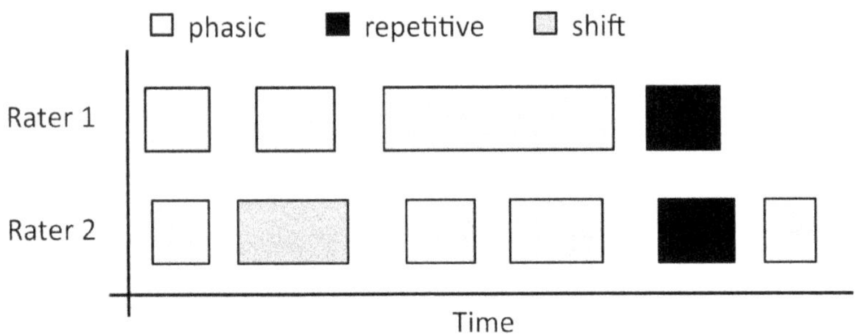

Figure 1 Example rating data used to illustrate the algorithm. The two tiers show the tags of two raters for the left hand.

Consider the first two tags given by the two raters (0 – 5 sec). Both tags are placed in the tier lh_Structure_R0 (criterion No. 1). They also both have the same value (i.e., *shift*), and a temporal overlap (criteria 2 & 3). Finally, the length of the temporal overlap covers more than 60% of the length of the longer

23 One cannot use the length of the shorter tag for overlap evaluation, because then short tags by one rater falling within very long tags of the other rater (as for instance in the case of the shift tags around 10 and 15 sec) would be erroneously classified as perfect agreement, although segmentation is very different between raters. Similarly, one cannot use less than 51% of the longer tag as a criterion, because this can result in tags entering agreement count erroneously more than once. Thus, "overlap > 51% of length of longer tag" is the smallest possible criterion for unambiguous results. For the present analysis, we chose to use 60% as overlap criterion, in order to have a more conservative and robust estimation of interrater agreement.

tag (criterion 4). Thus, all four criteria are fulfilled and the segment is therefore registered as an agreement in the 2 x 2 contingency table (see bottom row of Figure 2).

The next two tags given by the two raters (from 5 – 9 sec) do not fulfill criterion No. 2, because they have different annotation values (*phasic* vs. *shift*). Hence, there is no interrater agreement in this time segment, and the false positive *shift* movement seen by Rater 1 is added to the contingency table (see Figure 2).

Next, Rater 1 has seen a long *shift*, ranging from about 9 – 16 sec. Rater 2 has also seen a *shift*, but has used a different segmentation here (two shorter *shifts* instead of one long one). Should this be considered as an agreement? Criteria 1 – 3 are fulfilled here. What about criterion No. 4? Because segmentation is an important part of the decision process in the NEUROGES-ELAN system, the two tags by Rater 2 have to be evaluated separately. The algorithm matches the *shift* tag of Rater 1 with the first *shift* of Rater 2.[24] Next, it becomes evident that the overlap is less than 60% of the duration of the long *shift* tag by Rater 1. Therefore, this segment is classified as a false positive *shift* by Rater 1 (see)[25]. The second *shift* tag by Rater 2 does not have a corresponding tag to be matched with, therefore this segment is classified as a false positive shift by Rater 2.

Next, the *repetitive* tag of Rater 1 is matched with the *repetitive* tag of Rater 2. Since the value is different from the current value of interest (remember, we want to analyze agreement for *shift* movements), this segment is classified as negative agreement. In other words, both raters have agreed in *not* seeing a *shift* movement during this segment.

Finally, the last segment (where Rater 1 did not place any tag, whereas Rater 2 placed a *phasic* tag) is again classified as negative agreement. Again, both raters agreed here in not seeing a *shift* movement.

---

24 Matching always the first occurrence of equal annotations might be seen as overly conservative feature as it is perfectly conceivable that for example in the present case the second overlapping tag of Rater 2 might have a greater overlap with the tag from Rater 1 than the first overlapping tag. However, extending the proposed algorithm to include such cases has two negative consequences. First, it would dramatically increase the complexity of the algorithm. Second, it would break the symmetry as results would then depend on which rater is being used as a reference. With the present simpler and more conservative formulation this is not an issue.

25 Since there is no objective gold standard for segmentation here, it is in this case of course an arbitrary decision whether the false positive should be attributed to rater 1 or rater 2.

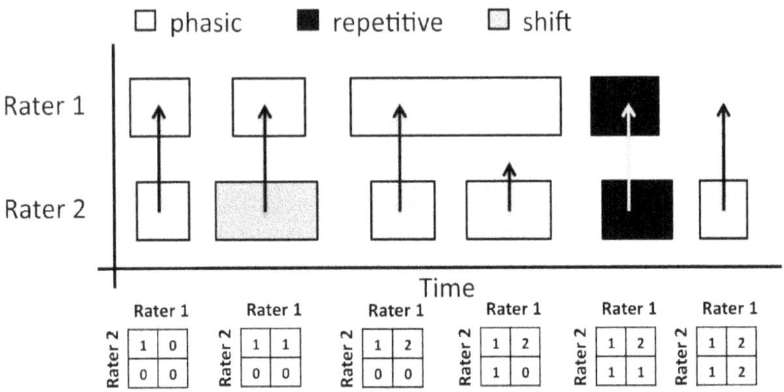

Figure 2 Scoring example for agreement counts of *shifts* vs. all other movement types. Arrows indicate which tags are matched with each other. Bottom row shows how the 2 x 2 contingency table is updated as the algorithm proceeds through the data.

To sum up the scores for *shift* movements, there is one segment of positive agreement, two segments of false positives on behalf of Rater 1, one segment of false positives on behalf of Rater 2, and finally two segments of negative agreement (see also the final contingency table in the bottom right corner of Figure 2).

Another example: Interrater agreement for *repetitive* movements

To further illustrate how the agreement count is performed, we now analyze agreement of *repetitive* movements vs. all other values for the example data set. The same tags as previously are matched with each other (see arrows in Figure 3), thereby creating the segments that are classified according to the 2 x 2 contingency table. Segments 1 – 4 are classified as negative agreements, because both raters agreed here in not seeing a movement of the value *repetitive*. Segment 5 is classified as positive agreement, and segment 6 as negative agreement. To sum up, there are five segments of negative agreement for this movement type, and one segment of positive agreement.

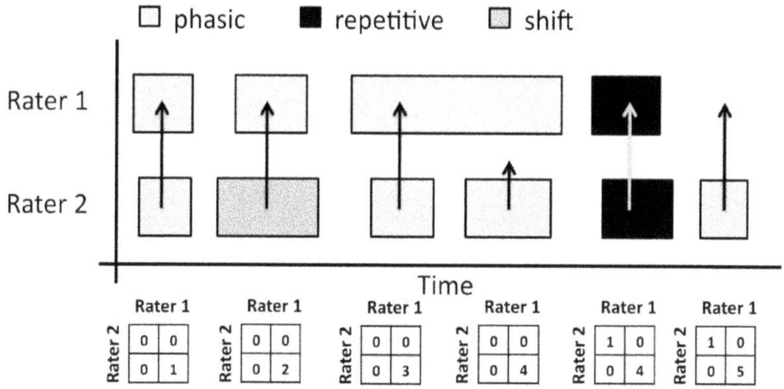

Figure 3 Scoring example for agreement counts of *repetitive* movements vs. all other movement types.

In this way, we calculated contingency tables for all values of interest, which allowed us to compute value-specific kappas as well as positive agreement indices.

15.3 Results

Concatenated StructureFocus annotations from two teams were used for the present analysis, resulting in a total of 76 min of annotated video material. Because one of the pre-requisites of bi-rater kappa is that the observations come from the same two raters (Crewson, 2005), agreement analysis were calculated separately for each team.[26] While Team 1 annotated a total of 23.30 min video and placed a total of 333 tags, Team 2 annotated more than twice as much (53.10 min) yielding a total of 1967 movement tags.

26 Please note that is not intended (nor particularly informative) to directly compare levels of agreement between teams, given that these two teams annotated movements from entirely different populations performing very different experimental paradigms.

Table 4 Data Basis

	Team 1 (JB and MR)	Team 2 (KH and MG)
Number of annotated videos (and participants)	15	44
Total length of annotated video segments	23 min 30 s	53 min 10 s
Mean video length (standard deviation)	93.31 s (18.75 s)	72.40 s (33.55 s)
Subjects & Topic	A sample of split-brain patients and matched healthy participants was videotaped while answering questions of the Wechsler-Adult Intelligence Scale (Tewes, 1994)	A sample of 40 patients with left or right hemisphere damage and 20 matched controls was videotaped during the narration of "Mr. Bean" movie clips
Movement Tags	333	1967

In a first analysis step, we analyzed how often the seven movement categories were detected in the two rating teams. Figure 4 shows the absolute number of tags for these categories, separately for each team. One result is that both teams show different frequency distributions. Whereas in Team 1, who rated videos showing participants responding to verbal items of an IQ test, most often *shift* movements were detected, the most frequently detected movement value in Team 2, who rated videos of patients and controls videotaped whilst narrating, was *phasic in space*.

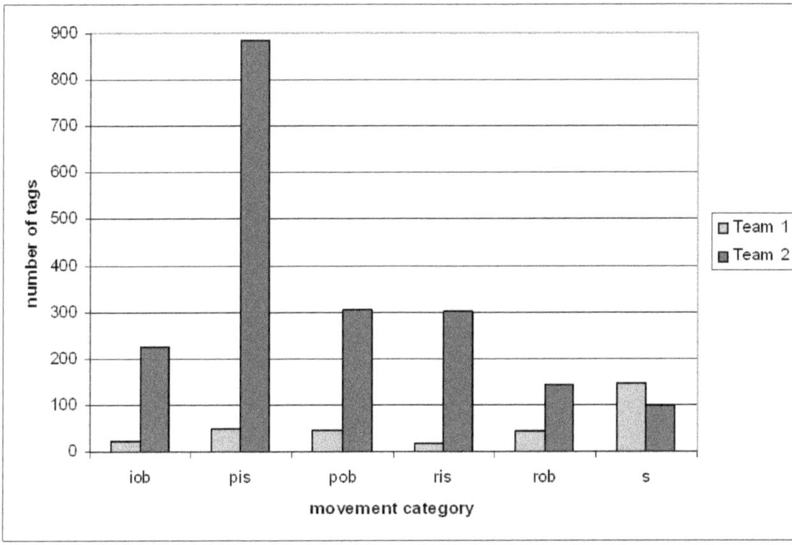

Figure 4 Frequency of StructureFocus values for both rating teams. The y axis represents the number of tags for each value, summed across all videos and both raters. Abbreviations: *irregular on body* (iob), *phasic in space* (pis), *phasic on body* (pob), *repetitive in space* (ris), *repetitive on body* (rob), *shift* (s). (Here, the value *on body* included the value on attached object.)

In a next analysis step, the value-specific kappas were calculated, using the previously described algorithm (see Figure 5). Team 1 had a mean kappa of about 0.4, whereas Team 2 (which analyzed much more data) had a mean kappa of about 0.6. Thus, all in all, interrater agreement can be described as fair. Please see below for a more detailed discussion of the obtained kappa values.

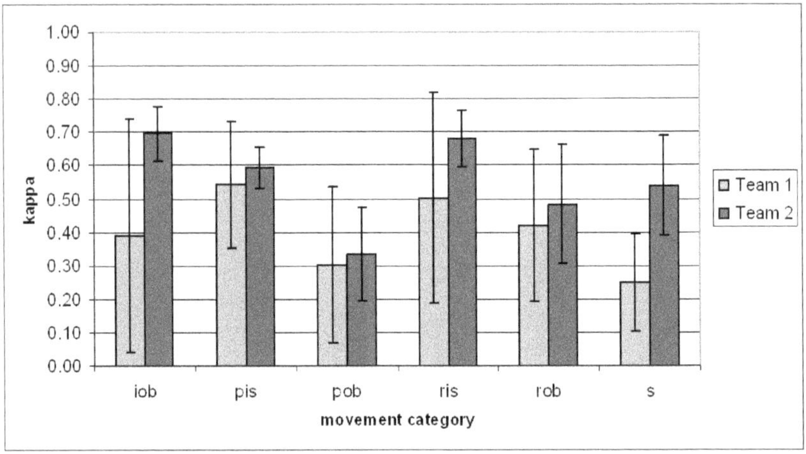

Figure 5 Cohen's kappa for the six StructureFocus values. Error bars represent 95% confidence intervals, which were determined using a non-parametric bootstrap algorithm (Graham & Bull, 1998).

For the kappa values described above, we used an overlap criterion of 60%. Of course, this can be criticized as an arbitrary setting, as any value between 51% and 100% could in principle have been used. We further explored the extent to which this parameter setting influences the obtained kappa values, by plotting the amount to which kappa decreases as the overlap criterion is increased (see Figure 6 and Figure 7). As can be seen from theses figures, a substantial drop in kappa values only occurs for values above 70% (and even more so for more extreme values above 80%). Below these values, there is a more or less stable plateau, where changing the overlap criterion (say to either 55% or 65%) does not have much impact on the obtained kappa values. Based on these data, we feel confident that our decision for a 60% criterion is a reasonable compromise between temporal precision and detection sensitivity.

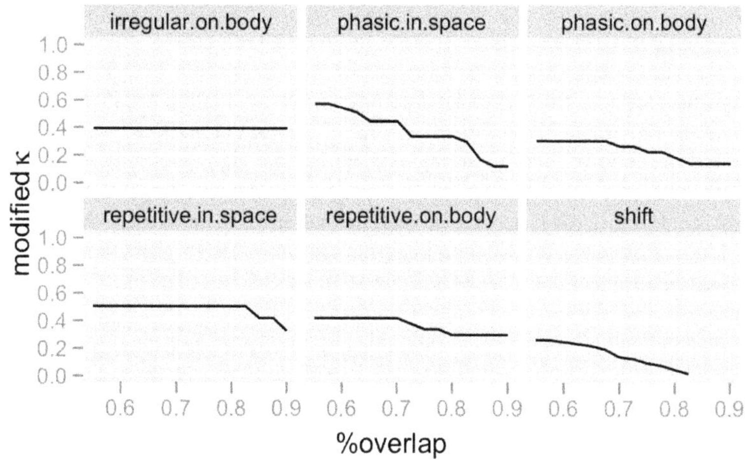

Figure 6 Team 1: Relationship between kappa and the % overlap criterion.

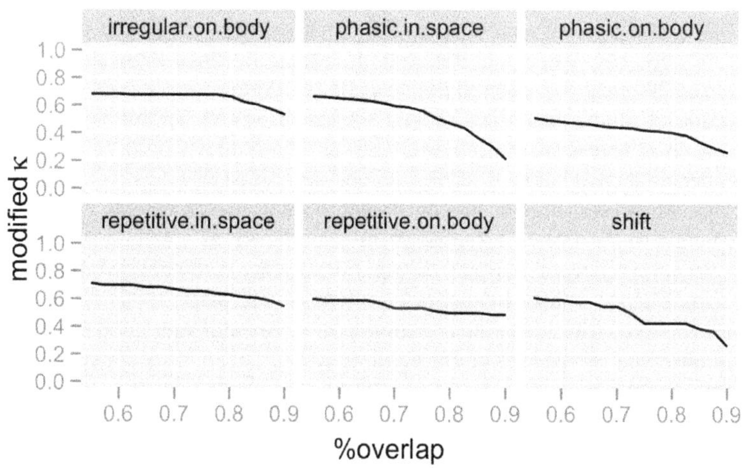

Figure 7 Team 2: Relationship between kappa and the % overlap criterion.

15.4 Discussion

Establishing interrater agreement is a crucial step to justify results obtained from annotated video-stream data. Here we present a novel approach that takes into account the interrelated problems of segmentation and annotation. Based on the analysis of two large datasets we were able to show that our algorithm obtains sensible data and is relatively robust against specific parameter choices, namely the percentage of overlap needed in order to score agreement.

An important aspect of determining interrater agreement is the number of observations required to yield statistically reliable agreement indices. As has been mentioned in the introduction, an insufficient sample size results in wide confidence intervals and thus, difficulties in drawing conclusions about the tool's reliability (cf. Jones, 2004). As can be seen in Figure 6, this is clearly the case for Team 1. For this team, confidence intervals are too wide to allow a conclusion about the reliability of the NEUROGES system for this population.

In the case of Team 2, confidence intervals are much narrower, and thus allow a more precise estimation of reliability for this population. In general, interrater agreement for this sample was fair (see Figure 7). For three of the six Structure-Focus values, somewhat higher (fair to moderate) degrees of reliability were observed (*iob*, *pis* & *ris*), whereas for the remaining three values, reliability was only slight to fair (*pob*, *rob* & *s*). The results for *rob* and *s* are, however, qualified by wide confidence intervals. With respect to the required sample size for reliability studies, Jones (2004) has suggested to sample enough data that all confidence intervals are smaller than 0.2. This requirement would be met by values *iob, pis*, *pob,* and *ris* in the case of Team 2. Each of these three values had at least 200 tags that entered the analysis (in Team 2, see Figure 7). Therefore, a rule-of thumb regarding sample size requirements for future reliability studies in the context of the NEUROGES-ELAN system would be to sample enough data that each value of interest comprises at least 200 tags.

Further, when one value occurs only seldom small disagreements will lead to large changes in the Cohen's kappa scores in particular as small occurrences of values can entail unequal marginal distributions for the contingency tables yielding to small kappa values (compare Feinstein & Cicchetti, 1990). This might also be a problem when obtaining small kappa values although good raw agreement is observed as the maximum possible kappa values also depends on the marginal distributions of the underlying contingency table (Banerjee, Capozzoli, McSweeney, & Shina, 1999; Cicchetti & Feinstein, 1990; Feinstein & Cicchetti, 1990). Similar, when the duration of annotations decreases changes in offsets and onsets might also stronger impact kappa values as for very brief movements it becomes more difficult to obtain the necessary overlap. As the calculation of Cohen's kappa requires at least two different values, the present algorithm also works only when there are at least two values in a category. Thus, the algorithm does not work for example for the Activation category. In conclusion, the measurement of interrater agreement depends always on multiple factors and sometimes it might be difficult to trace back the exact reason for why a particular Cohen's kappa value was obtained. Thus, calculation of the modified Cohen's kappa value does not relief one from investigating the raw data.

15.5 Further suggestions for future reliability studies

More often than not, users of the NEUROGES-ELAN system may find out that interrater agreement is initially disappointingly low. In such a case the users should make sure that low agreement scores are not due to simple slips and misses. Some of the more common systematic mistakes include (i) one rater places all of his tags in the wrong tier (e.g., lh_Structure_R0 instead of lh_Focus_R0) and (ii) confusion between raters about which hand is "left" and which is "right" (anatomical or specular?).

Besides these slips and misses, there are also other, more fundamental causes of rater disagreement. One source of disagreement is rater bias. For instance, within Team 2, it occurred 20 times that Rater 1 saw a *shift*, while Rater 2 did not. The reverse pattern occurred only 6 times, suggesting that Rater 1 had a stronger bias towards detecting *shift* movements. A statistical indicator of rater bias is a significant McNemar test.[27] While detecting rater bias is fairly simple, its elimination requires more effort, including renewed rater training.

A special case of rater bias is when raters apply different degrees of segmentation during the annotation process. As has been shown in the example during the introduction, one rater may see one long segment of a specific movement type, whereas the other rater sees the same time segment as multiple, shorter movements. If raters consistently disagree in their level of segmentation, rater agreement will of course be negatively affected. Such segmentation problems can be somewhat alleviated by renewed rater training.

One important fact to note that there can be no such thing as absolute reliability. Reliability is always defined with respect to a certain population (Jones, 2004; Shrout, 1998). It is therefore not possible to only rely on published reliability results when using the NEUROGES system for a new study. Because raters, experimental setting, and participants differ from project to project, each new study has to assess their own interrater reliability (see Jones, 2004, for a highly readable primer on the construction of reliability studies).

The final note of this chapter concerns the reliability of NEUROGES Module I. Most values achieved fair levels of interrater agreement, with kappa ranging between 0.48 and 0.68 (for Team 2). Although somewhat precise and significantly greater than zero, these agreement scores are of course far from perfect. However, it should be noted that the data were from the first studies applying the NEUROGES system. Since then the objectivity of the definitions and the quality of rater training has improved, and consequently, the interrater agreement has

27 A McNemar Test for 2x2 contingency tables is, for instance, provided by the Excel® Worksheet mentioned before.

improved (Chapter 16). Furthermore, Module I as compared to Modules II and III has the highest segmentation : annotation ratio. In Modules II and III, often the units from the previous category can be used directly. Thus, the process of segmentation units into subunits decreases and accordingly, the interrater agreement improves. Infact, if the interrater agreement is only or mainly determined by annotation and not by segmentation, much better agreement scores occur. This explains why in the field of gesture research, much greater agreement scores for annotations are typically reported (see, for instance, Broaders, Cook, Mitchell, & Goldin-Meadow, 2007). However, in these gesture studies, one person only first analyzes and segments the video data and subsequently only these selected segments of the video are then being rated by different raters (e.g., *Is the value of this segment X or Y?*). Note that segmentation is in such a case – unlike in the NEUROGES-ELAN system – not part of the rating process and therefore cannot contribute to rater disagreement. As is evident from the present work the initial process of segmentation can already cause large discrepancies between raters and thus should be included into the interrater agreement evaluation. These considerations give a new perspective on the agreement scores reported. Thus, the present analysis should be seen as a benchmark for future developments in assessing interrater agreement of the NEUROGES system and movement behaviour classification systems in general.

Acknowledgements

The present work has been funded by the Volkswagenstiftung through the project "Towards a grammar of gestures: Evolution, Brain, and Linguistic Structures" (Project-code. II/82175).

References

Banerjee, M., Capozzoli, M., McSweeney, L., & Shina, D. (1999). Beyond kappa: A review of interrater agreement measures. *The Canadian Journal of Statistics, 27*(1), 3-23.

Broaders, S.C., Cook, S.W., Mitchell, Z., & Goldin-Meadow, S. (2007). Making children gesture brings out implicit knowledge and leads to learning. *J Exp Psychol Gen, 136*(4), 539-550.

Cicchetti, D.V., & Feinstein, A.R. (1990). High agreement but low kappa: II. Resolving the paradoxes. *Journal of Clinical Epidemiology, 43*(6), 551-558.

Cohen, J. (1960). A coefficient of agreement for nominal scales. *Educational and Psychological Measurement, 20*, 37-46.

Crewson, P.E. (2005). Reader agreement studies. *AJR Am J Roentgenol, 184*(5), 1391-1397.

Feinstein, A.R., & Cicchetti, D.V. (1990). High agreement but low kappa: I. The problems of two paradoxes. *Journal of Clinical Epidemiology, 43*(6), 543-549.

Fleiss, J.L., Cohen, J., & Everitt, B.S. (1969). Large sample standard errors of kappa and weighted kappa. *Psychological Bulletin, 72*(5), 323-327.

Graham, P., & Bull, B. (1998). Approximate standard errors and confidence intervals for indices of positive and negative agreement. *J Clin Epidemiol, 51*(9), 763-771.

Jones, J.M. (2004). Reliability of nutritional screening and assessment tools. *Nutrition, 20*(3), 307-311.

Kraemer, H.C. (1992). Measurement of reliability for categorical data in medical research. *Stat Methods Med Res, 1*(2), 183-199.

Landis, J.R., & Koch, G.G. (1977). The measurement of observer agreement for categorical data. *Biometrics, 33*(1), 159-174.

Mackinnon, A. (2000). A spreadsheet for the calculation of comprehensive statistics for the assessment of diagnostic tests and interrater agreement. *Comput Biol Med, 30*(3), 127-134.

Shrout, P.E. (1998). Measurement reliability and agreement in psychiatry. *Stat Methods Med Res, 7*(3), 301-317.

Tewes, U. (1994). *HAWIE-R: Hamburg-Wechsler-Intelligenztest für Erwachsene Revision 1991* (2 ed.). Bern: Huber

Wirtz, M., & Kuschmann, M. (2007). Analyzing interrater agreement for categorical data using Cohen's kappa and alternative coefficients. *Rehabilitation (Stuttg). 46*(6), 370-377.

16. Recommendations for Assessing the Level of Interrater Agreement

Harald Skomroch

In the previous chapter, it was indicated that that calculating interrater agreement for segmentation and annotation results in worse agreement scores than calculating interrater agreement for annotation only. Thus, as compared to studies using the modified Cohen's Kappa, interrater agreement scores are generally higher when the annotations do not include segmentation processes (see, for instance, Broaders et al., 2007; Nicoladis et al., 1999), or when information different from movement, such as speech (e.g. a target word/phrase) is used to predefine units (see, for instance, Cocks et al., 2011; Duncan, 2002). The analysis of video taped hand movement behaviour with the NEUROGES is conducted without sound following seven subsequent steps, where the units created in the proceeding step partially predetermine the units used in the subsequent step. However, often new subunits have to be created by the raters individually. If interrater differences in the creation of these (sub-)units occur, these differences permeate to the following steps and affect the interrater agreement. This can be avoided by using units, which both raters have agreed on, as the basis for the next step. The present chapter investigates the impact differences during the segmentation process have on the interrater agreement. Based on the evaluation of previous studies and on the findings elicited by a filter, which excludes interrater differences in segmentations, it provides a recommendation to assess interrater agreement.

16.1 Interrater agreement in previous studies using the NEUROGES system

The interrater agreement depends on the complexity of the data and on the procedure, which is taken for analysis. The complexity of the data, in turn, is influenced by the setting as well as by inter-individual differences of the participants. Inter-individual differences may occur due to idiosyncratic features as well as due to mental or neurological disease. Further, the interrater agreement and the interpretation thereof are influenced by the quantity of data concerning one value. Nevertheless, the degree of interrater agreement also depends on the raters' proficiency and their ability to analyze consistently. All raters working on past material have been trained in applying NEUROGES on video data and they have met regularly for ongoing training and consensus.

In the paragraphs below, the interrater agreement scores for different rater dyads are shown for the NEUROGES categories Activation, Structure, concatenated StructureFocus, and Contact.

Table 1 Activation category: Compare Annotators ratio score mean for six rater dyads of five experiments

Rater Dyad	Mean
AB-KP	0.83
AB-MK	0.7
DD-DA	0.79
IH-MIK	0.845
IH-MK	0.73
RR-HS	0.781
Total	0.781

As illustrated in Table 1, the interrater agreement for the Activation category varied between 0.7 and 0.845 for the different dyads with a mean of 0.78 and a respective standard deviation of 0.05. The procedure to calculate interrater agreement for the Activation category has been described in Chapter 14.

Table 2 Structure category: Modified Cohen's kappa scores and raw agreement scores (in brackets) for the Structure values in seven experiments

Structure values		*phasic*	*repetitive*	*shift*	*aborted*	*irregular*
Experi-ment (number of sub-jects)	**Rater dy-ads**					
LEAS (n = 66)	AB-MK	0.52 (0.82)	0.56 (0.94)	0.49 (0.91)	0.20 (0.98)	0.47 (0.76)
	IH-MK	0.46 (0.78)	0.74 (0.95)	0.57 (0.92)	0.49 (0.99)	0.35 (0.73)
	CP-CK	0.48 (0.79)	0.42 (0.92)	0.35 (0.93)	0.1 (0.99)	0.5 (0.77)
HAWIE (n = 66)	AB-MK	0.48 (0.89)	0.71 (0.97)	0.59 (0.88)	0.22 (0.99)	0.27 (0.65)
	IH-MK	0.55 (0.86)	0.75 (0.97)	0.43 (0.82)	0.21 (0.98)	0.30 (0.70)
	CP-CK	0.44 (0.85)	0.38 (0.94)	0.39 (0.86)	0 (1.0)	0.52 (0.82)
Move-ment Scenes GO (n = 18)	IH-MiK	0.87 (0.97)	0.85 (0.98)	0.72 (0.96)	0.51 (0.96)	0.77 (0.99)
Move-ment Scenes VG (n = 18)	IH-MiK	0.74 (0.95)	0.80 (0.99)	0.61 (0.93)	0.58 (0.97)	0.70 (0.95)
Sylvester & Tweety (n = 60)	HS-RR	0.44 (0.76)	0.51 (0.87)	0.34 (0.91)	0.30 (0.92)	0.38 (0.83)
Mouse (n = 20)	DD-DB	0.41 (0.82)	0.51 (0.91)	0.52 (0.86)	0.28 (0.97)	0.49 (0.77)
AUVIS (n = 58)	MS-HS	0.61 (0.81)	0.61 (0.87)	0.75 (0.98)	0.42 (0.97)	0.68 (0.91)
	ES-HS	0.55 (0.79)	0.78 (0.94)	0.35 (0.97)	0.0 (0.99)	0.75 (0.9)
	IP-HS	0.67 (0.86)	0.59 (0.91)	0.71 (0.96)	0.44 (0.96)	0.71 (0.68)

Table 2 illustrates the interrater agreement for Structure values of 13 rater dyads in seven experiments. Except for the agreement scores for the experiment Movement Scenes, the scores seem to be relatively low ranging between 0.0 and 0.79.

The interrater agreement scores of the six experiments (all except AUVIS) were included in a Repeated Measures analysis with Structure value as a within-subject factor (with five levels: *phasic, repetitive, shift, aborted, irregular*). There was a significant effect of Structure ($F = 15.137$, $df = 4$; $p = .000$). Post hoc tests revealed that agreement for *repetitive* units was better than for *shift* ($p = 0.037$) units and for *aborted* units ($p = 0.00$). Agreement for *phasic* and *shift* units was also better than for *aborted* units ($p = 0.006$; $p = 0.005$).

A further analysis including experiment as a between-subjects factor, revealed no significant effect of Experiment although there was a trend indicating that the interrater agreement scores in Movement Scenes GO were better. This could be due to the circumstance that participants were asked to perform gestures on demand (stimuli) and the movement behaviour was more structured than in other experiments where participants conversed freely. Additionally, the scores for *repetitive, phasic,* and *irregular* appear to be slightly better for the AUVIS experiment. For this currently ongoing project, the procedure of analysis was different in that all *movement* units have been agreed upon before annotating on the level of Structure. Consequently, differences in the segmentation on the level of Activation did not permeate to the level of Structure. Still, agreement scores for *aborted* and *shift* units are relatively low. Simultaneously, the raw agreement for these values is high indicating that both raters agreed well on that a unit was **not** *aborted* or *shift.* Also these results reflect that *aborted* and, to a lesser extent, *shift* units occur infrequently.

The interrater agreement scores in Table 3 refer to the agreement for the concatenated Structure Focus values for ten rater dyads and eight experiments.

Table 3 Concatenated StructureFocus: Modified Cohen's kappa scores and raw agreement scores (in brackets) for the StructureFocus values in eight experiments

Structure Focus values / **Experiment**	**Rater dyad**	***phasic in space***	***phasic on body (incl. on attached object)***	***repetitive in space***	***repetitive on body (incl. on attached object)***	***irregu-lar-on body (incl. on attached object)***	***irregu-lar-within body***
HAWIE (n = 34)	AB-MK	0.52 (0.92)	0.27 (0.95)	0.73 (0.98)	0.64 (0.98)	0.30 (0.69)	0.34 (0.90)
	IH-MK	0.59 (0.89)	0.54 (0.96)	0.70 (0.98)	0.85 (0.99)	0.28 (0.79)	0.18 (0.82)
LEAS (n = 34)	AB-MK	0.53 (0.83)	0.57 (0.99)	0.57 (0.95)	0.81 (1.00)	0.52 (0.80)	0.28 (0.90)
	IH-MK	0.64 (0.79)	0.66 (0.99)	0.72 (0.96)	0.53 (0.98)	0.35 (0.84)	0.25 (0.81)
WAIS* (n = 15)	MR-MG	0.67 (0.91)	0.48 (0.89)	0.55 (0.94)	0.62 (0.94)	0.59 (0.90)	0.00 (1.00)
Sylvester & Tweety (n = 60)	RR-HS	0.46 (0.79)	0.35 (0.94)	0.57 (0.90)	0.40 (0.96)	0.44 (0.87)	0.12 (0.95)
Mr. Bean (n = 60)	KH-MG	0.61 (0.82)	0.50 (0.90)	0.67 (0.93)	0.53 (0.96)	0.71 (0.94)	0.00 (1.00)
Motion Scenes VG (n = 18)	IH-MiK	0.75 (0.96)	0.59 (0.99)	0.76 (0.98)	0.80 (1.00)	0.73 (0.97)	0.50 (0.97)
Motion Scenes GO (n = 18)	IH-MiK	0.88 (0.97)	0.66 (0.99)	0.86 (0.98)	0.59 (1.00)	0.79 (0.99)	0.64 (0.99)
Every-day Act. (n = 27)	R1-R2	0.46	0.39	0.44	0.34	0.59	0.80

For the experiments HAWIE, LEAS, Motion Scenes VG, Motion Scenes GO, and the Stroke Study, the same rater dyads were involved as for the Structure category. A visual comparison of the scores of interrater agreement for Structure values (Table 2) and the StructureFocus values (Table 3) reveals that whereas the scores improved for HAWIE and LEAS they did not improve so very much for the Motion Scenes VG, Motion Scenes GO, and the Stroke Study. Except for Motion Scenes VG and Motion Scenes GO, the interrater agreement scores for Structure Focus values varied between 0.4 and 0.7.

Interrater agreements on *irregular within body* varied much more (0.00 – 0.64) and appeared to be generally lower. When raters identify *within body* movements they have to rely on additional information other than where the hand acts. They need to distinguish, whether the motion serves to relax or contract muscles or joints, to a greater extent than for other Focus values. This information can be drawn from the criteria muscle contraction, anti-gravity position, and motion (see 5.1.2.1). Additionally, the Focus value *within body* occur sless often in many settings.

As shown in Table 4, the agreement scores for the Contact values *act on each other* and *act apart* happen to be consistently better for the three experiments analyzed.

Table 4 Contact category: Modified Cohen's kappa scores and raw agreement scores (in brackets) for the Contact values in three experiments

Contact values	***act as a unit***	***act on each other***	***act apart***
Motion Scenes VG (n = 11/18)	0.42 (.98)	0.90 (.98)	0.90 (.96)
Motion Scenes G0 (n = 11/18)	0.46 (.98)	0.73 (.99)	0.88 (.95)
Stroke Study (n = 20/60)	0.51 (.98)	0.80 (.94)	0.78 (.90)

The high scores for *act on each other* and *act apart* reflect that less segmentation has to be conducted when coding Module II. The 'to be coded' Contact units are generated by creating overlaps between right hand and left hand StructureFocus units, which often result in relatively small units that do not need to be subdivided further. The units have to be subdivided less often than *movement* units. High scores for the raw agreement on *act as a unit* again suggest that this value occurs less often. The establishment of interrater agreement for the value *act as a unit* appears to be more difficult as scores vary between 0.41 and 0.51.

16.2 Filter of segmentation processes and interrater agreement

In NEUROGES the analysis and the corresponding segmentation of movement behaviour becomes more and more fine grained after each step of coding. There is less possibility for further segmentation in Module II or III and most (sub-) units have to be created when annotating the Structure values.

In order to assess the agreement purely based on the raters' identification of the value, a filter was created, which excludes all units where segmentation differs, i.e., where the raters did not agree on the number of (sub-)units and/or the start and end of a given unit. The filter operates according to following restrictions:

a. The overlap between the units created by Rater 1 (R1) and Rater 2 (R2) is greater than 85% of the duration of the unit created by R1.
b. The overlap between the units created by R1 and R2 is greater than 85% of the duration of the unit created by R2.
c. Neither the unit of R1 nor the unit of R2 is shorter than 85% of the duration of the unit of the other Rater.
d. The overlap between the units created by R1 and R2 is smaller than 115% of the duration of the unit created by R1.
e. The overlap between the units created by R1 and R2 is smaller than 115% of the duration of the unit created by R1.
f. Neither the unit of R1 nor the unit of R2 is longer than 115% of the duration of the unit of the other Rater.

Consequently, the filter excludes all annotations for which R1 and R2 disagree about the segmentation to a larger degree as demonstrated in Figure 1. Only the 3rd and 4th units of R1 and R2 are considered after this filter as for these units both raters agree on where the structure units start and end. Additionally, those units that do not have an unambiguous pendant in the annotations of the other rater are excluded. This filter is not suitable to establish interrater agreement with respect to overall reliability. Rather, it is a tool to simulate a situation where movements units are predefined. The interrater agreement only refers to the choice of the value of any given unit. This procedure is frequently used in gesture research: either units are predefined by the experimenter, or the regions of interest are determined by "extra-behavioural" aspects such as speech. In contrast, NEUROGES gives attention to temporal aspects and the phenomena of segmentation itself, which is neglected in other methods. Additionally, in NEUROGES any movement is considered and annotated for differing values. In contrast, several other investigations focus on specific kinds of movements or gestures, such as gestures with iconic content, only (see for instance, Mol et al., 2009; Duncan, 2002)

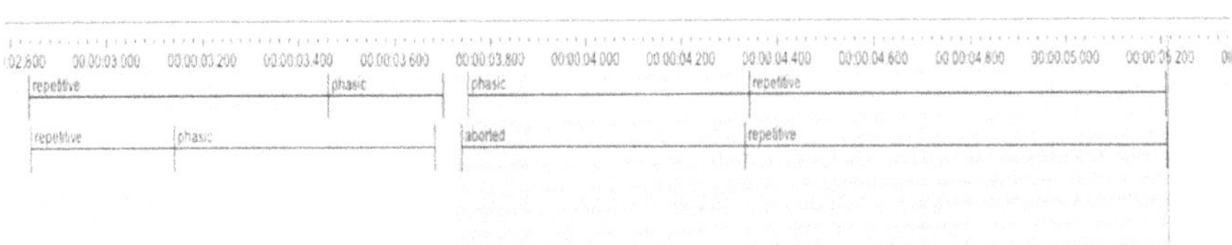

Figure 1 Units considered after filter

The filter was applied to the Structure annotations of the Stroke Study to exemplify the effects of the segmentation processes. In the analysis of the Stroke

Study, both raters annotated all steps of Module I and merged their transcriptions afterwards. This procedure implies that disagreements on the level of Activation to permeate to the Structure level. Table 5 shows the values of the modified Cohen's Kappa (see Chapter 15) for all annotations as well as for the filtered annotations.

Table 5 Comparison of modified Cohen's Kappa (Holle & Rein) pre and post filter

Value	**Modified Cohen's Kappa (raw agreement)**	**Modified Cohen's Kappa (raw agreement) after filter**	**Number of Units pre/post filter (33%)**
Irregular	0.38 (0.83)	0.79 (0.95)	557/155 (28%)
Phasic	0.46 (0.77)	0.85 (0.93)	832/380 (37%)
Repetitive	0.56 (0.88)	0.85 (0.95)	540/222 (41%)
Shift	035 (0.91)	0.75 (0.98)	263/50 (19%)
Aborted	0.36 (0.93)	0.84 (0.98)	204/52 (25%)

Only two thirds of the units passed the filter (33% remaining). *Phasic* and *repetitive* units were less affected than the other values. Simultaneously, the modified Cohen's Kappa values for each Structure value improved at least around 0.3 (e.g. for *repetitive*). As mentioned above, the values for *shift* and *aborted* after the filter can only be interpreted cautiously as the number of analyzed units is very low.

This exemplary analysis suggests two conclusions for assessing and interpreting the interrater agreements of NEUROGES codings according to the modified Cohen's Kappa (see Chapter 15). First, it highlights the impact and the potential difficulties arising when two observers segment human movement behaviour separately. In the case of the Structure values according to NEUROGES, this can be demonstrated by the following examples:

i. Both raters observe two complex phases (strokes), which do not differ in trajectory. Whereas Rater 1 observes a *rest position* in between the complex phases, Rater 2 does not. Accordingly, Rater 1 creates two *phasic* units and Rater 2 one *repetitive* unit.
ii. Both raters observe a *repetitive* complex phase. Whereas Rater 1 observes a retraction phase following this complex phase, Rater 2 creates an additional *phasic* unit as s/he observes an additional complex (e.g. volitional squeeze on the thigh) before the hand rests on the knee.

Consequently, one should emphasize during training the identification and analysis of complex hand movement behaviour (see Chapter 12). For analyzing strings of complex phases a high proficiency in detecting several (different) complex phases and distinguishing complex phases from transport/retraction phases appears to be necessary.

However, these results also indicate that the agreement for the NEUROGES Structure values is good when raters would code predefined units. According to Shroud (1998), the above post-filter scores are moderate to substantial, according to Landis and Koch (1977), they are even substantial to almost perfect. To agree on Structure values does not seem to be as difficult as to agree on the segmentation of movement. The segmentation, however, forms the basis for the value annotations. The differentiation between the Structure values as such is quite robust.

16.3 Recommendations for coding and consensus procedure

The juxtaposition of Kappa values demonstrates, that it is advisable to establish and guarantee consensus about designation of units for each coding step. Consequently, interrater agreement and consensus about the segmentation of movement should be established after each coding step before proceeding with the next step. The procedure for calculating the interrater agreement for the Activation category with the Compare Annotator function is outlined in Chapter 14, the procedure for all other categories with the Modified Cohen's Kappa is explained in Chapter 15.

First, the raters code the Activation category for the shared 25% of the data. Then they calculate the interrater agreement with Merged Compare Annotator function.

If the agreement for the Activation category is acceptable in analogy to previous studies, i.e., the Merged Compare Annotator value is > 0.75, the 100%-Rater continues to code the remaining 75% of the data. The value of > 0.75 is recommended based on the previous values presented in table 1.

If the agreement is not acceptable, i.e., < 0.75, the two raters should discuss their codings, if possible with the trainer. Based on these discussions, they should create consensus files of the 25 % of the data. Then, they should independently code another 25% of the data and calculate interrater agreement again. The 100%-Rater should only continue alone, if an agreement of > 0.75 was achieved. Otherwise, again consensus files have to be created.

For coding the Structure category, both raters use the *movement* units of the 100%-Rater or, if it applies, the consensus units in order to avoid that differences in segmentation in the Activation category permeate to the level of the Structure category.

First, the raters code the Structure category for the shared 25% of the data then they calculate the interrater agreement with the Modified Cohen's Kappa. If the agreement for the Structure category is acceptable, the 100%-Rater continues to code the remaining 75% of the data. It appears to be difficult to exactly define which scores are acceptable and which are not. Nevertheless, Table 6 is supposed to provide a guideline for good interrater agreement, which rater dyads should aim to establish after optimizing the procedure and consensus.

Table 6 Recommended Modified Cohen's Kappa interrater agreement scores for the Structure values

phasic	*repetitive*	*shift*	*aborted*	*irregular*
0.5 - 0.7	0.5 - 0.7	0.6	0.5	0.5 - 0.7

Note that these recommendations are estimations based on previous studies conducted by well trained raters and calculations on segmentation processes and that agreement can strongly depend on complexity and amount of data. If, for instance, interrater agreement for one participant is based on 45 seconds of data, in which this person performs only five units it is hard to establish the precise interrater agreement.

If the agreement is not acceptable, the two raters should discuss their codings, if possible with the trainer. Based on these discussions they should create consensus files of the 25 % of the data. Then, they should independently code another 25% of the data and then calculate the interrater agreement again. Quite often, it turns out that a large amount of differences are either caused by systematic differences in annotations or, on a smaller level, systematic differences occur when annotating a specific participant. In these cases, a general consensus should be obtained. The 100%-Rater can only continue alone, if an acceptable agreement was achieved or visual inspection suggests a good agreement. Before proceeding with the next step (Focus), the raters should create a consensus file, in which they agree on the annotations.

The procedure for the categories Focus, Contact, and Formal Relation is analogous to that for the category Structure. However, the agreement scores based on the modified Cohen's Kappa should be generally higher unless a very high raw agreement suggests that these values are relatively rare. In these cases it is also advisable to review the few occurrences of units of this value (e.g. *act as a unit*).

References

Broaders, S.C., Cook, S.W., Mitchell, Z., & Goldin-Meadow, S. (2007). Making children gesture brings out implicit knowledge and leads to learning. *J Exp Psychol Gen, 136*(4), 539-550.

Cocks, N. Dipper, L., Middleton, R., & Morgan, G. (2011). What can iconic gestures tell us about the language system? A case of conduction aphasia. *International Journal of Language and Communication Disorder, 46(4),* 423-436.

Duncan, S. (2002). Gesture, verb aspect, and the nature of iconic imagery in natural discourse. *Gesture.*183-206

Landis, J.R., & Koch, G. G. (1977). The measurement of observer agreement for categorical data. *Biometrics, 33*(1), 159-174.

Mol, L., Krahmer, E., & Swerts, M. (2009) Alignment in Iconic Gestures: Does it make sense? In Theobald, B-J. & Harvey, R. W. *The eighth international conference on auditory-visual speech processing, Norwich, United Kingdom.* 3-8.
Nicoladis, E., Maberry, R.I., & Genesee, F. (1999). Gesture and Early Bilingual Development. *Developmental Psychology. (2)*, 514 – 526.

Shrout, P.E. (1998). Measurement reliability and agreement in psychiatry. *Stat Methods Med Res, 7*(3), 301-317.

VI. Evaluating Data on Movement Behaviour

17. Statistical Evaluation and Data Presentation

Uta Sassenberg, Ingo Helmich

17.1 Introduction

In this chapter, we provide information on how to export, evaluate, and present NEUROGES-data. We first recommend which measures of hand movements can be analyzed in a meaningful way. Here, it is important to distinguish between (i) the frequency of movement values, (ii) the duration of movement values, and (iii) the proportion of time spent with movement values. Movement unit *frequency* is calculated as the mean number of value units per minute (number / minute) of the coded video duration. *Proportion of time* is calculated as the sum duration of all units of the coded video duration divided by time units (seconds / minute), and sum of *duration* of each units divided by the number of units (seconds / unit). These three measures provide information with different aims (see below). Second, we offer a step-by-step procedure for the export of the NEUROGES-data from ELAN. Finally, we report frequency, duration, and proportion of time of different hand movement values coded with the NEUROGES-system to offer reference data for adults for different types of study designs: (i) monologue-like descriptions of regular activities, such as making coffee, and (ii) interactive semi-standardized interview situations.

17.1.1 Different measures of body movements

Hand movement **frequency** (F) is the mean number of value units per minute. It is calculated to control the amount of movements that occur per minute (i.e., for each participant: the total number of units of one movement value divided by the duration in minutes of the participant's video sequence that was coded with NEUROGES-ELAN). **Duration** (D) describes the mean duration in seconds of each movement value unit (i.e., raw sum of duration in seconds divided by raw number, or the proportion of time divided by frequency). The third parameter for movement analysis is the **proportion of time** (PoT) as seconds of a certain value per video minute (i.e., raw sum of duration in seconds divided by the video duration in minutes). We chose to express this measure in this way rather than giving the percentage as an analogy to the frequency measure and because previous research also expressed duration measures in seconds. Table 1 illustrates these three measures.

Table 1 A fictitious example of hand movement analysis (two minutes, Module I). Hand movement behavior is calculated as frequencies (per minute of video), duration (seconds per unit) and proportion of time (per minute of video). S = seconds, rh = right hand, lh = left hand.

A participant speaks for 2 minutes and produces the following hand movements:	**Frequencies (number per minute of video)**	**Duration (seconds per unit)**	**Proportion of time (seconds per minute of video)**
3 *phasic in space* (2 with the right hand: 2.130s and 0.650s, 1 with the left hand: 1.550s)	1 rh *phasic in space*, 0.5 lh *phasic in space*	1.390s rh *phasic in space*, 1.550s lh *phasic in space*	1.390s rh *phasic in space*, 0.775s lh *phasic in space*

It is important to analyze the data in relative measures for different reasons. Within one study, coded video times differ. Even if the time was controlled for within one study, relative measures are important to compare movements amongst different studies. For this point it is also important to take care reporting explicitly what is included in the coded video sequence, e.g. including or excluding the time the experimenter speaks or the time the participants are presented with stimuli.

Depending on the research question, frequency, duration, or proportion of time should be used as the preferred measure for meaningful analyses – or a combination. Frequency is an important measure of how often a particular movement value occurs. *Phasic* movements are usually best reported as frequencies. The proportion of time is usually a better measure to evaluate *irregular* movements.

Note that the frequency and duration of Structure units cannot be calculated based on the StructureFocus units, as one Structure unit may be further divided into several StructureFocus units. E.g. in Step 3 Focus coding, one *phasic* unit may become one *phasic in space* unit, or it may become one *phasic in space* unit, one *phasic on body* unit, and one *phasic in space* unit. In the latter case, these *phasic* units add up to three, while originally in Step 2 Structure coding, there was only one *phasic* unit. Therefore, the frequency and duration of Structure units cannot be calculated based on StructureFocus data. The proportion of time, however, is a correct parameter that can be used to calculate the Structure based on StructureFocus data, as the proportion of time is not dependent on unit segmentation. Likewise, if one wishes to evaluate the Focus data alone, i.e., independent of the Structure, e.g. the question how much time is spent with *on body* movements (independent of whether they are *phasic*, *repetitive,* or *irregular*), one may calculate the proportion of time of a certain Focus value based on the StructureFocus values.

Duration can be used to investigate the time a movement value typically lasts (see 2.4). After introducing the reference values, presented later in this chapter, these points will become clearer.

17.1.2 Exporting NEUROGES-data from ELAN for statistical analysis

Here, we recommend how to export NEUROGES-data from ELAN (Version 4.1) to Excel (Microsoft Office 2008) as a preparation for further import into a statistical software (e.g. SPSS, IBM, SPSS Statistics). We provide a step-by-step description targeted to beginners for the use of NEUROGES-ELAN but we do assume a certain experience with Excel. Please note that there might be other and simpler ways to export the data, especially when other software is used and when software is further developed.

Open **ELAN** and choose File – Export Multiple Files As ▹ Tab-delimited Text…

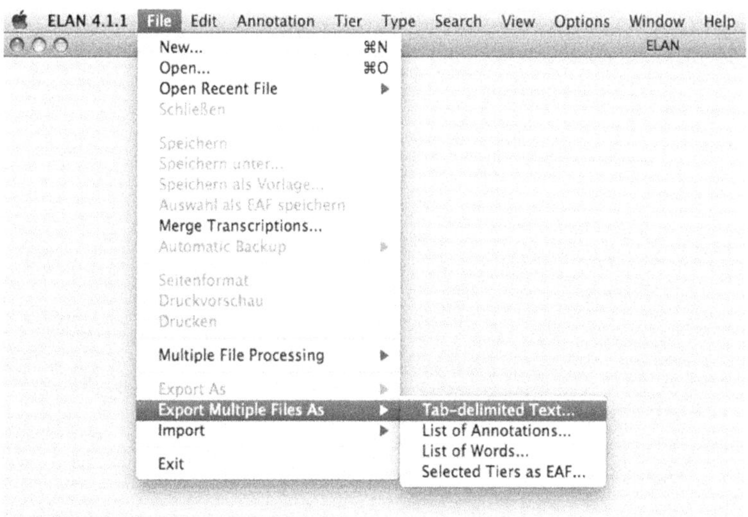

Figure 1 Export in ELAN

New Domain...: select all ELAN-files that you want to export (by highlighting them and clicking on arrows >> to make them appear in "Selected Files").
OK and save.

Export tiers as tab-delimited text: Select all tiers that you want to export[28].

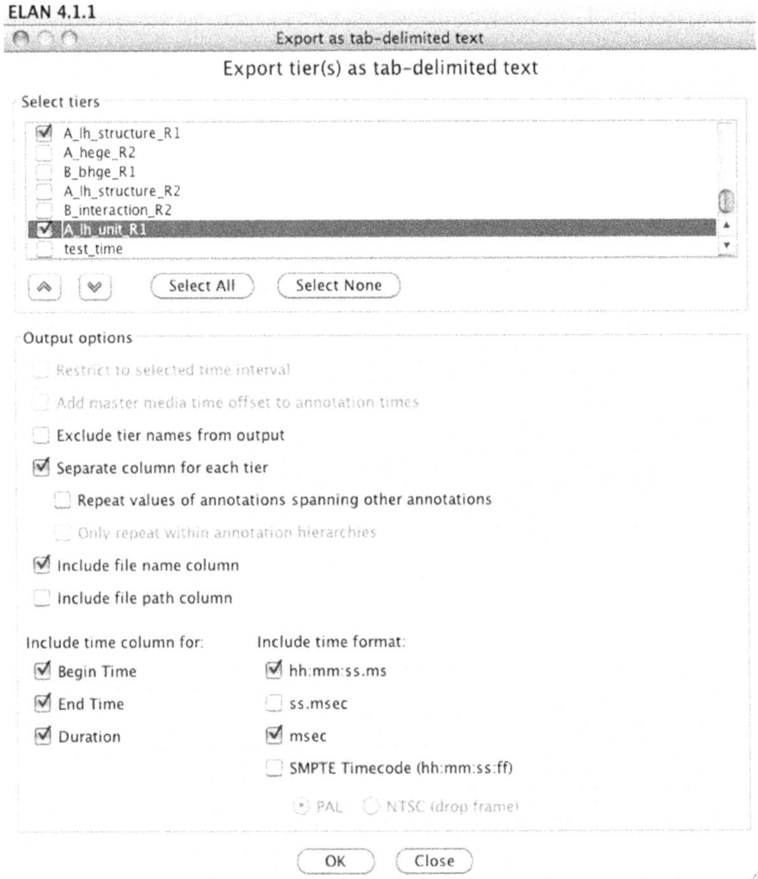

Figure 2 Select tiers and their output options in ELAN

28 Note that in Module I you cannot derive frequencies of Structure values from the tier StructureFocus (see above). Hence, if you analyze frequencies of Structure values and StructureFocus values, you will have to export both tiers.

Output Options:
Select the following (and deselect all others!): Separate column for each tier. Include file name column.

Include time column for:
3 Begin time
3 End time
3 Duration

Include time format:
3 hh:mm:ss.msec[29]
3 msec[30]

OK and save as a text file.

Open **Text** file: Select all, copy. Open new Excel-file: paste and save.

Within the **Excel** file: Tidy up your data.
Delete the following columns:
Begin time – msec
End time – msec
Duration – hh:mm:ss.msec

Change the column "File name" into "Participant number" or "Participant name":
Select the column "File". Edit – Replace…
For each participant, copy the file name and replace it with the participant number/name: Replace all.

Name Excel sheet (e.g., "Export") and save.

Create Pivot tables:
per tier 2 tables – one for frequencies (frequency of tier), one for duration of hand movements. This gives you the raw frequencies and raw durations. Save each pivot table within a new Excel sheet and name them.

Create a new Excel sheet for a summary of the raw data:
Create columns for the participants (copy and paste from one pivot table), the duration of the video in minutes (if you have it in seconds or milliseconds – change it), raw frequencies and raw durations of all exported tiers from the pivot tables.

Change durations in msec into durations in seconds.

29 This might be helpful for the beginning and end time if you want to look up a particular hand movement in your ELAN file.
30 This format will be used for durations of hand movements.

Copy the new table into another Excel sheet for creating relative frequencies and relative duration measures for further export into a statistical software:

Frequency: number / minutes of video registration
Duration: seconds / number
Proportion of time: seconds / minutes of video registration

17.1.3 Reference data for different contexts

Another aim of this chapter is to offer frequency, duration, and proportion of time of hand movement values of the NEUROGES coding system to serve as a reference frame for future studies. We only report StructureFocus values for Module I.

The three study designs reported here have the following points in common: The overall settings were psychological experiments. Video cameras were visible. There was one experimenter and one participant. Participants were not told beforehand that hand movements were the focus of the study. The adult German participants produced natural language with German as their first language. The studies are (i) monologue-like descriptions of regular activities, such as making coffee, and interactive semi-standardized interview situations with (ii) emotional scenarios (LEAS), and (iii) an intelligence test (HAWIE). They are described in detail in the Method section below. Differences between the study designs are presented in Table 2.

Table 2 Differences in the study design of the three experiments

	Regular activities	**LEAS**	**HAWIE**
Participants	n=27, female and male	n=17, male	n=17, male
Length of coded video	Approx. 2 minutes – only participant's speaking time	Approx. 14 minutes	Approx. 15 minutes
Coded video including/excluding experimenter	excluding	including	including
Experiment	Description of regular activities	Interview of emotional content	Interview of cognitive content
Assumed stress level	Lowest	Medium	Highest

17.2 Methods

17.2.1 Sample and procedure: description of regular activities (i)

27 German speakers participated for course credit or feedback (18 female, 9 male; aged 19 - 65 years, mean [*M*] = 28.2, standard deviation [*SD*] = 11). They all reported to be right-handed. At a later stage, 19 of the 27 participants completed the Edinburgh Handedness Inventory (EDI, Oldfield, 1971) and the Montreal Handedness Questionnaire (Crovitz & Zener, 1962). According to the EDI, all of the subsample were right-handed, and according to the Montreal Questionnaire, 10 were right-handed, and 9 ambidextrous.

Participants sat opposite the experimenter and a video-camera[31], and they were asked in random order to describe concretely and in detail four regular activities: *Making coffee* with a coffee machine, *Changing batteries* in an alarm clock, *Going by bus*, and *Ordering pizza* over the telephone. These activities are effective to elicit reliable written responses (Raisig, Welke, Hagendorf & van der Meer, 2009). The activities were chosen so that two were rated as frequent activities (making coffee, going by bus) and two as infrequent activities (changing batteries, ordering pizza; cf., Raisig et al., 2009). One frequent and one infrequent activity involved more manual behavior (making coffee, changing batteries) and one frequent and one infrequent activity involved less manual behavior (going by bus, ordering pizza). To limit the variability of responses, participants saw stimulus pictures showing the relevant object (e.g., a coffee machine) for each activity. On average, participants talked for about 2 minutes (*M* = 139 seconds; *SD* = 67) to describe all four regular activities (measured from the beginning to the end of their descriptions, i.e., excluding the time the experimenter asked for the descriptions). Figure 3 presents the pictures and an example description by one participant.

31 For a detailed description how to set up a hand movement research site see Appendix.

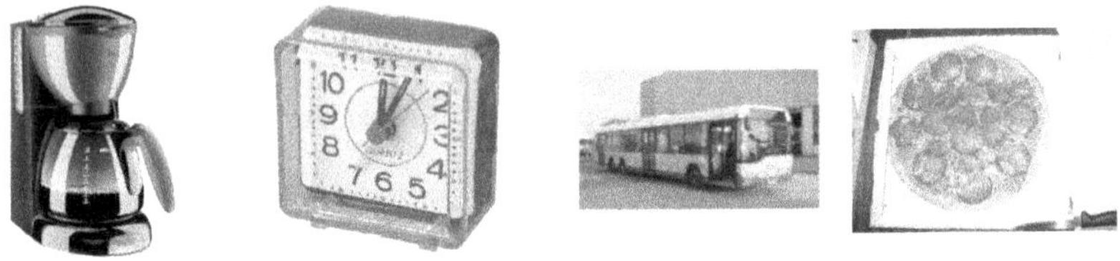

Making coffee *Changing batteries* *Going by bus* *Ordering pizza*

Changing batteries – German

P: Okay. Also erstmal nehm ich den Wecker hoch. Dann mach ich die Klappe unten auf wo die Batterie ja drinne ist.
E: Hmhm.
P: Dann pack ich die weg auf n sch- Nachttisch. Dann nehm ich die Batterie die ich vorher schon zurecht gelegt hab. Pack die rein.
E: Hmhm.
P: Und denn mach ich... nehm ich die Klappe wieder und mach zu und dann stell ich ihn wieder hin und stell ihn nochmal.
E: Hmhm.
P: Jo.

Changing batteries – English translation

P: Okay. Well first I pick up the alarm clock. Then I open the flap at the bottom in which the battery is.
E: Hmhm.
P: Then I put it away on the night table. Then I take the battery that I have already put in place. Insert it.
E: Hmhm.
P: And then I... I take the flap again and close it and then I put it [the alarm clock] back and set it [the alarm clock] again.
E: Hmhm.
P: Yeah.

Figure 3 Stimulus pictures and an example description by one participant in German with English translations (P = Participant; E = Experimenter).

17.2.2 Sample and procedure: semi-standardized interviews

17 German speakers participated in interview situations with (ii) emotional content and (iii) an intelligence test (sex: male; all right-handed according to the Edinburgh Handedness Inventory (Oldfield, 1971) and the Montreal Handedness Questionnaire (Crovitz & Zener, 1962); aged 20 - 59 years, $M = 36.2$, $SD = 12.5$). Participants sat opposite the interviewer in an interactive semi-standardized interview situation (same setting, one of two female interviewers). The participant and the interviewer were recorded by a video-camera without knowing that hand movements were the main objective of investigation (Figure 4).

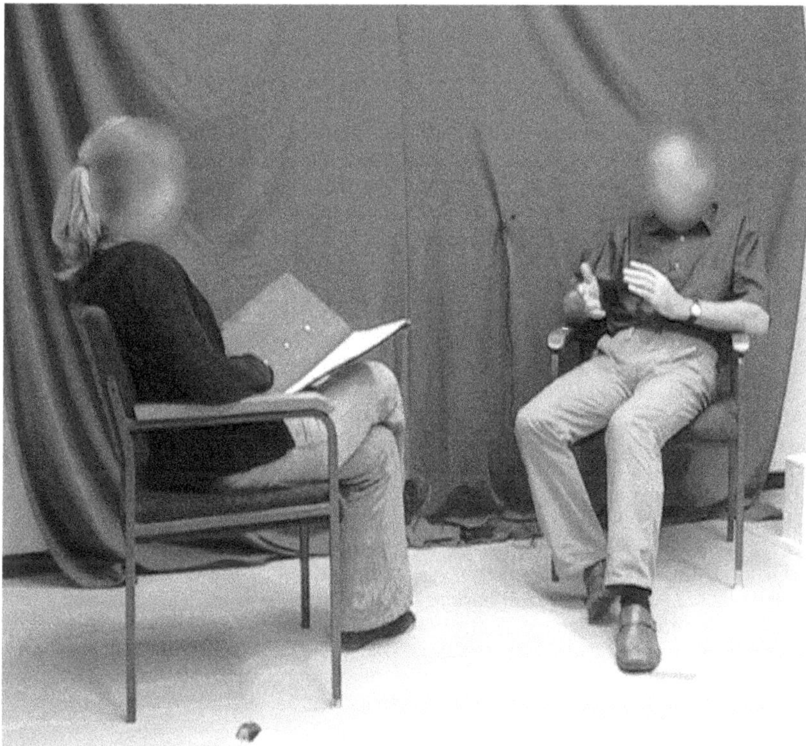

Figure 4 Semi-standardized interview situation of the experimenter (left) and the participant (right) in the semi-structured interviews.

During the interview, participants answered verbally to two different questionnaires: (ii) the Level of Emotional Awareness Scale (LEAS, part B) and (iii) the Hamburg-Wechsler Intelligence Scale for Adults (HAWIE).

With the LEAS, different states of sensitivity to internal emotional states can be identified. It shows the ability of people to be aware of their own feelings and to verbalize them (Lane et al., 1995). Table 3 presents an example interview situation by one participant. The mean duration of the LEAS-interview was 14 minutes (*M* = 14 min., *SD* = 4.32, *Minimum* = 08 min., *Maximum* = 22 min.). The HAWIE is a test to measure intelligence with eleven subcategories. We used three subcategories of the test: information, arithmetics, and similarities.

Table 3 Example question (E) and answer (P) of one scenario in the LEAS in German with English translations (P = Participant; E = Experimenter).

LEAS – German	*LEAS – English translation*
E: Sie wandern mit einem ortskundigen Führer durch die Wüste. Der Wasservorrat ist schon seit Stunden aufgebraucht. Die nächste Quelle ist auf der Karte des Führers noch drei Kilometer entfernt. Wie würden Sie sich fühlen? Wie würde der Führer sich fühlen?	E: You walk with a local guide through the desert. The water supply is used up for hours. The next source is according to the map of the leader still three kilometers away. How would you feel? How would the leader feel?
P: Ich hätte Durst. Auf jeden Fall. Ich würde mich aber ... ich würde mich jetzt aber nicht sehr unwohl fühlen, weil ich weiß dass ... da ist jemand der ist ortskundig ... der weiß wo's zur Quelle geht. Auch wenn's noch drei Kilometer sind, die wir zu wandern haben. Also eher wohl, auch, wenn ich vielleicht Durst hätte. Der Ortskundige hätte eher das Gefühl, da ist jemand, der ist ein bisschen abhängig von ihm ... und ... äh ... von daher ein gutes Gefühl hat sozusagen ihm zu helfen zur Quelle zu kommen. Oder auch ein bisschen Stolz. Ich kann mich ja ans ... also ich weiß wie man zur Quelle kommt. Er nimmt sozusagen mich an die Hand ... komm ... wir deixeln das ... musst keine Angst haben.	P: I would be thirsty. In any case. I would but ... I would not feel very uncomfortable now because I know that ... there is someone who has local knowledge ... who knows how you get to the source. Even if it's still three kilometers, which we have to walk. So rather well even if I might be thirsty. The local guide would tend to feel there is someone who is a bit dependent on him ... and ... uh ... therefore he has a good feeling to help him to get to the water. Or even a little pride. I can myself ... I know how to get to the source. He takes me by the hand, so to speak ... come on ... we manage this ... no need to have fear.

Table 4 presents an example by one participant. The mean duration of the HAWIE-interview was 15 minutes (*M* = 15 min., *SD* = 3.07, *Minimum* = 11 min., *Maximum* = 21 min.). In this context, the two tests are used to create scenarios of emotional and cognitive content.

Table 4. Example dialogue elicited by one question in the HAWIE in German with English translations (P = Participant; E = Experimenter).

HAWIE – German	*HAWIE – English translation*
E: Vögel legen Eier - welche Tiere noch?	E: Birds lay eggs - which animals too?
P: Hm ... das sind die Dinger, ja. Aja, also ich denke an Hühner oder Enten oder ... das sind ja ... äh ... ich weiß nicht ... zählt ... ist ein Huhn ein Vogel?	P: Hmm ... these are these things, yes. Yes, so I think of chickens or ducks, or ... those are ... uh ... I do not know ... counts ... is a chicken a bird?
E: Ja	E: Yes

P: In dieser Hinsicht schon ... da komm ich jetzt ins Schleudern. Ich komm jetzt nicht drauf. Wenn ich an Tiere denke. Weiß ich nicht.	P: In this regard ... I'm coming into a tailspin. I do not get it. When I think of animals. I do not know.
E: Lassen Sie sich ruhig Zeit.	E: Take your time.
P: Ja? Ich komm da immer wieder auf Vögel. Wenn ich an Strauss denke, der legt ja auch Eier. Aber heißt ja auch Vogelstrauss. Hm. Wie ist das bei Schlangen glaube ich. Eine gewisse Art von Schlangen.	P: Yes? I'm back to the birds again. When I think of ostrich, they lay eggs, too. But yes, it is called ostrich. Hm. How is it with snakes? A certain kind of snake.

17.2.3 Calculating interrater agreement

All videotapes were digitized, and hand movements were coded with NEUROGES within the environment of ELAN without sound. The coding for the monologue-like descriptions of regular activities was done with an earlier version of the NEUROGES system that combined within a single step StructureFocus values within Module I of the right hand and of the left hand (i.e., one tier for each hand).

In the monologue-like descriptions of regular activities two independent raters evaluated the participant's videotaped movement behavior. Rater 1 coded 100% of the data and rater 2 coded 25% (i.e., one description by each participant, selected at random). Interrater agreement was established on the data that had been coded by both raters. This resulted in 1.065 s (about 18 min) of coded descriptions by the two raters. Interrater agreement was established with the Modified Cohen's Kappa (Chpater 15). Note that in Module I, the modified Cohen's kappa does not only refer to the raters' agreement concerning StructureFocus but also to the agreement concerning the segmentation, i.e., the timeframes of the hand movement unit.

In interview situations with emotional and cognitive content (LEAS, HAWIE), three independent raters evaluated the participant's videotaped descriptions. Raters 1 and 2 each coded 50% of the data, i.e., half of the participants each. Each test of each participant was segmented into quarters depending on the video duration. Rater 3 coded 25% of all interviews to establish the interrater agreement (i.e., a quarter of each test per participant). The order in which raters 1 and 2 coded which test first, the order in which the quarters were coded, and the decision which quarter of a test was coded by rater 3 were all pseudo-randomized to avoid coding habituation effects. Table 5 presents the interrater agreement scores for the Activation category as measured with the Compare Annotator function (Chapter 14) in the description of regular activities and the interview situations of emotional and cognitive content (LEAS, HAWIE). Table

6 show the modified Cohen's Kappa scores according to Holle and Rein (Chapter 15) for the Structure and Focus categories.

Table 5 Interrater agreement (Compare Annotator) for the Activation category

Activation	Hand	Description task (N = 25)	LEAS (N = 17)	HAWIE (N = 17)
movement	Rh	-	.73 ± .19	.70 ± .23
	Lh	-	.67 ± .23	.70 ± .09

Table 6 Interrater agreement (Modified Cohen's Kappa) for the Structure and Focus categories

Structure	Focus	Description task (N = 25)	LEAS (N = 17)	HAWIE (N = 17)
phasic		-	.63	.55
	In space	.35	.64	.59
	On body	.35	.56	.49
repetitive		-	.75	.71
	In space	.51	.72	.71
	On body	.32	.74	.72
irregular		-	.45	.26
	Within body	.80	.37	.33
	On body	.50	.50	.30
shift		.43	.56	.50
aborted		.42	.46	.16

17.2.4 Statistical analyses

Analyses were performed on all hand movements displayed by the participants that were coded by the raters who coded 100% of the data[32]. Analyses are reported for Module I Units, Structure and Focus. For the monologue-like descriptions of regular activities the video duration excluded the experimenter's turns, and for the interview situations, the video duration included the experimenter's turns. **Frequency** analyses were performed on hand movement rates to control for differences in participant's description time (i.e., for each participant: the number of all hand movement units of one value divided by the participant's video duration). **Duration** per participant was analyzed (i.e., for each participant: the seconds per value unit) to gain insights about the duration of different values. **Proportion of time** was analyzed to provide reference data on how long a hand movement value was produced in relation to the overall description time (i.e., for each participant: the sum of the durations of all hand movements of one

32 In the description task: Rater 1; in the interview situations: Raters 1 and 2

category divided by the participant's video duration). For **frequency**, **duration,** and **proportion of time**, repeated measures analyses of variance (ANOVA's) were used with Greenhouse-Geisser corrections when the assumption of sphericity was violated. Multiple post hoc pairwise comparisons were corrected with Bonferroni corrections. Significant results are reported at an alpha-level of $p < .05$ (two-tailed); non-significant results are not reported. For **duration** in the description of daily activities, we offer descriptive analyses because of the considerable amount of missing values. We present comparisons and descriptives in the order from the most frequent unit value - independent of hand choice - to the least frequent and from the longest to the shortest, respectively.

17.3 Results

17.3.1 Descriptions of regular activities

Hand movement units of different values (StructureFocus) and hand choice are examined for differences concerning frequency, duration and proportion of time in descriptions of regular activities.

Table 7 Frequency distribution of hand movement values (StructureFocus) in the description of regular activities.

	StructureFocus							
Hand	*irregular on body*	*irregular within body*	*phasic in space*	*phasic on body*	*repetitive in space*	*repetitive on body*	*shift*	*aborted*
Lh	19/27	2/27	26/27	22/27	15/27	8/27	24/27	13/27
Rh	18/27	4/27	27/27	24/27	19/27	8/27	24/27	11/27

Frequency

To test whether participants produced value units with different frequency, we performed an 8 (StructureFocus: *phasic in space, phasic on body, repetitive in space, repetitive on body, irregular on body, irregular within, aborted, shift*) x 2 (hand: right, left) ANOVA on the mean frequency per minute of StructureFocus units (Fig. 5). There was a main effect of StructureFocus, $F(7,182) = 38.222$, $p < .001$. Pairwise comparisons confirmed that *phasic in space* units were produced more often than any other value (e.g. vs. *irregular on body* units, $MD = 4.557$, $SE = 1.025$, $p < .01$). *Irregular on body* units were produced more often than *aborted* units ($MD = 1.995$, $SE = 0.561$, $p < .05$), *irregular within body* units ($MD = 2.230$, $SE = 0.632$, $p < .05$), and *repetitive on body* units ($MD = 2.293$, $SE = 0.562$, $p < .05$). *Shifts* were produced more often than *aborted* units ($MD = 1.062$, $SE = 0.219$, $p = .01$) and *repetitive on body* units ($MD = 1.360$, $SE = 0.245$, $p < .001$). *Phasic on body* units were produced more often than *aborted* units ($MD = 0.705$, $SE = 0.201$, $p < .05$) and *repetitive on body* units ($MD = 1.003$, $SE = 0.190$, $p < .001$). *Repetitive in space* units were produced more often than *repetitive on body* units ($MD = 0.703$, $SE = 0.172$, $p < .05$). There was no main effect of which hand was used. There was an interaction effect between StructureFocus and choice of hand, $F(7,182) = 3.893$, $p < .05$.

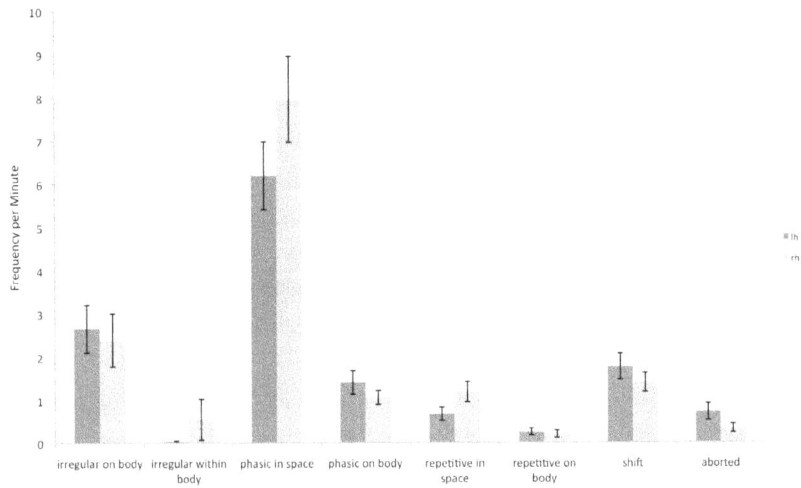

Figure 5 Frequency per minute of value units (StructureFocus) in the description of regular activities for the right and left hand. Error bars indicate the calculated standard error.

Duration

Due to the amount of missing data (Table 7), we report the observed value units and their durations descriptively (Fig. 6): *irregular on body* units were 3.83 seconds per unit (s/unit) (rh) and 3.70 s/unit (lh), *repetitive on body* units 2.39 s/unit (rh) and 3.02 s/unit (lh), *repetitive in space* units 2.13 s/unit (rh) and 2.39 s/unit (lh), *aborted* units 1.61 s/unit (rh) and 2.18 s/unit (lh), *irregular within body* units 2.26 s/unit (rh) and 0.85 s/unit (lh), *phasic in space* units 1.37 s/unit (rh) and 1.26 s/unit (lh), *phasic on body* units 1.07 s/unit (rh) and 1.06 s/unit (lh), *shift* units 2.18 s/unit (rh) and 0.92 s/unit (lh) long.

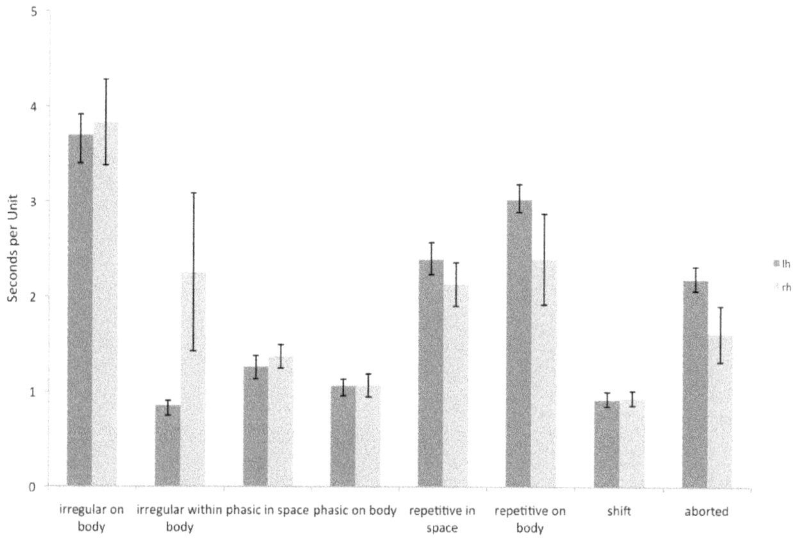

Figure 6 Duration of value units (StructureFocus) in the description of regular activities for the right and left hand. Error bars indicate the calculated standard error.

Proportion of Time

To test whether participants produced units with different proportions of time in the description of regular activities, we performed an 8 (StructureFocus: *phasic in space, phasic on body, repetitive in space, repetitive on body, irregular on body, irregular within, aborted, shift*) x 2 (hand: right, left) ANOVA on the proportion of time per minute of StructureFocus units (Fig. 7). There was a main effect of StructureFocus, $F(7,182) = 13.933$, $p < .001$. Pairwise comparisons confirmed that *irregular on body* units were produced for a longer proportion of time than *phasic on body* units ($MD = 8.653$, $SE = 2.448$, $p < .05$), *aborted* units ($MD = 8.861$, $SE = 2.546$, $p = .05$), *irregular within body* units ($MD = 9.270$, $SE = 2.651$, $p < .05$), and *repetitive on body* units ($MD = 9.334$, $SE = 2.498$, $p < .05$). *Phasic in space* units were produced for a longer proportion of time than all other unit values apart from *irregular on body* units (e.g. vs. *repetitive in space*: $MD = 6.985$, $SE = 1.015$, $p < .001$). There was no main effect of the choice of hand. There was an interaction effect between StructureFocus and choice of hand, $F(7,182) = 2.921$, $p < .05$.

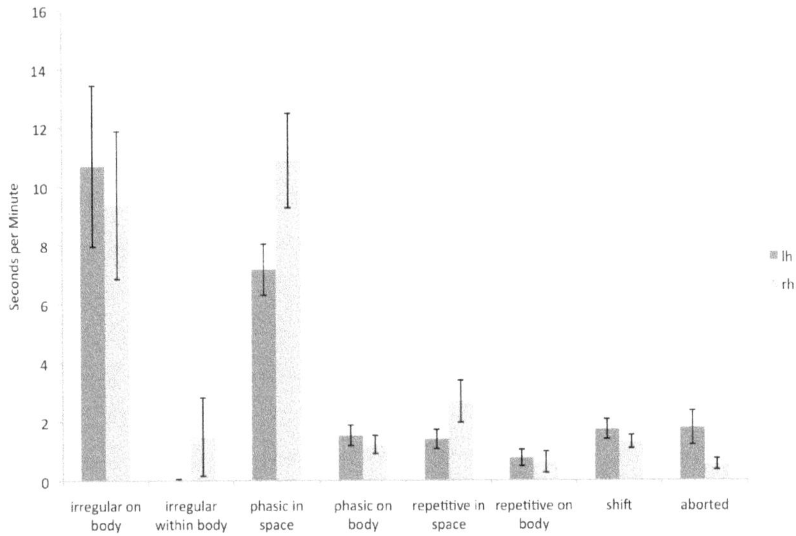

Figure 7 Proportion of time in seconds per minute of value units (StructureFocus) in the description of regular activities for the right and left hand. Error bars indicate the calculated standard error.

17.3.2 Semi-structured interview on emotional scenarios (LEAS)

Hand movement units of different values (StructureFocus) and hand choice are examined for differences concerning frequency, duration and proportion of time in the interview situation.

Table 8 Frequency distribution of hand movement values (StructureFocus) in the LEAS interview situation.

	StructureFocus							
Hand	*irregular on body*	*irregular within body*	*phasic in space*	*phasic on body*	*repetitive in space*	*repetitive on body*	*shift*	*aborted*
Lh	17/17	16/17	17/17	16/17	16/17	11/17	17/17	12/17
Rh	17/17	17/17	17/17	13/17	16/17	10/17	17/17	10/17

Frequency (LEAS)

To test whether participants produced value units with different frequencies in the LEAS interview situation, we performed an 8 (StructureFocus: *phasic in space, phasic on body, repetitive in space, repetitive on body, irregular on body, irregular within body, aborted, shift*) x 2 (hand: *right, left*) ANOVA on the frequency per minute of StructureFocus values (Fig. 8). There was a main effect of StructureFocus, $F(2.580, 41.275) = 34.903$, $p < .001$. Pairwise comparisons confirmed that *irregular on body* units were the units produced most often, significantly more often than *phasic on body* units ($MD = 2.433$, $SE = .324$, $p < .001$), *repetitive in space* units ($MD = 1.937$, $SE = .381$, $p < .01$), *repetitive on body* units ($MD = 2.491$, $SE = .342$, $p < .001$), *irregular within body* units ($MD = 1.637$, $SE = .436$, $p < .05$), *aborted* units ($MD = 2.499$, $SE = .340$, $p < .001$) and *shifts* ($MD = 1.871$, $SE = .300$, $p < .001$). *Phasic in space* units were the second most, significantly more frequent than *phasic on body* units ($MD = 2.187$, $SE = .209$, $p < .001$), *repetitive in space* units ($MD = 1.691$, $SE = .208$, $p < .001$), *repetitive on body* units ($MD = 2.245$, $SE = .231$, $p < .001$), *irregular within body* units ($MD = 1.391$, $SE = .297$, $p < .01$), *aborted* units ($MD = 2.253$, $SE = .222$, $p < .001$) and *shifts* ($MD = 1.625$, $SE = .196$, $p < .001$). The third most common units were *irregular within body*, produced more often than *phasic on body* units ($MD = .796$, $SE = .212$, $p < .05$), *repetitive on body* units ($MD = .853$, $SE = .201$, $p < .05$) and *aborted* units ($MD = .862$, $SE = .209$, $p < .05$). *Shifts* were produced more often than *phasic on body* units ($MD = .563$, $SE = .097$, $p < .01$), *repetitive on body* units ($MD = .620$, $SE = .099$, $p < .001$) and *aborted* units ($MD = .628$, $SE = .109$, $p < .01$). *Repetitive in space* units, the fourth most common StructureFocus, were produced more often than *aborted* units ($MD = .562$, $SE = .142$, $p < .05$). There was neither main effect of which hand was used nor an interaction between the choice of hand and StructureFocus.

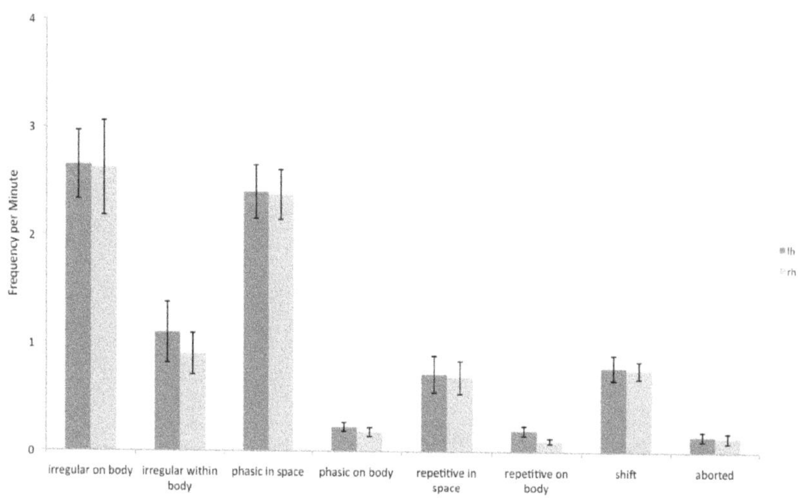

Figure 8 Frequency per minute of value units (StructureFocus) in the LEAS interview situation for the right and left hand. Error bars indicate the calculated standard error.

Duration (LEAS)

As there was less missing data (Table 8) than in the previous study of monologue-like descriptions of regular activities, for the LEAS interview situation, we performed an 8 (StructureFocus: *phasic in space*, *phasic on body*, *repetitive in space*, *repetitive on body*, *irregular on body*, *irregular within body*, *aborted*, *shift*) x 2 (hand: *right*, *left*) ANOVA on the duration of StructureFocus values (Fig. 9). For this calculation missing values were treated as "zeros". There was a main effect of StructureFocus, $F(3.311, 52.968) = 8.617$, $p < .001$. Pairwise comparisons confirmed that *irregular on body* units were produced for the longest duration (5.8 s/unit (rh) and 6.01 s/unit (lh)), significantly longer than *irregular within body* units ($MD = 3.391$, $SE = .691$, $p < .01$), *phasic in space* units ($MD = 3.796$, $SE = .766$, $p < .01$), *phasic on body* units ($MD = 3.048$, $SE = .805$, $p < .05$), *repetitive on body* units ($MD = 3.739$, $SE = .908$, $p < .05$) and *shifts* ($MD = 3.930$, $SE = .894$, $p < .05$). *Repetitive in space* units showed the second longest duration, 3.64 s/unit (rh) and 3.62 s/unit (lh), differing significantly from *phasic in space* units ($MD = 1.520$, $SE = .384$, $p < .05$). There was neither main effect of hand nor an interaction between the choice of hand and StructureFocus.

Calculating the duration of units for the "real data" (without replacing the missing values by "zeros"), durations for StructureFocuses change as follows (Figure 10), from the longest to the shortest: *irregular on body* (5.8 s/unit (rh) and 6.01 s/unit (lh), *aborted* (4.1 s/unit (rh) and 4.45 s/unit (lh), *repetitive in space* (3.86 s/unit (rh) and 3.85 s/unit (lh), *repetitive on body* (3.06 s/unit (rh) and 3.92 s/unit (lh), *phasic on body* (3.50 s/unit (rh) and 3.22 s/unit (lh), *irregular within body* (2.82 s/unit (rh) and 2.34 s/unit (lh), *phasic in space* (2.10 s/unit (rh) and 2.12 s/unit (lh) and *shifts* (1.90 s/unit (rh) and 2.06 s/unit (lh).

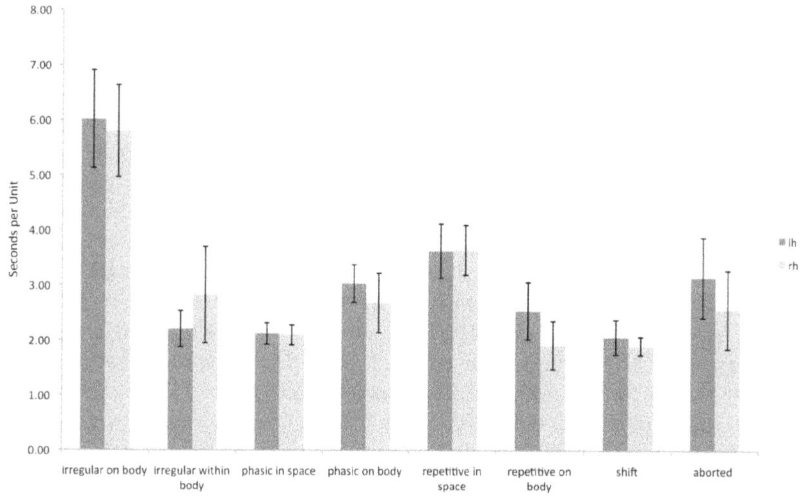

Figure 9 Duration of value units (StructureFocus) in the LEAS interview situation for the right and left hand. Error bars indicate the calculated standard error. Missing values were replaced with "zeros".

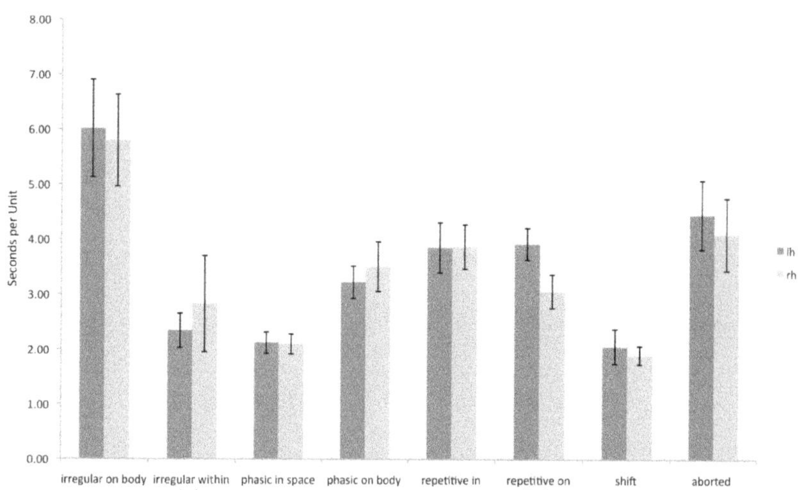

Figure 10 Duration of value units (StructureFocus) in the LEAS interview situation for the right and left hand for the "real data" (without replacing the missing values by "zeros"). Error bars indicate the calculated standard error.

Proportion of Time (LEAS)

To test whether participants produced value units of different proportions of time in the LEAS interview situation, we performed an 8 (StructureFocus: *phasic in space*, *phasic on body*, *repetitive in space*, *repetitive on body*, *irregular on body*, *irregular within body*, *aborted*, *shift*) x 2 (hand: *right*, *left*) ANOVA on the proportion of time per minute of StructureFocus values (Fig. 11). There was a main effect of the StructureFocus of unit, $F(1.412, 22.598) = 28.332$, $p < .001$. Pairwise comparisons confirmed that *irregular on body* units were produced for most of the time, significantly longer than *phasic in space* units ($MD = 10.458$, $SE = 2.261$, $p < .01$), *phasic on body* units ($MD = 15.038$, $SE = 2.479$, $p < .001$), *repetitive in space* units ($MD = 12.999$, $SE = 2.719$, $p < .01$), *repetitive on body* units ($MD = 15.112$, $SE = 2.522$, $p < .01$), *irregular within body* units ($MD = 13.297$, $SE = 2.380$, $p < .01$), *aborted* units ($MD = 15.025$, $SE = 2.553$, $p < .01$) and *shifts* ($MD = 14.270$, $SE = 2.404$, $p < .01$). *Phasic in space* units were produced the second-longest, significantly longer than *phasic on body* units ($MD = 4.581$ s/min, $SE = .622$, $p < .001$), *repetitive on body* units ($MD = 4.655$, $SE = .690$, $p < .001$), *aborted* units ($MD = 4.567$, $SE = .693$, $p < .001$) and *shifts* ($MD = 3.812$, $SE = .604$, $p < .001$). *Shifts* were produced more often than *phasic on body* units ($MD = .769$, $SE = .202$, $p < .05$). There was neither main effect of hand, nor an interaction between the choice of hand and StructureFocus.

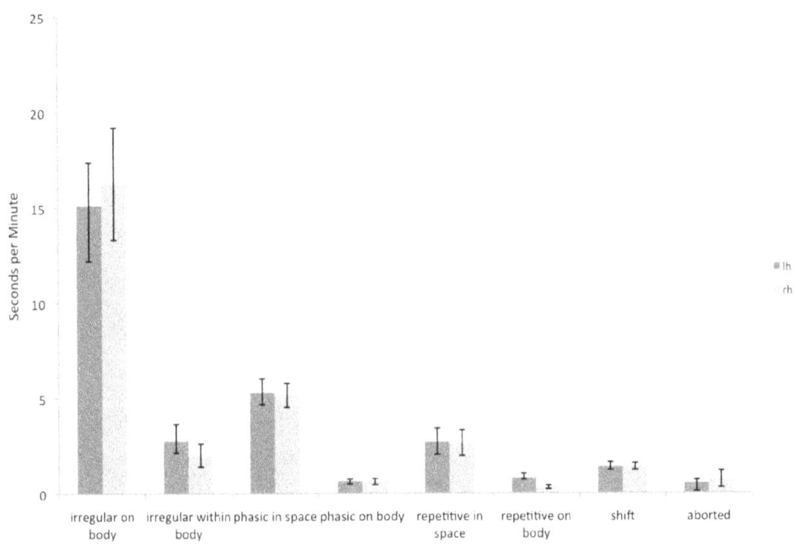

Figure 11 Proportion of time in seconds per minute of value units (StructureFocus) in the LEAS interview situation for the right and left hand. Error bars indicate the calculated standard error.

17.3.3 Semi-structured interview with intelligence test (HAWIE)

Table 9 Frequency distribution of hand movement values (StructureFocus) in the HAWIE interview situation.

	StructureFocus							
Hand	*irregular on body*	*irregular within body*	*phasic in space*	*phasic on body*	*repetitive in space*	*repetitive on body*	*shift*	*aborted*
Lh	16/17	16/17	17/17	16/17	14/17	16/17	17/17	12/17
Rh	17/17	16/17	17/17	15/17	14/17	12/17	17/17	7/17

Frequency (HAWIE)

To test whether participants produced value units of different frequency in the HAWIE interview situation, we performed an 8 (StructureFocus: *phasic in space, phasic on body, repetitive in space, repetitive on body, irregular on body, irregular within body, aborted, shift*) x 2 (hand: right, left) ANOVA on the frequency per minute of StructureFocus values (Fig. 12). There was a main effect of the StructureFocus, $F(2.267, 36.274) = 31.723$, $p < .001$. Pairwise comparisons confirmed that *irregular on body* units, the most often produced unit StructureFocus in the HAWIE situation, were more often produced than *phasic in space* units ($MD = 1.377$, $SE = .328$, $p < .05$), *phasic on body* units ($MD = 2.201$, $SE = .355$, $p < .001$), *repetitive in space* units ($MD = 2.251$, $SE = .330$, $p < .01$), *repetitive on body* units ($MD = 2.350$, $SE = .335$, $p < .001$), *irregular within body* units ($MD = 1.580$, $SE = .349$, $p < .05$), *aborted* units ($MD = 2.448$, $SE = .327$, $p < .001$) and *shifts* ($MD = 1.264$, $SE = .332$, $p < .05$). *Phasic in space* units were produced the second most, significantly more often than *phasic on body* units ($MD = .823$, $SE = .105$, $p < .001$), *repetitive in space* units ($MD = .874$, $SE = .096$, $p < .001$), *repetitive on body* units ($MD = .972$, $SE = .096$, $p < .001$) and *aborted* units ($MD = 1.071$, $SE = .100$, $p < .001$). *Irregular within body* units differed in their frequencies from *repetitive in space* units ($MD = .671$, $SE = .161$, $p < .05$), *repetitive on body* units ($MD = .770$, $SE = .169$, $p < .01$) and *aborted* units ($MD = .868$, $SE = .172$, $p < .01$). *Shifts* were produced more often than *phasic on body* units ($MD = .937$, $SE = .152$, $p < .001$), *repetitive in space* units ($MD = .987$, $SE = .196$, $p < .01$), *repetitive on body* units ($MD = 1.086$, $SE = .163$, $p < .001$) and *aborted* units ($MD = 1.184$, $SE = .183$, $p < .001$). There was neither main effect of which hand was used, nor an interaction between the choice of hand and StructureFocus.

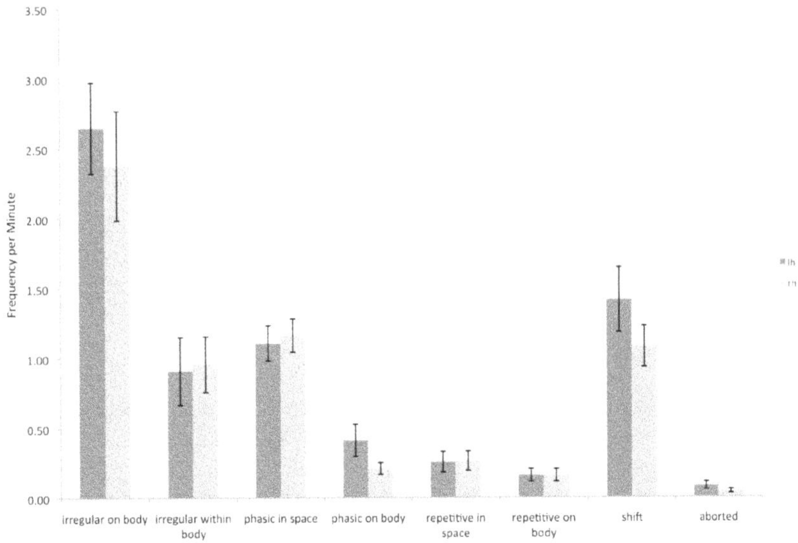

Figure 12 Frequency per minute of value units (StructureFocus) in the HAWIE interview for the right and left hand. Error bars indicate the calculated standard error.

Duration (HAWIE)

As there were less missing values (Table 9) than in the study of descriptions of regular activities, we performed an 8 (StructureFocus: *phasic in space*, *phasic on body*, *repetitive in space*, *repetitive on body*, *irregular on body*, *irregular within body*, *aborted*, *shift*) x 2 (hand: right, left) ANOVA on the duration of StructureFocus values (Fig. 13). For this calculation missing values were treated as "zeros". There was a main effect of StructureFocus, $F(3.720, 59.519) = 8.566$, $p < .001$. Pairwise comparisons confirmed that *irregular on body* units were produced for the longest duration (5.59 s/unit (rh) and 5.59 s/unit (lh)), significantly longer than *irregular within body* units ($MD = 3.632$, $SE = .652$, $p = .001$), *phasic in space* units ($MD = 3.224$, $SE = .632$, $p < .01$), *shifts* ($MD = 3.363$, $SE = .624$, $p < .01$) and *aborted* units ($MD = 2.746$, $SE = .647$, $p < .05$). Calculating the duration of units for the "real data" (without replacing the missing values by "zeros") presented in table 8, durations for the StructureFocuses change as follows (Fig. 14), from the longest to the shortest: *irregular on body* units were 5.59 s/unit (rh) and 5.94 s/unit (lh), *aborted* units 6.18 s/unit (rh) and 3.65 s/unit (lh), *repetitive on body* units 5.11 s/unit (rh) and 5.13 s/unit (lh), *repetitive in space* units 3.21 s/unit (rh) and 4.44 s/unit (lh), *phasic on body* units 3.64 s/unit (rh) and 3.56 s/unit (lh), *phasic in space* units 2.43 s/unit (rh) and 2.31 s/unit (lh), *shifts* 2.22 s/unit (rh) and 2.23 s/unit and *irregular within body* units 1.98 s/unit (rh) and 2.18 s/unit (lh) long.

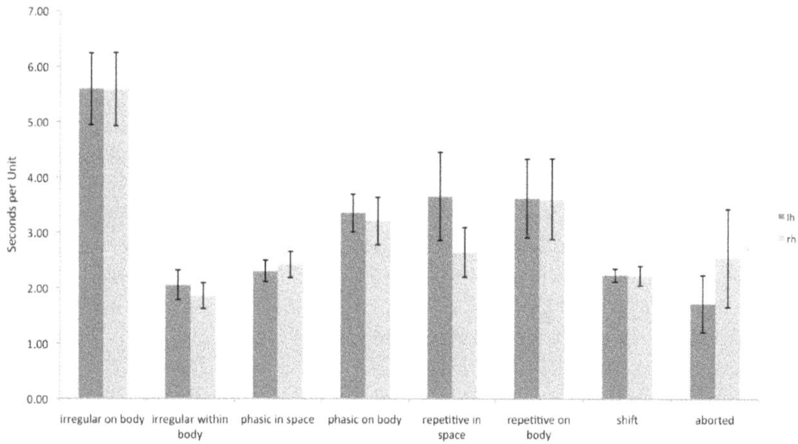

Figure 13 Duration of value units (StructureFocus) in the HAWIE interview situation for the right and left hand. Error bars indicate the calculated standard error. Missing values were replaced with "zeros".

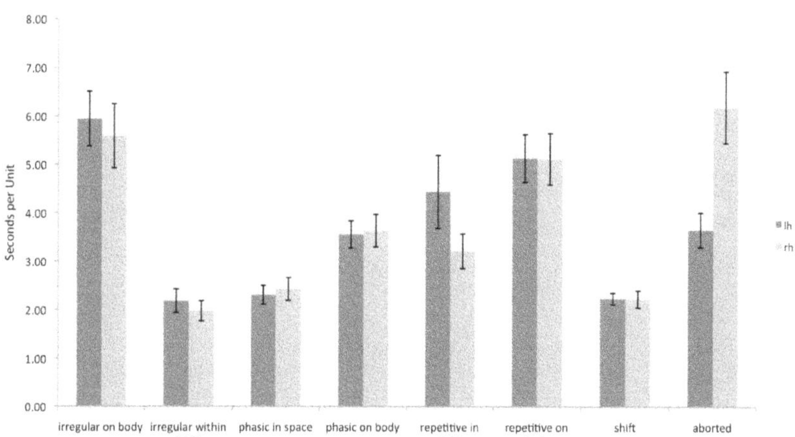

Figure 14 Duration of value units (StructureFocus) in the HAWIE interview situation for the right and left hand for the "real data" (without replacing the missing values by "zeros"). Error bars indicate the calculated standard error.

Proportion of Time (HAWIE)

To test whether participants produced units with different proportions of time in the HAWIE interview situation, we performed an 8 (StructureFocus: *phasic in space, phasic on body, repetitive in space, repetitive on body, irregular on body, irregular within body, aborted, shift*) x 2 (hand: right, left) ANOVA on the proportion of time per minute (Fig. 15). There was a main effect of the StructureFocus, $F(1.164, 18.622) = 24.752$, $p < .001$. Pairwise comparisons confirmed that *irregular on body* units were produced most of the time, significantly longer than *phasic in space* units ($MD = 12.661$, $SE = 2.705$, $p < .01$), *phasic on body* units ($MD = 14.015$, $SE = 2.797$, $p < .01$), *repetitive in space* units ($MD = 14.093$, $SE = 2.596$, $p < .01$), *repetitive on body* units ($MD = 14.424$, $SE = 2.737$, $p < .01$), *irregular within* units ($MD = 13.141$, $SE = 2.731$, $p < .01$), *aborted* units ($MD = 14.981$, $SE = 2.689$, $p < .01$) and *shifts* ($MD = 12.560$, $SE = 2.648$, $p < .01$). *Shifts* showed the second-longest duration, significantly longer than *phasic on body* units ($MD = 1.456$, $SE = .376$, $p < .05$), *repetitive on body* units ($MD = 1.865$, $SE = .365$, $p < .01$) and *aborted* units ($MD = 2.421$, $SE = .340$, $p < .001$). *Phasic in space* units were produced longer than *repetitive on body* units ($MD = 1.763$, $SE = .245$, $p < .001$) and *aborted* units ($MD = 2.320$, $SE = .272$, $p < .001$). *Irregular within body* units were produced longer than *aborted* units ($MD = 1.840$, $SE = .462$, $p < .05$). There was neither main effect of the choice of hand, nor an interaction between the choice of hand and StructureFocus.

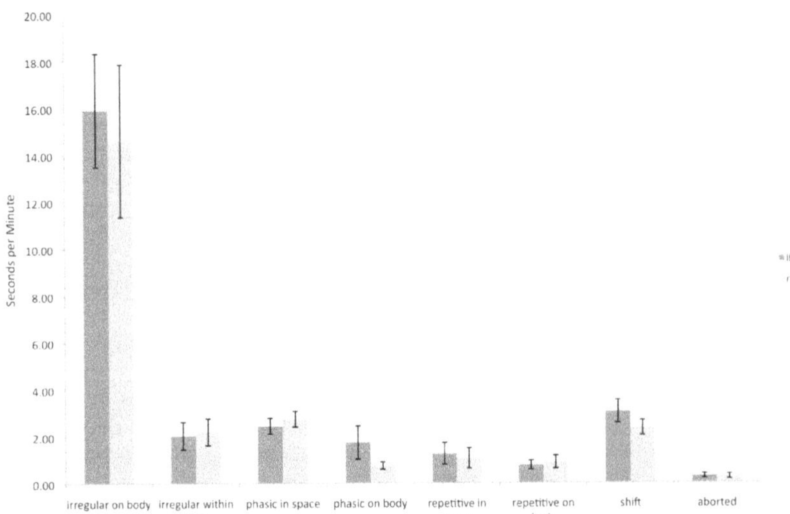

Figure 15 Proportion of time in seconds per minute of value units (StructureFocus) in the HAWIE interview situation for the right and left hand. Error bars indicate the calculated standard error.

17.4 Discussion

The present chapter is reported with two aims in mind. The first is to supply steps how to export and evaluate NEUROGES-data. The second aim is to provide reference data coded with the NEUROGES system in situations common to hand movement studies, namely monologue-like descriptions of regular activities and interactive semi-standardized interview situations. Apart from providing reference data, we shall discuss the obtained values and elaborate on the theoretical approaches.

17.4.1 Description of regular activities

The frequency of hand movements, providing information about which hand movement value is used the most, differed depending on the StructureFocus value. As expected for a descriptive task, *phasic in space* hand movements were produced most often. *Irregular on body* units, *shifts*, and *repetitive in space* units were produced with medium frequency. *Aborted, irregular within body,* and *repetitive on body* units were produced least frequent.

The choice of hand showed differences in the StructureFocus values. Reporting hand preferences of spontaneous hand movement behavior may be considered as the direct correlate of neuronal activation of the contralateral hemisphere of the moving hand (see 2.5). While there was a preference for the right hand for communicative hand movements (*phasic* and *repetitive in space*), there was a preference for the left hand in *on body* movements (*irregular*, *phasic* and *repetitive on body)* as well as for *shifts* and *aborted* units. Reporting the proportion of time of the StructureFocus value is of certain interest because *irregular* movements, in particular, tend to last longer than the units of other Structure values. *Irregular* units seem to start and end by chance and involuntarily, serving for auto-regulative reasons. Here, the proportion of time differed depending on the StructureFocus value: *Phasic in space* and *irregular on body* hand movements were produced for the longest and about equal in time. *Repetitive in space* and *on body, phasic on body, shifts* and *aborted* units were produced for a medium proportion of time. *Irregular within body* units were observed for a very short time and only for the right hand. The same proportion of time of *phasic in space* and *irregular on body* units in this experimental task might be caused by two reasons: first, the task was to describe regular activities resulting in *phasic in space* units for most of the time. Second, hand movements during the speaking time of the experimenter were excluded. Consequently, we do not know which Structure value was executed during this time. To evaluate the movement behavior during certain experimental situations in general, this needs to be further examined. Depending on the StructureFocus, we could also observe a difference in the choice of hand. Most of the time, communicative units (*phasic* and *repetitive in space*) were produced with the right hand. *On body* units (*irregular*, *phasic*, and *repetitive on body*) as well as *shift* and *aborted* units showed the opposite pattern. These hand movements revealed a preference for the left hand. As outlined in Subsection 2.5.3, several neuropsychological studies reported a left hand preference for *on body* hand movements ("self-touch", "grooming and fidgeting") as compared to a right hand preference for communicative hand movements ("free movements", "symbolic hand movements"), which are most often executed in space from the body (Blonder et al., 1995; Dalby et al., 1980; Kimura, 1973a, 1973b; Lavergne & Kimura, 1987; Saucier & Elias, 2001). This pattern of hand preference seems to be quite stable over the life span. It is even evident in babies aged 1 to 6 months (Trevarthen, 1996). The relative left hand preference for on body hand movements might indicate a right hemisphere activity (Hampson & Kimura, 1984; Verfaellie, Bowers, & Heilman, 1988), which is well compatible with psychological states of emotional stress and a need for internal regulation.

The duration also differed depending on the StructureFocus value. As expected, *irregular* and *repetitive* units were longer than *phasic* units. They were from longest to shortest: *irregular, repetitive, aborted, phasic*, and *shifts*.

17.4.2 Semi-structured interview on emotional scenarios (LEAS)

Frequencies of hand movements differed significantly depending on their value in the LEAS interview. The most frequent StructureFocus values were *irregular on body* units. For nearly the same amount and not significantly differing in their frequency from *irregular on body*, *phasic in space* units occurred in this experimental interview situation. The frequency of both values differed significantly from all other StructureFocus values. *Repetitive in space, irregular within body* units, and *shifts* were produced for a medium amount, *repetitive on body, phasic on body* and *aborted* units were produced the least. Narrations of the participants in the LEAS interview situation mainly contained three distinctions: describing (i) the participant's own feelings, (ii) the feelings of the second person and also (iii) giving explanatory details about the lifelike situation (the "stage") they put themselves and the second imaginary person in.

The high amount of *irregular on body* units differing significantly from all other StructureFocus values (except *phasic in space* units) is assumed to be caused by the large emotional content in the LEAS interview situation. The participants were asked to describe their own feelings to the interviewer and further, they had to empathize with someone else's feelings and describe those as well. *Irregular* body-focused hand movements are believed to have self-regulating functions (Ekman, Friesen, 1969) and are increased in stressful situations, negative emotional experiences or the more personal the topic becomes (Sousa- Poza und Rohrberg 1977; Freedman und Bucci 1981; Ulrich 1977) (see also Subsction 2.1.2). According to our findings, it can be assumed that during the LEAS interview situation the participants had to deal with strong emotional experiences that caused the high amount of *irregular on body* hand movements. To cope with this mental arousal, participants tried to compensate unconsciously, but effectively by *irregular on body* hand movements, as Freedmann and Bucci (1981) already postulated and Lausberg and Kryger (2011) further evaluated. It must be mentioned that participants rarely experienced this experimental situation before which might have influenced their emotional activation and therefore had an effect on the amount of body-focused activity. Another aspect that might have influenced *irregular* unit values is the fact that videos were coded for the whole time including the experimenter speaking time.

The high amount of *phasic in space* hand movements might be caused by the "interactive" and "communicative" interview situation in which the participants were asked to describe lifelike emotional situations to the interviewer (see Table 3 for one example). Participants often described not only their and the other person's feelings, they also created a "stage" and introduced imaginary details about their own or its participating person's situations before going into the emotional details. *Phasic* and *repetitive in space* hand movements are understood to be the classical communicative hand movement values that reflect conceptual processes as the gestural formation of a thought (Lausberg & Kryger, 2011). Therefore, *phasic in space* hand movements seem to offer the most compatible hand movement value to create and describe an imaginary scenario in a communicative way. In this experiment *phasic in space* hand movements are used extensively differing significantly from *repetitive in space* hand movements. Therefore, it can be assumed that the image, the participants were trying to explain, was very clear in their minds and did not need to be emphasized by an increased amount of *repetitive in space* hand movement units. To validate these hypotheses, additional data will be needed taking together hand movements and its synchronized speech content.

Neither significant differences were observed concerning the choice of hand nor any interaction effects of value and hand. This indicates that during the LEAS interview, no right hand preference for any kind of hand movement could be observed, not even for communicative hand movements like *phasic* or *repetitive in space* and despite the fact that all participants were right-handed. Furthermore, although not significant but still noteworthy, for any hand movement value during the LEAS interview we observed a trend towards a greater use of the left hand (Figure 8), also for the communicative hand movements. This might be due to the greater right hemispheric engagement in the description of emotional scenarios and is in line with the observations of Moscovitch and Olds (1982) regarding the fact that the more personal a topic, the greater the left-hand-use for communicative hand movements.

For the proportion of time of hand movements in the LEAS interview, *irregular on body* hand movements were produced for the longest period differing significantly from all other values (Figure 11). *Phasic in space*, *repetitive in space*, *irregular within body* hand movements and *shifts* were produced for a medium, *phasic on body*, *repetitive on body* and *aborted* hand movements were produced for the shortest time. The long proportion of time of *irregular* units fits well with the previous frequency analysis and also with the kinematic analysis of the

Structure values (Chapter 6). *Irregular* units, as already mentioned in the discussion of the description task, tend to last longer than the communicative hand movement Structures (*phasic, repetitive*) because they are missing the transport phase, the complex phase, and the retraction phase. *Irregular* hand movements do not demand a wide movement space as, for example, *phasic in space* hand movements who have a clear start and end point do. They usually take place in the same location, over a longer time period, e.g. "finger-kneading". Therefore it is important to distinguish in the analysis of hand movements the Structure value and to report frequencies as well as the proportion of time for the values.

Again, there were neither significant influences by the choice of hand nor any interaction effects of hand and unit value. Also, and in contrast to the description task, there was no clear right-hand preference for the communicative hand movements, even though all subjects were right-handed. This leads to the assumption that the spontaneously preferred hand, as a correlate for the current state of mind and its hemispheric lateralized functions, was influenced by the high emotional activation triggered by the LEAS interview situation that could be observed in the increased use of the left hand.

The duration of hand movement units in the LEAS interview situation was similar to the durations observed in the description task. *Irregular on body* and *repetitive in space* hand movements were the longest and *phasic in space* the shortest hand movements observed. The similar duration of values in different experiments shows that this facet of hand movement seems to be stable over different experimental settings. But as noted in Figure 9, 10 and table 8, *aborted* hand movements could not be observed in many participants. If the data is reported for the real values ($n_{aborted}$ = 10 (rh), $n_{aborted}$ = 12 (lh), table 8, figure 10), *aborted* units show the second longest duration after *irregular on body* units. The characteristic of this Structure value is the abortion of the movement after the preparation phase. The stopped hand movement might be retracted instantly or held for some time (here, 6.18 s/unit (rh) and 3.65 s/unit (lh)) leading to the assumption that the participant in the moment of an *aborted* hand movement hit upon an idea, but could not process his thought to an ultimate concept. Therefore, it might be a Structure value showing a person's uncertainty to figure out a cognitive formulated concept. Because this Structure value could not be observed in all participants, further studies would be needed to evaluate this phenomenon.

17.4.3. Semi-structured interview with intelligence test (HAWIE)

In the HAWIE interview, the most frequent StructureFocus value was *irregular on body* that differed significantly from all other values. *Phasic in space, irregular within* units and *shifts* were produced with a medium frequency and *phasic on body, repetitive on body* and *aborted* units were produced the least. The HAWIE interview measures intelligence, in this case by three chosen subcategories information, arithmetic and similarities. For the participants this test induces on the one hand a cognitively demanding as well as a stress inducing task. Participants were obliged to give correct answers to the questions that forced them to give a serious consideration about each topic. Knowing facts and communicating the responses resulted in a high amount of *phasic in space* hand movements. Not knowing the correct answer induced a highly stressful situation resulting in a high amount of *irregular on body* hand movements differing significantly from all other hand movement values. In line with Berridge et al. (1999), who could show that grooming attenuates in the right hemisphere of rats the prefrontal dopamine response to stress, subjects here seemed to cope with the emotional stress of the HAWIE interview by moving continuously in a body-focused manner, e.g. by kneading their hands, touching their face, etc. In human studies it is documented that spontaneous self-touch in the face due to unpleasant sounds increases the activity of beta and theta waves in the EEG (Grunwald and Weiss, submitted) that could explain the self-regulating effect of *on body* focused hand movements. Further, the HAWIE interview evoked a high amount of *shifts*. This Structure value is associated with a change of subject or a change of psychological states (see Subsection 5.1.2.2). The high amount of *shifts* (Figure 12) indicates a restless behavior of the participants due to the stressful situation of answering the questions correctly. The participants seemed to be anxious in solving the task, although they had to give serious consideration to each question. Significant differences in the choice of hands were not observed in the HAWIE but the data shows a trend of more left-hand-use for body-focused hand movements and an increased right-hand-use for the communicative hand movements. A right hand preference can be explained by the knowledge of facts and quick responses of the participants associated with more communicative hand movements towards the experimenter. The left hand preference was observed mainly for hand movements associated with arousal such as *shifts* and *irregular on body* hand movements possibly indicating a higher right hemispheric involvement due to the stress during experimental task. In the HAWIE interview, the highest proportion of time of hand movements was taken by *irregular on body* units. This differs significantly from all other hand movement values. *Phasic in space, irregular within body* units and *shifts* were produced for a medium, *phasic on body, repetitive on body* and *aborted* units were produced for the shortest proportion of time. The long proportion of time for *irregular on body* units compared to all other hand movement values fits with the nature of the movement Structure, since, as mentioned previously, *irregular* hand movements occur over a longer period. This is in line with the observations in the frequencies of the HAWIE interview. The long proportion of time of *shifts* (as long as *phasic in space* hand movements) confirms the subject's indisposition that results in a restless demeanor. The choice of hand was similar to the data observed in the frequencies. Durations of hand movements in the HAWIE interview situation were similar to the durations observed in the description task and in the LEAS interview situation. *Irregular on body* hand movements showed the longest duration, followed by *aborted* and *repetitive on body* units. But as mentioned before, *aborted* units had a high quantity of missing values.

17.4.4 Summary

While the description task is characterized in its frequencies by *phasic in space* units with the right hand, the LEAS and HAWIE showed increased *irregular on body* focused units accompanied by greater left hand use. Further, the LEAS interview situation showed the same amount of *phasic* and *irregular in space* units, while the HAWIE interview situation was characterized by *irregular in space* units and *shifts*. The fact that the speaking time of the experimenter was included in the LEAS and HAWIE experiments and not in the description task should not be disregarded. Excluding all hand movements during the speaking time of the experimenter might lead to less *irregular on body* units. This needs to be further evaluated by analyzing the data during the speaking time of the experimenter in the description task. Therefore, it is necessary to be careful when choosing the kind of experimental setup (see also Part IV) as well as the participants who will be compared to each other. Here, we focused on offering standard values of different experiments on hand movement behaviour to enable further standardized research in this scientific direction. In all, these results show that the context and the demanding task influence Structure, Focus and hand preference of hand movements and provide first standard values for designs with narratives and interview situations for further hand movement research. The findings are relevant for different disciplines of gesture research, such as computer science and neuropsychological research with patients. They strongly suggest that specific values are characterized by a specific duration (see also 2.4) that could contribute to a more natural appearance of artificial agents' gestural behavior when hand movement behavior is modeled in computer science. Furthermore, if the duration of hand movement values is reliable for healthy adults, it might be a better indicator for "normal" or "abnormal" hand movement behavior than hand movement frequency because frequency differs substantially between healthy individuals (Feyereisen, 1991). Therefore, with the offered values of these three experiments and future work with NEUROGES, it will be possible to refer to standardized hand movement values and collect coherent data of hand movements, to enable further research to make precise distinctions between varying values and the standard.

Acknowledgements

The regular activities study was funded by doctoral grants from *Studienstiftung des deutschen Volkes* and Berlin School of Mind and Brain. We gratefully thank Diana Funke for her help in designing the study, for collecting the data, and for her work as one of the raters. The semi-standardized interview study was funded by the *Deutsche Forschungsgemeinschaft* (German Research Foundation) within the Cluster of Excellence (302) "Languages of Emotion" (Project 307 "Implicit emotional processing"). We gratefully thank our colleagues of the "Berlin Alexithymia Inventory (Project 109) for their help in designing the study and collecting the data. Furthermore, we thank Monika Kryger and Anna Berger for their work as two of the three raters.

References

Alibali, M.W. (2005). Gesture in spatial cognition: Expressing, communicating, and thinking about spatial information. *Spatial Cognition and Computation, 5*(4), 307-331.

Berridge, C.W., Mitton, E., Clark, W., & Roth, R.H. (1999). Engagement in a Non-Escape (Displacement) Behaviour Elicits a Selective and Lateralized Suppression of Frontal Cortical Dopaminergic Utilization in Stress. *Synapse*, 32, 187-197.

Blonder, L.X., Burns, A.F., Bowers, D., Moore, R.W., & Heilman, K.M. (1995). Spontaneous Gestures Following Right Hemisphere Infarct. *Neuropsychologia, 33*, 203-213.

Cohen, J. (1960). A Coefficient of Agreement for Nominal Scales. *Educational and Psychological Measurement, 20*(1), 37-46.

Crovitz, H.F., & Zener, K. (1962): A group-test for assessing hand and eye-dominance. *American Journal of Psychology*, *75*, 271-6.

Dalby, J.T., Gibson, D., Grossi, V., & Schneider, R.D. (1980). Lateralized hand gesture during speech. *Journal of Motor Behavior, 12*, 292-297.

Ekman, P., Friesen W.V. (1969). The repertoire of non-verbal behavior. *Semiotica*, 1, 49-98.

Feyereisen, P. (1991). Brain Pathology, Lateralization, and Nonverbal Behavior. In: Feldman, R.S., Rimé, B. (Eds.) *Studies in Emotion and Social Interaction. Fundamentals of Nonverbal Behavior*, pp. 31–70. Cambridge University Press, Cambridge.

Freedman, N. (1972). The Analysis of Movement Behavior during the Clinical Interview. In: Siegman, A.W., Pope, B. (Eds.). *Studies in Dyadic Communication*, pp. 153-175. Pergamon, New York.

Freedman, N., & Bucci, W. (1981). On kinetic filtering in associative monologue. *Semiotica*, 34(3/4), 225-249.

Freedman N. & Hoffman S.P. (1967). Kinetic Behaviour in Altered Clinical States: Approach to Objective Analysis of Motor Behaviour during Clinical Interviews. *Perceptual Motor Skills, 24*, 527-539.

Grundwald, M., & Weiss, T. (submitted). Emotional Stress and Facial Self-Touch Gestures.

Hampson, E., & Kimura, D. (1984). Hand Movement Asymmetries during Verbal and Nonverbal Tasks. *Canadian Journal of Psychology, 38*, 102-125.

Kimura, D. (1973a). Manual Activity during Speaking - I. Right-Handers. *Neuropsychologia, 11*, 45-50.

Kimura, D. (1973b). Manual Activity during Speaking - II. Left-Handers. *Neuropsychologia, 11*, 51-55.

Kita S., de Condappa O., & Mohr C. (2007). Metaphor explanation attenuates the right-hand preference for depictive co-speech gestures that imitate actions. *Brain Language*, 101(3), 185-97.

Lane R.D., Kivley L.S., Du Bois A., Shamasundara P., & Schwart G.E. (1995). Levels of emotional awareness and the degree of right hemispheric dominance in the perception of facial emotion. *Neuropsychologia*, 33(5), 525-538.

Lausberg H., & Kita S. (2003). The content of the message influences the hand choice in co-speech gestures and in gesturing without speaking. *Brain Language*, 86(1), 57-69.

Lausberg, H., & Kryger, M. (2011). Gestisches Verhalten als Indikator therapeutischer Prozesse in der verbalen Psychotherapie: Zur Funktion der Selbstberührungen und zur Repräsentation von Objektbeziehungen in gestischen Darstellungen. *Psychotherapie-Wissenschaft, 1*, 41-55.

Lausberg, H., & Slöetjes, H. (2009). Coding Gestural Behaviour with the NEUROGES-ELAN System. *Behavior Research Methods, 41*(3), 841-849.

Lausberg, H., Zaidel, E., Cruz, R.F., & Ptito, A. (2007). Speech-Independent Production of Communicative Gestures: Evidence from Patients with Complete Callosal Disconnection. *Neuropsychologia, 45*(13), 3092-3104.

Lavergne, J., & Kimura, D. (1987). Hand Movement Asymmetry during Speech: No Effect of Speaking Topic. *Neuropsychologia, 25*, 689-693.

McNeill, D. (1992). Hand and Mind: What Gestures Reveal about Thought. *University of Chicago Press, Chicago.*

Miller K., & Franz E.A.(2005). Bimanual gestures: expressions of spatial representations that accompany speech processes. *Laterality*, 10(3), 243-65.

Moscovitch, M., & Olds, J. (1982). Asymmetries in spontaneous facial expressions and their possible relation to hemispheric specialization. *Neuropsychologia*, 20 (1), 71-81.

Oldfield, R.C. (1971). The assessment and analysis of handedness: the Edinburgh inventory. *Neuropsychologia,* 9(1): 97-113.

Raisig, S., Welke, T., Hagendorf, H., & van der Meer, E. (2009). Insights into Knowledge Representation: The Influence of Amodal and Perceptual Variables on Event Knowledge from Memory. *Cognitive Science, 33*, 1252-1266.

Saucier DM, Elias LJ. (2001). Lateral and sex differences in manual gesture during conversation. *Laterality*, 6(3), 239-45.

Sousa-Poza, J.F., & Rohrberg, R. (1977). Body movements in relation to type of information (person- and non-person oriented) and cognitive style (field dependence). *Hum Commun Res*, 4(1), 19-29.

Sousa-Poza J.F., Rohrberg R., & Mercure A. (1979). Effects of type of information (abstract-concrete) and field dependence on asymmetry of hand movements during speech. *Percept Mot Skills*, 48(3 Pt 2), 1323-30.

Trevarthen, C. (1996). Lateral Asymmetries in Infancy: Implications for the Development of the Hemispheres. *Neuroscience & Biobehavioral Reviews, 20*, 571-586.

Ulrich, G. (1977). Untersuchungsinstrumente. Videoanalytische Methoden zur Erfassung averbaler Verhaltensparameter bei depressiven Symptomen. *Pharmakopsychiatrie*, 10, 176-82.

Ulrich G. (1980). Hand movements of depressed patients in an interview situation: behavioral and physiological aspects. *Nervenarzt*, 51(5), 294-301.

Verfaellie, M., Bowers D., & Heilman K.M. (1988). Hemispheric Asymmetries in Mediating Intention, but not Selective Attention. *Neuropsychologia, 26*, 52-531.

18. Evaluating NEUROGES Data on Interaction

Hedda Lausberg, Daniela Dvoretska, and Monika Kryger

18.1 Background of the NEUROGES Interaction Coding

Since long it has been documented that interaction partners show a temporal attunement concerning their verbal utterances. This phenomenon was described as ‚turn-taking' by Sacks et al. (1974). The interactive partners' temporal attunement, however, is not limited to verbal interaction but it has also been observed in movement behaviour such as synchronous position *shifts* or synchronous *on body* movements (Condon & Ogston, 1966; Davis, 1982; LaFrance, 1982). It is noteworthy that these temporal attunements happen beyond the interactive partners' awareness, i.e., they are generated implicitly. Dysfunctions of interactive attunement were demonstrated in mental disease (Condon & Brosin, 1969), and in disturbed mother-child interaction (Kestenberg, 1965a; Kestenberg, 1965b; Kestenberg, 1967; Kestenberg & Sossin, 1979; Bebee et al. 1982). While these observations open interesting perspectives on mechanisms of implicit interpersonal regulation, little empirical research has been conducted in this field due to the lack of economic methods.

Another aspect of behavioural coordination concerns the formal congruency of positions and gestures between the interaction partners. Interaction partners imitate the specific forms of their body and arm positions (Bernieri, Davis, Rosenthal, & Knee, 1994; La France, 1982; La France & Broadbent, 1976). Even yawning and laughing are imitated (Provine, 1986, 1992). Subsequent research in the field of imitation stated that copying the movement pattern of the interaction partner belongs to the basic human needs (Chartrand & Bargh, 1999). The greater the similarity between two persons' body positions and body movements, the more likely it is that they interact without conflicts. Indeed, it was shown that the interpersonal coordination is linked to the level of the rapport, empathy, and agreement. People who like each other are more similar in their body configuration and movements than those who dislike each other. Dyads working on a task with highly synchronized movements mostly judged their rapport as harmonic (Bernieri, 1988). Students who showed the same body and arm configuration as their teacher showed a greater involvement, agreement, and rapport with the teacher (La France, 1982). The tendency to adopt behaviours, body positions, or movement patterns of interaction partners has been claimed to have major evolutionary significance. This behaviour served a "social glue" function, which binds people together and creates harmonious relationships, which in turn are very influential factors in an individual's ability to survive and reproduce (Lakin et al., 2003).

18.2 Rationale of the NEUROGES Interaction Coding

18.2.1 The Kinesic Turn-Taking category

In turn-taking research the categories Gap and Overlap are used to investigate the temporal relation between the partners' verbal utterances (Sacks et al. 1974; Weilhammer & Rabold, 2005). Following this approach, in NEUROGES interaction coding it is distinguished whether partner A starts moving **before** partner B ends his/her movement, or whether partner A starts moving **after** partner B ended his/her movement. Accordingly, the category Kinesic Turn-taking has two values: (i) *subsequent*, and (ii) *overlapping*.

The logic of the system implies that two aspects of the temporal interaction are analysed: the relation from A to B, and the relation from B to A. Thus, the Kinesic Turn-Taking category assessment delivers four scores: A>B *subsequent*, A>B *overlapping*, B>A *subsequent*, and B>A *overlapping*.

The temporal interaction analysis can be conducted for discrete movements in any NEUROGES category. Discrete movement units are those with a defined duration, i.e., *phasic, repetitive, shift,* and *aborted* units. *Irregular* movements are potentially continuous. Thus, as they are potentially ongoing, they cannot constitute turns.

The beginning of a turn is the beginning of the first discrete unit that is displayed partially or completely by partner A alone, i.e., the beginning of the unit may start while B still moves. Analogously, the end of a turn is the end of the last discrete unit that is displayed partially or completely by partner A alone, i.e., the unit may end when B has already started moving. Accordingly, a turn comprises one or more discrete movement unit(s) of partner A that (s)he displays while partner B does not display discrete movement units. However, as stated above at the beginning and end of such a term, there may be overlapping movement activity of the two partners. In case of *overlapping* hand movements, the partners act simultaneously, and in case of *subsequent* units, there are gaps between the partners' movement units. With this method the temporal relation between the partners' Activation units, the Structure units, the Focus units, etc, can be investigated.

18.2.2 The Formal Matching category

Furthermore, in NEUROGES interaction coding the categorical relation between the partners' movements can be assessed. This method reveals whether the partners perform simultaneous movements of the same value or whether they perform simultaneous movements of a different value. As examples, simultaneously both partners perform a *repetitive on body* movement, or one performs a *phasic in space* movement while the other performs an *irregular on body* movement. Accordingly, the category Formal Matching has two values: (i) *same value*, and (ii) *different value*.

18.3 Analysis of interactive processes with the NEUROGES system

18.3.1 Kinesic Turn-taking in psychotherapy

Lausberg (2007, 2011) examined the interactive patterns in three patient-therapist dyads. One dyad was video-taped during a consultation interview (dyad J., patient with somatoform complaints). The other two dyads were registered during psychodynamic psychotherapy (dyads F. and B., patients with eating disorders), with two sessions for each dyad. The temporal interaction was investigated with the NEUROGES system, including hand/arm, head, foot/leg and trunk movements. The Kinesic Turn-taking procedure (see below) was applied to the discrete units of the Structure category. Continuous *irregular* units were excluded.

Table 1 shows the percentages (and in brackets the absolute numbers) of *subsequent* and *overlapping* turn-takings.

Table 1 Percentages and absolute numbers of *subsequent* and *overlapping* turn-takings in 5 therapist-patient interactions

	Subsequent Turn-takings	**Overlapping Turn-takings**
Patient-Therapist Dyad J., consultation interview		
patient takes turn (n=39 turn-takings)	80% (31)	20% (8)
therapist takes turn (n=39)	59% (23)	41% (16)
Patient-Therapist Dyad F., psychotherapy session 1		
patient takes turn (n=79)	65 % (51)	35% (28)
therapist takes turn (n=78)	68 % (53)	32% (25)
Patient-Therapist Dyad F., psychotherapy session 18		
patient takes turn (n=99)	66% (65)	34% (34)
therapist takes turn (n=98)	75% (74)	25% (24)
Patient-Therapist Dyad B., psychotherapy session 4		
patient takes turn (n=59)	75% (44)	25% (15)
therapist takes turn (n=60)	82% (49)	18% (11)

Patient-Therapist Dyad B., psychotherapy session 22		
patient takes turn (n = 25)	28% (7)	72% (18)
therapist takes turn (n = 24)	54% (13)	46% (11)
Mean ± standard deviation	**61,88 ± 15.96**	**38.13 ± 15.96**

In Figure 1 for dyad J., the distribution of the durations between the therapist's unit endings and the patient's unit beginnings is given (Fig. 1 a) and vice versa, the distribution of the durations between the patient's unit endings and the therapist's unit beginnings (Fig. 1 b). The intervals on the x-axis show the duration in seconds between the end of partner A's unit and the beginning of partner B's unit. Positive numbers represent *subsequent* turn-takings. Negative numbers represent *overlapping* turn-takings.

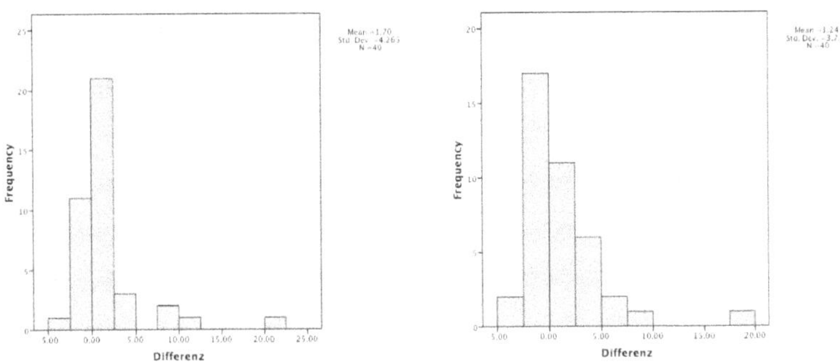

Figure 1a Patient J.'s turn-taking: Time intervals in seconds between the beginning of the patient's unit and the end of the therapist's unit. Frequency distribution of *subsequent* turns (intervals with positive numbers) and *overlapping* turns (intervals with negative numbers).
Figure 1b Therapist J.'s turn-taking: Time intervals in seconds between the beginning of the therapist's unit and the end of the patient's unit. Frequency distribution of *subsequent* turns (intervals with positive numbers) and *overlapping* turns (intervals with negative numbers).
(Figure 1 was first published in: Balint 2011; 12(1): 15-24; DOI: 10.1055/s-0030-1262617.)

In Figure 2 for patient F., the frequency distribution of the *overlapping* and *subsequent* turn-takings is shown for the psychotherapy sessions 1 and 18.

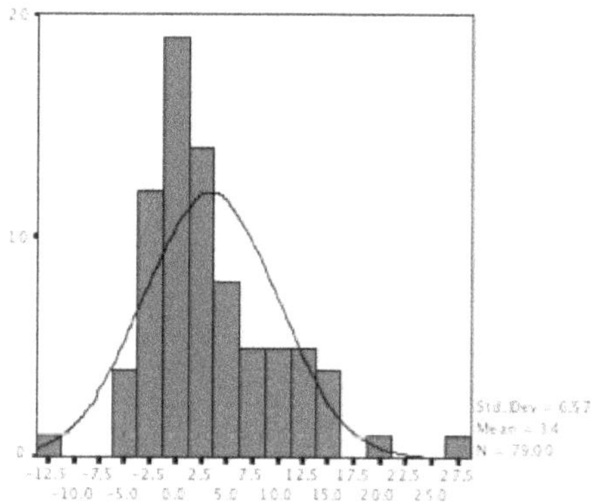

Figure 2a Patient F.'s turn-taking in psychotherapy session 1

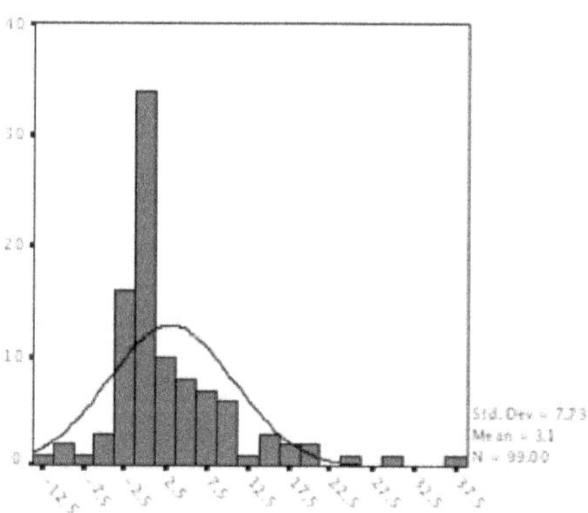

Figure 2b Patient F.'s turn-taking in psychotherapy session 18

In Figure 3 for therapist F., the frequency distribution of the *overlapping* and *subsequent* turn-takings is shown for the psychotherapy sessions 1 and 18.

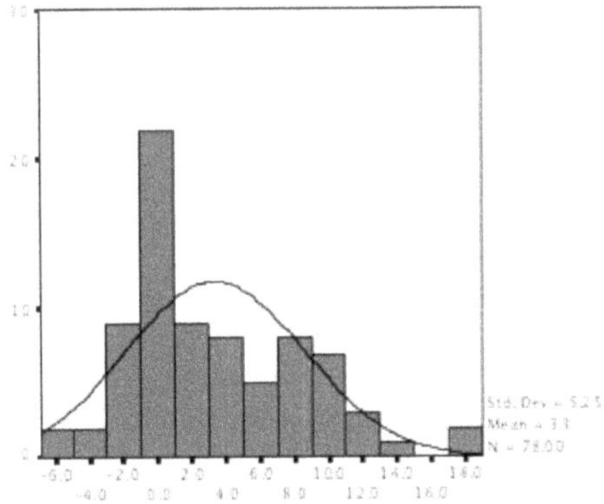

Figure 3a Therapist F.'s turn-taking in psychotherapy session 1

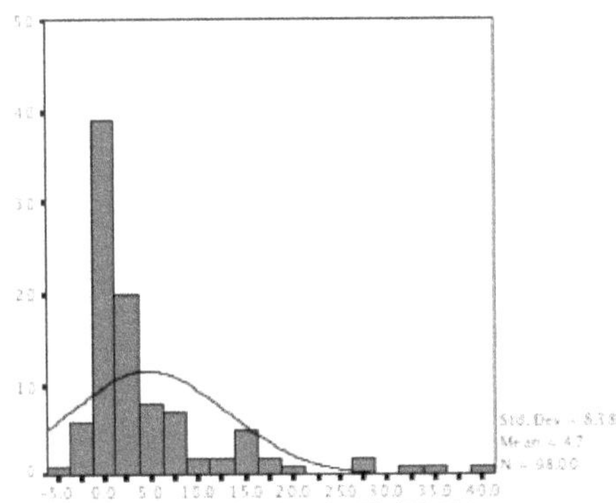

Figure 3b Therapist F.'s turn-taking in psychotherapy session 18

The data suggest that the discrete movements of interactive partners do not occur randomly, but that they are temporally inter-related. If one partner starts to move, it is most likely that she/he starts to move when the other partner has finished or is about to finish his/her movement. The distribution of the duration between the kinesic turns of the interaction partners is comparable to the distribution of time intervals reported for verbal turn-takings (Weilhammer & Rabold, 2005). However, most importantly, the kinesic turn-taking is **not** a mere reflection of verbal turn-taking, since not only gestures that accompany speech were analyzed but **all** discrete movements, i.e., also *on body* movements such as self-touches, *within body* movements such as bouncing with the foot, positions *shifts*, etc. The regularity of the kinesic turn-taking suggests that the interactive partners' movement units are implicit reactions to the each other, i.e., on the kinesic level, there is an ongoing interaction that is independently of the verbal interaction.

In the present data on psychotherapy sessions / consultation, about 2/3 of the turns were *subsequent* turns while about 1/3 was *overlapping*. The high frequency of *subsequent* turns relative to *overlapping* ones may reflect the specific settings of psychotherapy and consultation, in which both partners are engaged in listening to each other. Furthermore, the data reveal different developments in psychotherapy. In dyad F., the turn-taking patterns were similar in the sessions 1 and 18. Thus, one could assume that the quality of their relation remained stable during the course of psychotherapy. In contrast, in dyad B. from session 4 to 22, the patient displayed a substantial increase of *overlapping* turn-takings. This possibly indicates an increase in her engagement in interaction in the course of the psychotherapy.

18.3.2 Kinesic Turn-taking and rapport

Dvoretska et al. (2013) examined the temporal kinesic interaction in view of the intra-dyadic rapport (self-rating - Interaction Quality Questionnaire and observer rating; Denissen, 2005) and the personality characteristics (Neo-FFI; Borkenau & Ostendorf, 1993). The interactions of 40 same-sex dyads (20 male dyads, 20 female dyads, mean age 24,1 ± 3,9 years) were videotaped during interaction. The partners' movement behavior was evaluated with the NEUROGES system, including hand/arm, head, foot/leg and trunk movements. Thus, all body movements accompanying the conversation were coded. In order to control for if the temporal relations of the interactive partners' movement behaviour are by chance phenomena, control dyads were generated by randomly combining the data of two participants who did not interact with each other in the real experimental setting. The interactive behaviour was assessed with the Kinesic Turn-Taking Procedure (see below).

Longer overlaps were found in the control group as compared to the experimental group. Furthermore, in the experimental group, as compared to the control group, the partners showed significantly more *synchronous* movements of their left hand movements, i.e., both started to move the left hand within 0.1 seconds. Furthermore, in the experimental group, significantly more *subsequent* head movements were found than in the control group, and less *synchronous* ones. With regard to the quality of rapport, in the group with the better rapport, there were less *overlapping* right hand *in space* movements and less *overlapping on body* movements. In the better rapport group there were also significantly more *overlapping* head movements.

The significant differences between experimental und control groups confirmed that the movements of two conversation partners do not occur randomly in time, but show a distinct intra-dyadic temporal coordination. As the left hand is predominantly controlled by the right hemisphere, the data suggest that the right hemisphere contributes to *overlapping* movements of the two partners. In contrast, head movements showed a similar turn-taking pattern as reported for verbal utterances. Thus, kinesic interaction seems to take place on (at least) two levels: (i) in line with verbal turn-taking, and (ii) on a kinesic level independently of the verbal turn-taking. The first aspect can be explained by the coordination with the verbal interaction and the second by the partners' attempt to show agreement and understanding with each other.

18.3.3 Formal Matching and therapeutic relationship

In two patients with eating disorders, hand movement behaviour was investigated in the course of 25-sessions lasting psychotherapies (Kryger, 2010). The two patients were treated by the same psychotherapist. For each patient two video-taped 50-minute sessions were selected that had been evaluated with the STEP concerning the clarification of the motivation, active support in problem solving, and therapeutic relationship. In patient A, the 2nd session with a low STEP score and the 18th with a high STEP score were selected, whereas in patient B the 15th and 16th sessions with similar STEP scores were chosen. The patients' and therapist's hand movement behaviour was evaluated with the NEUROGES system. Here the Formal Matching procedure (see below) was employed, which - in contrast to the Kinesic Turn-Taking procedure - includes the irregular units.

In patient A's session 2, 18% of the time of simultaneous hand movements of patient and therapist were spent with movements of the same StructureFocus value, e.g. both simultaneously performed a *shift*. 82% of the time simultaneous movements was spent with different values, e.g. the patient performed an *irregular on body* movement and the therapist a *phasic in space* movement. In contrast, in patient A's session 18, in 31 % of the time of simultaneous movements the patient and the therapist displayed movements of the same value. Qualitatively, there was a decrease from session 2 to 18 in simultaneous *irregular* and *repetitive on body* movements and an increase in simultaneous *phasic in space* movements. In patient B, sessions 15 and 16 with similar STEP values showed similar proportions of simultaneous patient and therapist hand movements of the same value.

Notably, the interactive pattern of the first 5 minutes roughly predicted the pattern of the whole session. This supports the assumption of Ambady and Rosenthal (1992) who claimed that a short segment, e.g. only 30 seconds, of an interaction can have the same validity as a longer one. Furthermore, the analysis of the within-session hand movement behaviour profiles revealed clear interactive patterns. The data suggest that in psychotherapy a higher proportion of simultaneous hand movements that are of the same value are associated with a good quality of the session, whereas a higher proportion of simultaneous hand movements of different values are associated with a worse quality of the session.

18.3.4 Summary

To summarize, the studies on Kinesic Turn-Taking evidence that the interactive partners' discrete movements do not occur randomly, but that they are temporally inter-related. If one partner starts to move, it is most likely that she/he starts to move when the other partner has finished or is about to finish his/her movement. Most importantly, the turn-taking in movement behaviour is **not** a mere reflection of verbal turn-taking, since the turn-taking patterns apply to **all** discrete body movements. Thus, on the kinesic level, there is an ongoing interaction independently of the verbal turn-taking. Future research will clarify whether the high proportion of *subsequent* turn-takings in the present data are psychotherapy-specific or if they represent general turn-taking patterns in interaction.

A better intra-dyadic rapport correlates positively with a higher amount of *subsequent* turn-takings as compared to *overlapping* turn-takings. It is noteworthy that the different parts of the body seem to follow different turn-taking patterns.

The investigation of Formal Matching revealed that in psychotherapy a higher proportion of simultaneous hand movements that are of the same StructureFocus value are associated with a good quality of the session. In contrast, a higher proportion of simultaneous hand movements of different StructureFocus values are associated with a worse quality of the session.

18.4 Procedures in NEUROGES-ELAN

18.4.1 The Kinesic Turn-Taking category

The Kinesic Turn-taking is assessed as (i) *subsequent*, or (ii) *overlapping.* We suggest two procedures to achieve these values. In the first one the turn-taking is evaluated on a global level, i.e., all hand movements are considered, regardless of the particular relations between the hands (A_rh – B_rh, A_lh – B_lh, A_rh – B_lh, A_lh – B_rh). The second procedure allows an exploration of the finer levels.

18.4.2 Procedure for calculating Kinesic Turn-Taking with SPSS

1. For calculating the turn-taking you need to export the Structure values, since only the discrete movement units are considered (*phasic*, *repetitive*, *shift*, and *aborted*). Export the file as tab-delimited text in msec.
   File > Export Multiple Files As Tab-delimited Text
   Select tiers: *A_rh_Structure_RX, A_lh_Structure_RX, B_rh_Structure_RX, B_lh_Structure_RX.* Select the time columns **Begin Time** and **End Time**, and for a time format select **msec**.

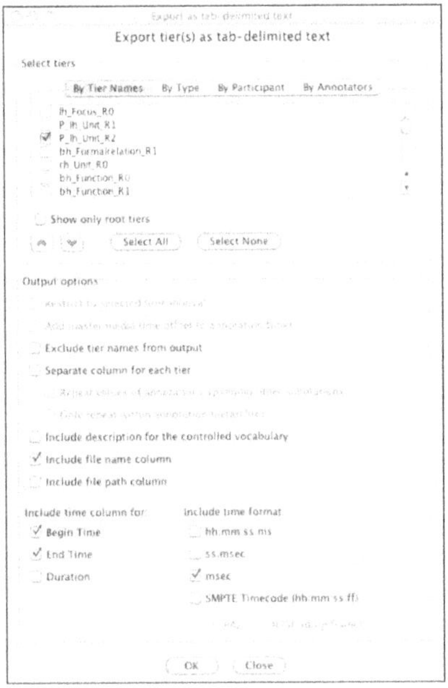

2. Save the text file and then open it in SPSS.

3. Name the variables *subject*, *begin*, *end*, *move,* and *case.*

4. Sort the data by *move* in an ascending way: **Data > Sort Cases.**

5. Highlight all rows containing *irregular* units and delete them.

6. Sort the data by *case* and *begin*: **Data > Sort Cases.**

7. From the menus choose: **Transform > Recode into Different Variables**. Select the variable *subject*. Enter *partner* as an output variable name. Click **Old and New Values**. Recode all movements of person A in “1” and of person B in “2”. (*A_rh_Structure_RX* = 1, *A_lh_Structure_RX* = 1, *B_rh_Structure_RX* = 2, *B_lh_Structure_RX* = 2)

8. Copy the variable *partner*. Name the new variable *copy_partner*.

9. Shift the values in the variable *copy_partner* one cell down. (Cut the values, than paste them one cell down).

10. From the menus choose: **Transform > Compute Variable**. Enter the name of the new variable into the box **Target variable**: *partner_turn*. Compute: *partner – copy_partner*. The values "1" and "-1" indicate now the partner, who takes the turn. "1" denotes that partner B takes turn and "-1" that partner A takes turn. In the "0" cases there was no switch between the partner's moves.

Turn-taking is defined as a beginning of a movement unit relative to the movement of the partner. In an overlapping turn-taking partner A begins to move during the movement of partner B (or vice versa). In a subsequent turn-taking the movement of partner A (or partner B) starts after the end of a partner's movement. So the turn-takings (TT) of partner A are calculated to the following formula: **TT_A = Begin_A – End_B**, and for partner B accordingly: **TT_B = Begin_B – End_A.** To compute these relations with SPSS both subtraction values must be in a same row. To achieve this proceed as follows accordingly:

11. Copy the variable *end.* Name the new variable *copy_end.* Shift the values in *copy_end* one cell down (cut the values, then paste them one cell down).

12. Copy the variable *case*. Name the new variable *copy_case*. Shift the values in *copy_case* one cell down. For the further procedure the values must be (convert to) numerical.

13. Calculate the turn-taking. From the menus choose: **Transform > Compute Variable**. Enter the name of the new variable: *turn_taking*. Compute: (*begin – copy_end*) / 1000. Select the function **IF**. Activate the field **Include if case satisfies condition**: *case - copy_case* = 0. Continue and click on **OK**. Now you have the overlapping time between two movements in seconds. Negative values represent the overlapping time of two movements and positive values represent the time interval between the end of a movement and the begin of the subsequent partner's move.

14. Delete the first and the last row.

15. To filter the valid turn-takings from the menus choose: **Transform > Recode into Same Variable**. Choose the *turn_taking* variable. Select the function: **If**. Activate the field **Include if case satisfies condition**: Give the formula: *partner_turn* = 0 and click on Next. Click **Old and New Values**. Recode **All other values** to **System missing values**.

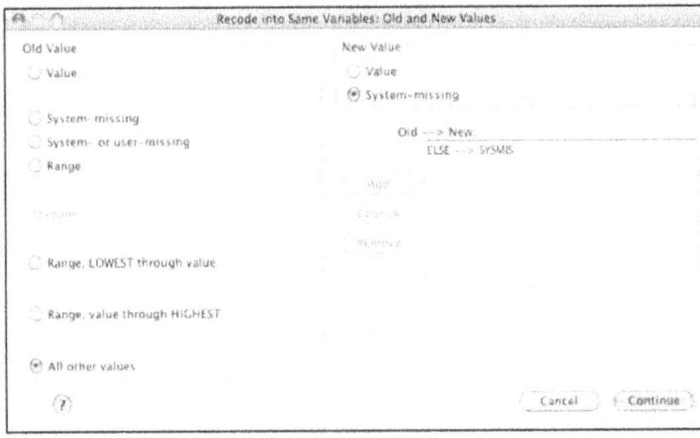

Now only the values for the switches between the partner's moves are left in the *turn-taking* variable.

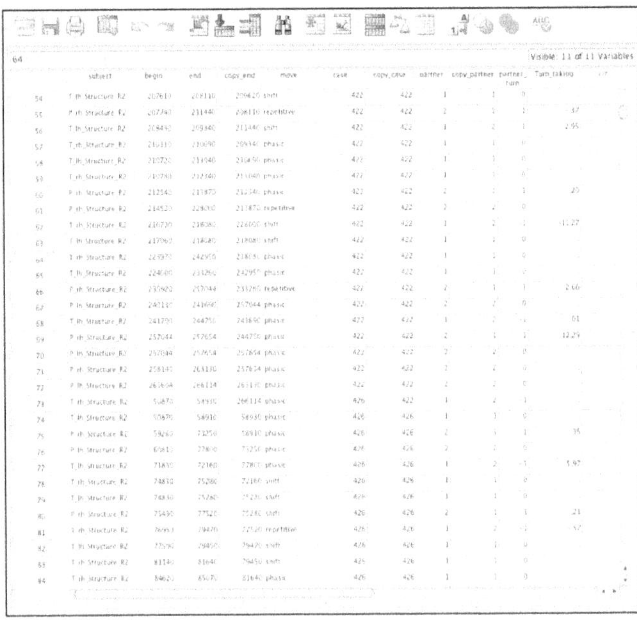

16. For graphic presentation of the turn-taking choose from the menus: **Graphs > Legacy Dialogs > Histogram**. Choose the variable *turn_taking*. Check the box **Display normal curve** and click **OK**.

17. If you need to adjust the scaling: open the diagram editor with double-click on the histogram.

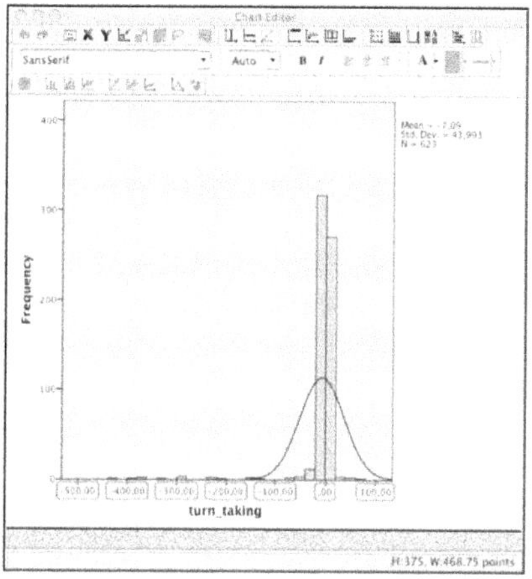

18. Double-click on the scaling values opens a new edit window:

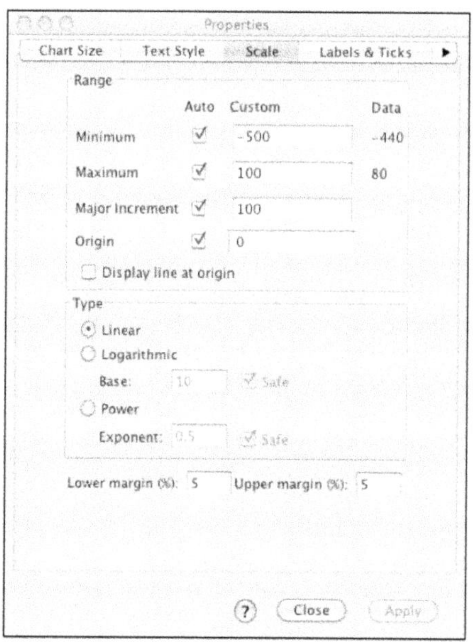

18.4.3 Procedure for calculating Interactive Overlap

The advantage of this procedure is that it is less hypothesis-bound. All units are considered. As an example, this method provides information how how much time both partners spent with the (same) behaviour. The only disadvantage is that no precise data about the time between the end of a unit and the beginning of the next unit can be obtained. To achieve the interactive overlap values, proceed as follows:

1. Open the file in ELAN.

2. From the menu choose **Tier -> Create Annotations from Gaps**
   Select the source tier. It can be on Activation, Atructure, or Focus level, or any other level you want to explore. Choose **Specific value**. Name it: *rest.* Click **OK**. Repeat this for all relevant tiers. **Close** the window.

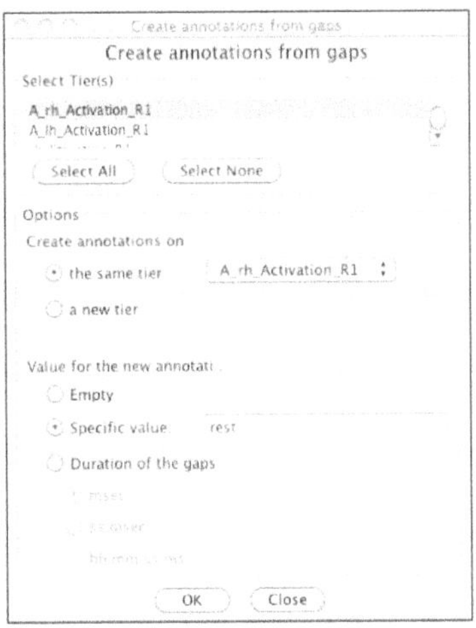

3. If you have coded only a part from the video (e. g. only the first 5 minutes), delete the *rest*-units for the first and after the last movement unit, or adjust their length to the length of the coded part. Otherwise there will be two long *rest*-units at the beginning and the end of the coded section.

4. Choose **Tier -> Create Annotations from Overlaps (Classic)**
   Select the 2 source tiers.

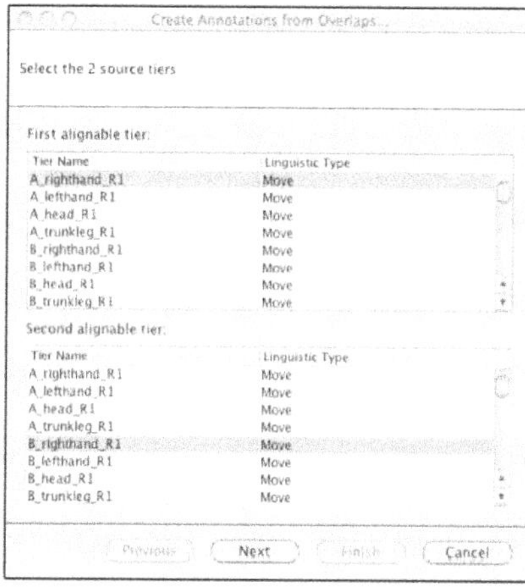

Name the destination tier, e.g. *A_rh_B_rh_equal_overlap* (A and B refer to the participants).
Select a linguistic type: **Notes**.
Select the options: **Concatenate the values of overlapping annotations** and **Only process if the overlapping annotations have the same value.**

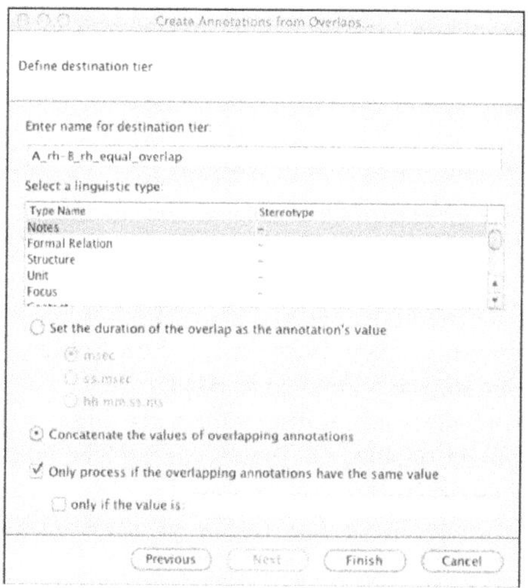

Click **Finish**.

5. Repeat the previous steps for the relations A_left hand – B_left hand, A_right hand – B_left hand, and A_left hand – B_right hand.

6. For better clarity, you can delete the *rest*-units in the source tiers.
Choose **Tier -> Remove Annotations or Value.**
Select the source tiers. Choose: **Annotations where value is ...** *rest.* Click **OK.**

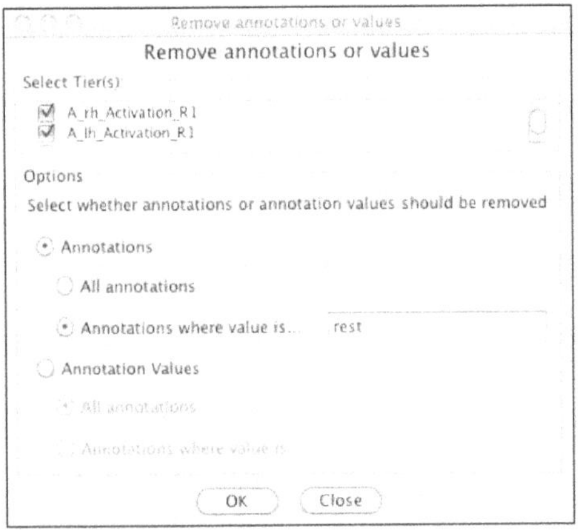

7. The overlap of the movement units represents the overlapping turn takings. The overlap of the rest units represents the subsequent turn takings.

8. Under **View -> Annotation Statistics** you can see the values of occurrences and duration, from which you can calculate the proportion of overlapping and subsequent turn takings to the movements of each participant.

9. The option **Create Annotations from Overlaps** is also available for multiple file processing. If you analyze more than one file, do step 1 – 4 for all files separately and then choose **File -> Multiple File Processing -> Annotations from Overlaps**.

10. **Select files from domain > New Domain... > Add Folder... /Add File...**
Select the tiers to overlap (see 5.) and go to **Next**.
Choose the option **And their annotation values are equal** and go to **Next**.
Enter the name of the destination tier (see 5.) and select **Notes – free values** for a linguistic type. Go to **Next.**
Select the option: **Concatenate the values of overlapping annotations**. Click **Finish.**

18.4.4 The Formal Matching category

The Formal Matching is assessed as (i) *same value*, or (ii) *different value*. To achieve these values, proceed as follows:

First, determine the complete overlap. This procedure determines how often and how long simultaneous movement generally occurs in the interaction. Specific values of the gestures are not considered at this point. Since the coding in Module 1 is done separately for both hands, now several steps are necessary to merge the movements of the right and left hand.

1. Use the function **Create annotations from overlaps** and choose the tiers A_rh_Focus right-hand-tier of Person A and of Person B. Possible tier-name: *rh_rh*.

2. (see above) Choose left-hand-tier of Person A and Person B. Possible tier-name: *lh_lh*.

3. Use the function **Merge tiers** and merge the two new tiers of Step 1 and 2. The results are all annotations of the movements, which happened simultaneously with the same hand. Possible tier-name: *homo_overlap*.

4. (See Step 1 and 2) Choose right-hand-tier of Person A and left-hand-tier of Person B. Possible tier-name: *rh_lh*.

5. Choose left-hand-tier of Person A and right-hand-tier of Person B. Possible tier-name: *lh_rh*.

6. (See Step 3) **Merge** the tiers of Step 4 and 5. The results are all annotations of movements, which happened simultaneously with the contralateral hand. Possible tier-name: *hetero_overlap*.

7. **Merge** the tiers *homo_overlap* and *hetero_overlap*. The results are all annotations of movements, which happened simultaneously. Possible tier-name: *complete_overlap*.

Determine the overlaps of units with the same Structure or StructureFocus value

To analyze the actual quality of simultaneous movements, all overlaps in the same gestural category should be established.

Repeat Steps 1 to 7 by using the option **Only process if the overlapping annotations have the same value**.

It is necessary to give these new tiers other names so that they differ from the tiers coded before. Possible tier-name: *SV_rh_lh* (SV for same value).

Determine the overlaps of units with different Structure or StructureFocus values

To get an additional variable that gives information about the degree of quality of simultaneous movements, all overlaps in different gestural categories can be identified.

1. Export the tiers *complete_overlap* and *SV_overlap* into the program Microsoft Excel.

2. *Substract SV*_overlap from *complete_overlap.*

In this way all overlaps of movement occurring simultaneously in a different gestural category can be gathered. Possible tier-name: *DV_overlap* (DV for different value). The three values *complete_overlap*, *SV_overlap* and *DV_overlap* can be put into a procentual relation to each other now.

Determine overlaps for specific values

To get more distinguished information about the *SV_overlap*, the program ELAN provides the possibility to identify overlaps for specific values. It can be detected in which values overlaps occur often and in which they occur rarely. Furthermore, this function can be used for analysis, focussing on one value only, e.g. *irregular on body*.

1. Accomplish Steps 1 to 7 using the option: **Only process if the overlapping annotations have the same value**.

2. Additionally use the option: **Only if the value is: ...** and enter the gestural category you want to analyze.

References

Ambady, N., & Rosenthal R. (1992): Thin slices of expressive behavior as predictors of interpersonal consequences: A meta-analysis. *Psychological Bulletin, 111*, S.256-274.

Beebe, B., Gerstman, L., & Carson, B. (1982). Rhythmic Communciation in the Mother-Infant Dyad. In: Davis M. Interaction Rhythms. New York: Human Sciences Press, 79-100.

Bernieri, F.J. (1988). Coordinated movement and rapport in teacher-student interactions. *Journal of Nonverbal Behavior, 12,* 120-138.

Bernieri, F.J., & Rosenthal, R. (1991). Interpersonal coordination: behaviour matching and interactional synchrony. In R. S. Feldmann & B. Rimé (Eds.), *Fundamentals of nonverbal behaviour* (pp. 401-432). Cambridge, England: Cambridge University Press.

Bernieri, F.J., Davis, J., Rosenthal, R., & Knee, C. (1994). Interactional synchrony and rapport: Measuring synchrony in displays devoid of sound and facial affect. *Personality and Social Psychology Bulletin, 20*(3), 303-311.

Borkenau, P., & Ostendorf, F. (1993). *NEO-Fünf-Faktoren-Inventar (NEO-FFI) nach Costa und McCrae.* Göttingen: Hogrefe.

Bouhuys, A.L., & Sam, M.M. (2000). Lack of coordination of nonverbal behaviour between patients and interviewers as a potential risk factor to depression recurrence: vulnerability accumulation in depression. *Journal Affective Disorders ; 57*: 189-200.

Chartrand, T.L., & Bargh, J.A. (1999). The chameleon effect: The perception-behavior link and social interaction. *Journal of Personality and Social Psychology, 76*, 893-910.

Condon, W.S., & Ogston, W.D. (1966). Sound film analysis of normal and pathological behaviour patterns. *The Journal of Nervous and Mental Disease; 143(4)*, 338-347.

Condon, W.S., & Brosin, H.W. (1969). Micro Linguistic-Kinesic Events in Schizophrenic Behaviour. In: McQuown, N. A. (ed.): The natural history of an interview. Chicago: University of Chicago, 812-837.

Davis, M. (1982). Interaction Rhythms: Periodicity in Communicative Behavior. New York: Human Sciences Press.

Davis, M. (1986). Nonverbal Behavior Research and Psychotherapy. In: Stricker, G., Keisner, R. H. (eds.): From Research to Clinical Practice. New York: Plenum Press.

Denissen, J. (2005). Understanding and being understood: The impact of intelligence and dispositional valuations on social relationships (*doctoral dissertation, Humboldt-University, 2005*), from http://edoc.hu-berlin.de/dissertationen/ denissen-jacobus-josephusadrianus-2005-07-08/PDF/Denissen.pdf

Dvoretska, D., Denissen, J., & Lausberg, H. (2013). Kinesic Turn Taking and Mutual Understanding in Interactive Dyads. Conference Proceedings, TiGeR 2013, 06 / 2013, Tilburg.

Kestenberg, J. (1965a). The role of movement patterns in development I. *The Psychoanalytic Quarterly, 24(1)*, 1-36.

Kestenberg, J. (1965b). The role of movement patterns in development II. *The Psychoanalytic Quarterly, 24(4)*, 515-63.

Kestenberg, J. (1967). The role of movement patterns in development III. *The Psychoanalytic Quarterly, 26(3)*, 356-409

Kestenberg, J, & Sossin, M. (1979). The Role of Movement Patterns in Development II. New York: Dance Notation Bureau.

La France, M., &. Broadbent, M. (1976). Group rapport: Posture sharing as a nonverbal indicator. *Group and Organization Studies, 1,* 328-333.

La France, M. (1982). Posture Mirroring and Rapport. In: Davis, M. Interaction rhythms: Periodicity in Communicative Behavior. New York: Human Sciences Library.

Lakin, J.L., Jefferis, V.E., Cheng, C.M., & Chartrand, T.L. (2003): The chameleon effect as social glue: evidence for the evolutionary significance of nonconscious mimicry. *Journal of Nonverbal Behaviour, 27*, S. 145-162.

Lausberg, H. (2007). When we speak, we gesture – How gesture reflects and affects individual and interactive cognitive processes. Unpublished paper presented at the Scientific Colloquium of the Center of Lifespan Psychology, Max Planck Institute for Human Development, Berlin.

Lausberg, H., & Kryger, M. (2011). Gestisches Verhalten als Indikator therapeutischer Prozesse in der verbalen Psychotherapie: Zur Funktion der Selbstberührungen und zur Repräsentation von Objektbeziehungen in gestischen Darstellungen. *Psychotherapie-Wissenschaft, 1*, 41-55.

Lausberg, H. (2011). Das Gespräch zwischen Arzt und Patientin: Die bewegungsanalytische Perspektive. *Balint Journal 12*, 15-24.

Provine, R.R. (1986). Yawning as a stereotyped action pattern and releasing stimulus. *Ethologie, 72,* 109-122.

Provine, R.R. (1992). Contagious laughter: Laughter is a sufficient stimulus for laughs and smiles. *Bulletin of the Psychonomic Society, 30,* 1-4.

Sacks, H, Schegloff, E.A., & Jefferson, G. (1974). A simplest systematics for the Organisation of Turn Taking for Conversation. *Languages, 50*, 696-735.

Scheflen, A.E. (1964). The significance of posture in communication systems. *Psychiatry, 27,* 316-331.

Scheflen, A.E. (1973). Communicational Structure: Analysis of a Psychotherapy Transaction. Bloomington: Indiana University.

Weilhammer, K., & Rabold, S. (2005). Durational Aspects in Turn Taking. *Psychonomic Bulletin and Review 12(6).*

www.ingramcontent.com/pod-product-compliance
Ingram Content Group UK Ltd.
Pitfield, Milton Keynes, MK11 3LW, UK
UKHW020122290926
15471UKWH00003B/220

9 783631 582497